Learning Disabilities Sourcebook, 3rd Edition

Leuk...

Live...

Lung...

Medi...

Men's Health Concerns Sourcebook, 2nd Edition

Mental Health Disorders Sourcebook, 4th Edition

Mental Retardation Sourcebook

Movement Disorders Sourcebook, 2nd Edition

Multiple Sclerosis Sourcebook

Muscular Dystrophy Sourcebook

Obesity Sourcebook

Osteoporosis Sourcebook

Pain Sourcebook, 3rd Edition

Pediatric Cancer Sourcebook

Physical & Mental Issues in Aging Sourcebook

Podiatry Sourcebook, 2nd Edition

Pregnancy & Birth Sourcebook, 2nd Edition

Prostate & Urological Disorders Sourcebook

Prostate Cancer Sourcebook

Reconstructive & Cosmetic Surgery Sourcebook

Rehabilitation Sourcebook

Respiratory Disorders Sourcebook, 2nd Edition

Sexually Transmitted Diseases Sourcebook,
   3rd Edition

Sleep Disorders Sourcebook, 3rd Edition

Smoking Concerns Sourcebook

Sports Injuries Sourcebook, 3rd Edition

Stress-Related Disorders Sourcebook, 2nd Edition

Stroke Sourcebook, 2nd Edition

Surgery Sourcebook, 2nd Edition

Thyroid Disorders Sourcebook

Transplantation Sourcebook

Traveler's Health Sourcebook

Urinary Tract & Kidney Diseases & Disorders
   Sourcebook, 2nd Edition

Vegetarian Sourcebook

Women's Health Concerns Sourcebook, 3rd Edition

Workplace Health & Safety Sourcebook

Worldwide Health Sour...

FOR REFERENCE

Do Not Take From This Room

...n Health Series

...Violence Information for
   Teens

Accident & Safety Information for
   Teens

Alcohol Information for Teens, 2nd
   Edition

Allergy Information for Teens

Asthma Information for Teens, 2nd
   Edition

Body Information for Teens

Cancer Information for Teens

Complementary & Alternative
   Medicine Information for Teens

Diabetes Information for Teens

Diet Information for Teens, 2nd Edition

Drug Information for Teens, 3rd Edition

Eating Disorders Information for Teens,
   2nd Edition

Fitness Information for Teens, 2nd
   Edition

Learning Disabilities Information for
   Teens

Mental Health Information for Teens,
   3rd Edition

Pregnancy Information for Teens

Sexual Health Information for Teens,
   2nd Edition

Skin Health Information for Teens, 2nd
   Edition

Sleep Information for Teens

Sports Injuries Information for Teens,
   2nd Edition

Stress Inf...

D1053093

Adolescent Health
SOURCEBOOK

Third Edition

Health Reference Series

Third Edition

Adolescent Health
SOURCEBOOK

Basic Consumer Health Information about Adolescent Growth and Development, Puberty, Sexuality, Reproductive Health, and Physical, Emotional, Social, and Mental Health Concerns of Teens and Their Parents, Including Facts about Nutrition, Physical Activity, Weight Management, Acne, Allergies, Cancer, Diabetes, Growth Disorders, Juvenile Arthritis, Infections, Substance Abuse, and More

Along with Information about Adolescent Safety Concerns, Youth Violence, a Glossary of Related Terms, and a Directory of Resources

Edited by
Amy L. Sutton

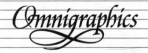

P.O. Box 31-1640, Detroit, MI 48231

Bibliographic Note
Because this page cannot legibly accommodate all the copyright notices, the Bibliographic Note portion of the Preface constitutes an extension of the copyright notice.

Edited by Amy L. Sutton

Health Reference Series

Karen Bellenir, *Managing Editor*
David A. Cooke, MD, FACP, *Medical Consultant*
Elizabeth Collins, *Research and Permissions Coordinator*
Cherry Edwards, *Permissions Assistant*
EdIndex, Services for Publishers, *Indexers*

* * *

Omnigraphics, Inc.
Matthew P. Barbour, *Senior Vice President*
Kevin M. Hayes, *Operations Manager*

* * *

Peter E. Ruffner, *Publisher*

Copyright © 2010 Omnigraphics, Inc.

ISBN 978-0-7808-1140-9

Library of Congress Cataloging-in-Publication Data

Adolescent health sourcebook : basic consumer health information about adolescent growth and development, puberty, sexuality, reproductive health, and physical, emotional, social, and mental health concerns of teens and their parents, including facts about nutrition, physical activity, weight management, acne, allergies, cancer, diabetes, growth disorders, juvenile arthritis, infections, substance abuse, and more; along with information about adolescent safety concerns, youth violence, a glossary of related terms, and a directory of resources / edited by Amy L. Sutton. -- 3rd ed.
    p. cm.
    Summary: "Provides basic consumer health information about the physical, mental, and emotional health and development of adolescents. Includes index, glossary of related terms, and other resources"--Provided by publisher.
    Includes bibliographical references and index.
    ISBN 978-0-7808-1140-9 (hardcover : alk. paper) 1. Teenagers--Health and hygiene. 2. Adolescent psychology. 3. Consumer education. 4. Adolescence. I. Sutton, Amy L.
    RJ140.A335 2010
    616.8900835--dc22

                                                          2010031436

∞

Table of Contents

Visit www.healthreferenceseries.com to view *A Contents Guide to the Health Reference Series*, a listing of more than 15,000 topics and the volumes in which they are covered.

Part II: Staying Healthy during Adolescence

Part III: Puberty, Sexuality, and Reproductive Health

Part IV: Common Health Concerns of Teens and Their Parents

Part V: Emotional, Social, and Mental Health Concerns in Adolescents

Part VIII: Violence against Adolescents

Preface

About This Book

During adolescence, as teenagers transition into adulthood, they experience significant physical, mental, and emotional changes. The choices they make as they grapple with increased independence can have profound ramifications on well-being. Teens who become involved in unhealthy or risky behaviors—such as inactivity, unbalanced eating, substance abuse, unprotected sexual activity, or dangerous driving—may find themselves at risk for long-term, even life-long, health consequences. In addition, because social connections are so critical during the adolescent years, the demands of friendships, peer pressure, and other relationship stresses can complicate healthy decision-making processes.

Adolescent Health Sourcebook, Third Edition, offers parents and teens basic information about growth and development during adolescence and related safety issues. It discusses the importance of routine medical care, adequate nutrition, physical activity, and sleep. It offers facts about reproductive development and the health consequences of sexual decisions. It also describes many of the most common health problems that affect adolescents, including acne, allergies, asthma, diabetes, and infections. Emotional, social, and mental health concerns—including depression, anxiety disorders, self-injury, suicide, and addictions—are also discussed. The book concludes with a glossary of related terms and a directory of resources for additional help and information.

How to Use This Book

This book is divided into parts and chapters. Parts focus on broad areas of interest. Chapters are devoted to single topics within a part.

Part I: An Overview of Adolescent Health discusses the physical, mental, and emotional components of adolescent well-being. Facts about brain development during the teen years, the role of risk taking during the transition to adulthood, and the challenges of parent-teen communication are also included.

Part II: Staying Healthy during Adolescence explores strategies teens can take to promote good health. These include getting recommended vaccinations, eating right, exercising, limiting caffeine use, managing weight, and avoiding sleep deprivation.

Part III: Puberty, Sexuality, and Reproductive Health provides detailed information about gender-related concerns. For males, these issues include testicular self-exams, disorders of the testes, and gynecomastia (male breast development). For females, topics include menstruation and the menstrual cycle, breast and pelvic exams, and vaginal yeast infections. This part also offers information about sexual orientation, sexually transmitted diseases, sexual abstinence, birth control, and teen pregnancy.

Part IV: Common Health Concerns of Teens and Their Parents discusses chronic health conditions that may affect adolescents. These include acne, allergies, asthma, cancer, diabetes, growth disorders, juvenile arthritis, and infectious diseases spread in schools.

Part V: Emotional, Social, and Mental Health Concerns in Adolescents identifies stresses, pressures, and disorders that interfere with a teen's ability to function at home, work, and school, including depression, anxiety disorders, attention deficit hyperactivity disorder, bipolar disorder, eating disorders, self-injury, obsessive-compulsive disorder, schizophrenia, tics, and Tourette syndrome. Information about the risk factors and warning signs of adolescent suicide is also included.

Part VI: Substance Abuse and Adolescents provides information about why teens are susceptible to addiction and discusses risk factors and treatment strategies for the most commonly abused substances, including nicotine, alcohol, marijuana, prescription medications, and inhalants.

Part VII: Adolescent Safety Concerns offers advice on preventing adolescent injuries and accidents. Teens and parents will find information on reducing the risk of motor vehicle accidents, avoiding online sexual solicitation and electronic aggression, and averting problems with body piercings, tattoos, and other skin issues. Tips on staying safe at work and preventing sports injuries are also included.

Part VIII: Violence against Adolescents identifies factors that protect teens against violence, such as family support, academic achievement, and community infrastructure. Adolescent aggression, which may take the form of bullying, hazing, choking games, dating violence, abusive violence, sexual assault, and gang-related activity, is discussed. This part also includes suggestions for families dealing with the aftermath of violence and trauma.

Part IX: Additional Help and Information provides a glossary of important terms related to adolescence. A directory of organizations that provide health information to teens and their parents and a list of hotlines and referral services specifically for teens in trouble are also included.

Bibliographic Note

This volume contains documents and excerpts from publications issued by the following U.S. government agencies: Centers for Disease Control and Prevention (CDC); Environmental Protection Agency (EPA); Federal Interagency Forum on Child and Family Statistics (FORUM); Federal Trade Commission (FTC); Human Resources and Services Administration (HRSA); National Cancer Institute (NCI); National Diabetes Education Program (NDEP); National Institute of Alcohol Abuse and Alcoholism (NIAAA); National Institute of Arthritis and Musculoskeletal and Skin Diseases (NIAMS); National Institute of Child Health and Human Development (NICHD); National Institute of Diabetes and Digestive and Kidney Diseases (NIDDK); National Institute of Justice (NIJ); National Institute of Mental Health (NIMH); National Institute on Deafness and Other Communication Disorders (NIDCD); National Institute on Drug Abuse (NIDA); National Youth Anti-Drug Media Campaign/Office of National Drug Control Policy (ONDCP); National Youth Violence Prevention Resource Center (NYVPRC); Office on Women's Health (OWH); Substance Abuse and Mental Health Services Administration (SAMHSA); U.S. Department of Health and Human Services (HHS); and the U.S. Food and Drug Administration (FDA).

In addition, this volume contains copyrighted documents from the following organizations and individuals: A.D.A.M., Inc.; American College of Sports Medicine; American Heart Association, Inc.; American Psychological Association; Anxiety Disorders Association of America;

Center for Young Women's Health Children's Hospital Boston; Children's Mercy Hospital Section of Adolescent Medicine; Cincinnati Children's Hospital Medical Center; Cleveland Clinic Foundation; Crimes Against Children Research Center; DHE, LLC; Guttmacher Institute; Hazing-Prevention.org; Hormone Foundation; Immunization Action Coalition; National Campaign to Prevent Teen Pregnancy; National Collaborative for Hazing Research and Prevention; National Institute on Media and the Family; National Meningitis Association; National Safety Council; National Youth Network; Nemours Foundation; Newton Youth Commission; Palo Alto Medical Foundation; Partnership for a Drug-Free America; Penn State Cooperative Extension; Planned Parenthood Federation of America, Inc.; Lynn E. Ponton; SIECUS, the Sexuality Information and Education Council of the United States; Testicular Cancer Resource Center; University of Florida; and the Virginia Department of Motor Vehicles.

Full citation information is provided on the first page of each chapter or section. Every effort has been made to secure all necessary rights to reprint the copyrighted material. If any omissions have been made, please contact Omnigraphics to make corrections for future editions.

Acknowledgements

Thanks go to the many organizations, agencies, and individuals who have contributed materials for this *Sourcebook* and to medical consultant Dr. David Cooke and document engineer Bruce Bellenir. Special thanks go to managing editor Karen Bellenir and research and permissions coordinator Liz Collins for their help and support.

About the Health Reference Series

The *Health Reference Series* is designed to provide basic medical information for patients, families, caregivers, and the general public. Each volume takes a particular topic and provides comprehensive coverage. This is especially important for people who may be dealing with a newly diagnosed disease or a chronic disorder in themselves or in a family member. People looking for preventive guidance, information about disease warning signs, medical statistics, and risk factors for health problems will also find answers to their questions in the *Health Reference Series*. The *Series*, however, is not intended to serve as a tool for diagnosing illness, in prescribing treatments, or as a substitute for the physician/patient relationship. All people concerned about medical symptoms or the possibility of disease are encouraged to seek professional care from an appropriate health care provider.

A Note about Spelling and Style

Health Reference Series editors use *Stedman's Medical Dictionary* as an authority for questions related to the spelling of medical terms and the *Chicago Manual of Style* for questions related to grammatical structures, punctuation, and other editorial concerns. Consistent adherence is not always possible, however, because the individual volumes within the *Series* include many documents from a wide variety of different producers and copyright holders, and the editor's primary goal is to present material from each source as accurately as is possible following the terms specified by each document's producer. This sometimes means that information in different chapters or sections may follow other guidelines and alternate spelling authorities. For example, occasionally a copyright holder may require that eponymous terms be shown in possessive forms (Crohn's disease *vs.* Crohn disease) or that British spelling norms be retained (leukaemia *vs.* leukemia).

Locating Information within the Health Reference Series

The *Health Reference Series* contains a wealth of information about a wide variety of medical topics. Ensuring easy access to all the fact sheets, research reports, in-depth discussions, and other material contained within the individual books of the *Series* remains one of our highest priorities. As the *Series* continues to grow in size and scope, however, locating the precise information needed by a reader may become more challenging.

A Contents Guide to the Health Reference Series was developed to direct readers to the specific volumes that address their concerns. It presents an extensive list of diseases, treatments, and other topics of general interest compiled from the Tables of Contents and major index headings. To access *A Contents Guide to the Health Reference Series*, visit www.healthreferenceseries.com.

Medical Consultant

Medical consultation services are provided to the *Health Reference Series* editors by David A. Cooke, MD, FACP. Dr. Cooke is a graduate of Brandeis University, and he received his M.D. degree from the University of Michigan. He completed residency training at the University of Wisconsin Hospital and Clinics. He is board-certified in Internal Medicine. Dr. Cooke currently works as part of the University of Michigan Health System and practices in Ann Arbor, MI. In his free time, he enjoys writing, science fiction, and spending time with his family.

Our Advisory Board

We would like to thank the following board members for providing guidance to the development of this *Series*:

Health Reference Series Update Policy

The inaugural book in the *Health Reference Series* was the first edition of *Cancer Sourcebook* published in 1989. Since then, the *Series* has been enthusiastically received by librarians and in the medical community. In order to maintain the standard of providing high-quality health information for the layperson the editorial staff at Omnigraphics felt it was necessary to implement a policy of updating volumes when warranted.

Medical researchers have been making tremendous strides, and it is the purpose of the *Health Reference Series* to stay current with the most recent advances. Each decision to update a volume is made on an individual basis. Some of the considerations include how much new information is available and the feedback we receive from people who use the books. If there is a topic you would like to see added to the update list, or an area of medical concern you feel has not been adequately addressed, please write to:

Editor
Health Reference Series
Omnigraphics, Inc.
P.O. Box 31-1640
Detroit, MI 48231
E-mail: editorial@omnigraphics.com

Part One

An Overview of Adolescent Health

Chapter 1

Statistics on Adolescent Health in the United States

Adolescence is a period of accelerated growth and change that bridges the complex transition from childhood to adulthood. The second decade of life is often a turbulent period in which adolescents experience hormonal changes, physical maturation, and, frequently, opportunities to engage in risk behaviors. The patterns of behavior they adopt may have long-term consequences for their health and quality of life. Because of the rapid physical, cognitive, and emotional developments that take place during this age period, adolescence is also a time when many health problems may first emerge.

Overweight

Overweight and obesity have serious health consequences among adolescents, increasing the risk of high cholesterol, hypertension, and diabetes. Diet, physical inactivity, genetic factors, environment, and health conditions all contribute to overweight in adolescents.

- In 2001–2004, 17% of adolescents 12–19 years of age were overweight. The percentage of adolescents who are overweight has more than tripled since 1980.

- The percentage of adolescents who are overweight varies by race, Hispanic origin, and gender. In 2001–2004, non-Hispanic

Excerpted from "Adolescent Health in the United States, 2007," by the Centers for Disease Control and Prevention (CDC, www.cdc.gov), December 2007.

black female adolescents were more likely to be overweight than non-Hispanic white and Mexican-American female teenagers. Among male adolescents, there were no significant differences in overweight by race and Hispanic origin.

- Overweight adolescents have a 70% chance of becoming overweight or obese adults. This probability increases to 80% if at least one parent is overweight or obese. Overweight or obese adults are at risk for a number of health problems including heart disease, type 2 diabetes, high blood pressure, and some forms of cancer. Type 2 diabetes, previously considered an adult disease, has increased in children and adolescents.

Suicide Ideation and Attempts

In 2004, suicide was the third leading cause of death among adolescents 13–19 years of age. In addition, many teenagers seriously consider suicide without attempting it, or they attempt but do not complete suicide. Factors influencing suicidal thoughts may include depression, feelings of hopelessness or worthlessness, and a preoccupation with death. Factors that may contribute to adolescent's attempting suicide include a history of previous suicide attempts, a family history of suicide, alcohol or drug abuse, and a stressful life event or loss. Substance abuse or dependence can escalate suicidal thoughts to suicide attempts.

- In 2005, about one fifth of all high school students reported seriously considering suicide or attempting suicide during the previous 12 months. About one half of all students who seriously considered suicide actually attempted suicide (8% of all students). About 2% of all students reported having an injurious suicide attempt that resulted in an injury, poisoning, or overdose that was treated by a doctor or nurse.

- Female students were substantially more likely to consider suicide than male students in all racial or ethnic and grade level subgroups.

- Among students in grades 9–11, female students were significantly more likely to attempt suicide than male students were. There was no significant difference in the rate of suicide attempts between male and female students in 12th grade. In contrast, the rate of completed suicides was significantly higher for male adolescents than for female adolescents.

- Among female students, Hispanic students were significantly more likely to report a suicide attempt than non-Hispanic white or black students were. No difference by race and ethnicity was present among male students.

- In 2005, 20% of male students and 37% of female students reported feeling so sad or hopeless almost every day for 2 or more consecutive weeks during the past 12 months that they stopped doing some usual activities.

Alcohol-Related Emergency Department Visits

Alcohol is the most widely used drug among youth and causes serious and potentially life-threatening problems for adolescents and young adults. Research indicates that drinking is associated with risk-taking and sensation-seeking behavior, and alcohol has disinhibiting effects that may increase the likelihood of unsafe activities. In 1984, the Uniform Drinking Age Act mandated reduced federal transportation funds to those states that did not raise the minimum legal drinking age to 21; by 1988, all states had increased the legal drinking age to 21 years.

The National Hospital Ambulatory Medical Care Survey (NHAMCS) collects data on alcohol-related visits to hospital EDs. In the NHAMCS, an ED visit was considered alcohol-related by reviewing the ED record, including the patient's reason for the ED visit and the diagnoses and the injury codes recorded.

- During 2002–2004, there were, on average each year, over 230,000 alcohol-related ED visits among underage adolescents 14–20 years of age. Alcohol-related ED visits among underage adolescents accounted for 2% of all ED visits for this age group.

- Alcohol-related ED visit rates differed by gender and age for both underage and legal drinkers. Visit rates among males were higher than those among females. Alcohol-related ED visit rates increased with age from early to late adolescence and remained at that level through young adulthood.

- In 2002–2004, rates for older male adolescents 18–20 years of age were more than twice those of younger male adolescents 14–17 years of age, and rates for older female adolescents were more than three times those of younger female adolescents. Alcohol-related ED visit rates did not differ significantly between young adults who had reached legal drinking age and late adolescent drinkers 18–20 years of age.

- Most (89%) alcohol-related ED visits resulted in patients being treated and released from the ED; 5% of patients were admitted to inpatient units, and a small number of patients were transferred to other health facilities, left before being seen, or left against medical advice.

Death Rates

Deaths are categorized by the cause of death: injury or natural causes (natural is a term similar to noninjury that is used to categorize causes of death).

- Injuries cause more than twice as many deaths among adolescents as do natural causes. For the period 2002–2004, almost 13,000 adolescents died annually from injuries compared with about 5,000 adolescents who died from natural causes; that is, 71% of all deaths among adolescents 10–19 years of age were caused by an injury. The proportion of deaths that were due to injury increased with age, from 42% at 10 years of age to 80% at 18 years of age.

- Death rates varied by gender. In 2002–2004, the injury death rate for males 10–19 years of age was 2.6 times that of females, whereas the death rate for natural causes for male adolescents was 1.3 times that for females.

- Among male adolescents, death rates for natural causes exceeded those for injury among male adolescents 10–11 years of age. Beginning at 12 years of age, injury death rates exceeded natural cause death rates at each age through 19 years, and the difference increased with age. Among male adolescents 19 years of age, the injury death rate was almost 15 times the rate of those 10 years of age. Compared with death rates for injuries, death rates for natural causes increased more slowly with age. Among male adolescents 19 years of age, the natural cause death rate was about 2.5 times that of males 10 years of age.

- Among female adolescents 10–13 years of age, death rates for natural causes exceeded those for injuries; among females 14–19 years of age, injury death rates were higher than natural cause death rates. Injury death rates for female adolescents did not increase as sharply with age as did the rates for male adolescents. Among female adolescents 19 years of age, the injury death rate was six times the rate for females 10 years of age, whereas the natural cause death rate doubled between ages 10 and 19 years.

- In 2002–2004, unintentional injuries constituted the majority of injury deaths: 63% among male adolescents and 78% among female adolescents. For both sexes, the proportion of injury deaths that were unintentional declined with age, whereas homicide and suicide deaths increased with age.

Motor Vehicle-and Firearm-Related Deaths

Motor vehicle traffic-related injuries and firearm-related injuries are the two leading causes of injury death among adolescents 10–19 years of age.

- For the period 2002–2004, motor vehicle traffic-related injuries were the leading cause of injury death for adolescents 10–19 years of age (averaging 6,360 deaths per year), followed by injuries from firearms (averaging 2,740 per year).Together, these two causes accounted for 51% of all deaths and 72% of all injury deaths for adolescents. By comparison, malignant neoplasms, the leading natural cause of death for this age group, accounted for 7% of all deaths.

- For motor vehicle traffic-related injury deaths, rates increased markedly with age for male and female adolescents. Notably, between ages 15 and 16 years, the rates for males and females doubled. A similar increase at these ages was noted in the ED visit rates for motor vehicle traffic-related injuries.

- Disparities by race and ethnicity were apparent in rates of death from motor vehicle injuries for male and female adolescents. Among males and females, motor vehicle injury rates were highest among American Indian or Alaska Native adolescents and lowest among Asian or Pacific Islander adolescents.

- The high rates of death from motor vehicle traffic-related injuries are partially attributable to risk behavior among adolescents. In 2005, almost 29% of high school students reported that in the previous 30 days, they rode in a car with a driver who had been drinking alcohol, and 15% reported that they drove after drinking alcohol. Ten percent of students surveyed had rarely or never worn seatbelts when riding in a car or truck driven by someone else.

- The risk of a motor vehicle crash is particularly high during the first year that teenagers are eligible to drive. The presence of teenage passengers increases the crash risk of unsupervised teenage drivers, and the risk also increases with the number of teenage passengers. A crash is considered speeding-related if the driver was charged with a speeding-related offense or if an officer indicated that racing, driving too fast for conditions, or exceeding the posted speed limit was a contributing factor to the crash. Among male drivers 15–20 years of age who were involved in fatal crashes in 2003, 39% were speeding at the time of the crash.

- Firearm-related injury death rates also increase substantially with age; the rate for males 19 years of age was 59 times the rate for those 10 and 11 years of age. In contrast, the firearm death rate for 19-year-old females was nine times the rate for 11-year-old females.

- Differences exist in firearm-related injury death rates by race and ethnicity for male and female adolescents. Rates were remarkably higher among black adolescents than among other racial and ethnic groups. Firearm-related injury death rates were lower for non-Hispanic white and Asian- or Pacific-Islander adolescents compared with other race and ethnicity groups.

Health Care Coverage

Access to and use of health care services for adolescents is dependent, to a great degree, on the ability to pay for services. Compared with their insured counterparts, the uninsured are more likely to lack a usual source of care, have unmet health care needs, and go without contact with a physician during the course of the year.

- Family income is a key factor in the likelihood that an adolescent will be uninsured. The large majority of poor and near poor adolescents under age 19 are eligible for public coverage through Medicaid or State Children's Health Insurance Program (SCHIP). Nonetheless, in 2005, one fifth of adolescents in families below the poverty level had no health insurance, compared with 8% of adolescents in families with income at twice the poverty threshold or greater.

- Adolescents 18–19 years of age are more likely to be uninsured than younger adolescents, reflecting lower rates of both public and private coverage.

Chapter 2

Key Indicators of Adolescent Well-Being

Demographic Background

- In 2008, there were 73.9 million children ages 0–17 in the United States (or 24% of the population) down from a peak of 36% at the end of the "baby boom" (1964). Children are projected to remain a fairly stable percentage of the total population through 2021, when they are projected to compose 24% of the population.

- Racial and ethnic diversity in the United States continues to increase over time. In 2008, 56% of U.S. children were White, non-Hispanic; 22% were Hispanic; 15% were Black; 4% were Asian; and 5% were of other races. The percentage of children who are Hispanic has increased faster than that of any other racial or ethnic group, growing from 9% of the child population in 1980 to 22% in 2008.

Family and Social Environment

- In 2008, 67% of children ages 0–17 lived with two married parents, down from 77% in 1980.

This chapter contains text excerpted from "America's Children: Key National Indicators of Well-Being," by the Federal Interagency Forum on Child and Family Statistics (www.childstats.gov), 2009. Text under the heading "Student Health and Academic Achievement" is excerpted from a document of the same title by the National Center for Chronic Disease Prevention and Health Promotion, part of the Centers for Disease Control and Prevention (CDC, www.cdc.gov), March 10, 2010.

- The nonmarital birth rate in 2007 was 53 births per 1,000 unmarried women ages 15–44 years. The nonmarital birth rate has increased annually since 2000–2002, when it was relatively stable at 44 births per 1,000. In 2007, 40% of all births were to unmarried women, the highest percentage ever reported. This percentage has increased from 34% in 2002.

- In 2008, 19% of children were native children with at least one foreign-born parent, and 3% were foreign-born children with at least one foreign-born parent. Overall, the percentage of all children living in the United States with at least one foreign-born parent rose from 15% in 1994 to 22% in 2008.

- In 2007, 21% of school-age children spoke a language other than English at home and 5% of school-age children both spoke a language other than English at home and had difficulty speaking English.

- In 2007, the adolescent birth rate was 22.2 per 1,000 young women ages 15–17, up from the 2006 rate of 22.0 per 1,000. This was the second consecutive year of increase in this rate after dropping by almost half from 1991 to 2005.

Economic Circumstances

- In 2007, 18% of all children ages 0–17 lived in poverty, an increase from 17% in 2006. Among children living in families, the poverty rate was also 18% in 2007.

- The percentage of children who had at least one parent working year round, full time was 77% in 2007, down from 78% in 2006.

- The percentage of children living in households with very low food security among children increased from 0.6% in 2006 to 0.9% in 2007. In these households, eating patterns of one or more children were disrupted and food intake was reduced below a level considered adequate by caregivers.

Health Care

- In 2007, 89% of children had health insurance coverage at some point during the year, up from 88% in 2006. The number of children without health insurance at any time during 2007 was 8.1 million (11% of all children).

- In 2007, 77% of children ages 19–35 months had received the recommended combined six-vaccine series. Reporting for this combined six-vaccine series began in 2002, and percentages have steadily increased from 66%.

- In 2007, 77% of children ages 2–17 had a dental visit in the past year. In 2003–2004, 25% of children ages 2–17 had untreated dental caries (cavities), an increase from 21% in 1999–2002.

Physical Environment and Safety

- In 2007, 66% of children lived in counties in which one or more air pollutants were above allowable levels. Ozone is the pollutant that is most often above the allowable levels as defined by the Primary National Ambient Air Quality Standards.

- Children's exposure to secondhand smoke, as indicated by blood cotinine levels, dropped between 1988–1994 and 2005–2006. Overall, 51% of children ages 4–11 had cotinine in their blood in 2005–2006, down from 88% in 1988–1994. In 2005, 8% of children ages 0–6 lived in homes where someone smoked regularly, down from 27% in 1994.

- In 2007, 43% of households with children had one or more of three housing problems: physical inadequacy, crowding, or a cost burden of more than 30% of income. This percentage increased from 30% in 1978. The percentage of households with children with severe cost burdens—where more than half of income is spent for housing—rose from 6% to 16% over the same period.

- In 2005–2006, the leading causes of initial injury-related emergency department (ED) visits among adolescents ages 15–19 were being struck by or against an object or person (26 visits per 1,000); motor vehicle traffic crashes (24 visits per 1,000); and falls (22 visits per 1,000), altogether accounting for about half of all injury-related ED visits for this age group.

Behavior

- Heavy drinking declined from the most recent peaks of 13% in 1996 to 8% in 2008 for 8th grade students, from 24% in 2000 to 16% in 2008 for 10th grade students, and from 32% in 1998 to 25% in 2008 for 12th grade students.

Education

- In 2007, 89% of young adults ages 18–24 had completed high school with a diploma or an alternative credential such as a general education development (GED) certificate. The high school completion rate has increased slightly since 1980, when it was 84%.

- In 2007, 67% of high school completers enrolled immediately in a 2-year or 4-year college. Between 1980 and 2007, the rate of immediate college enrollment has trended upward from 49% to 67%; however, the rate has fluctuated from year to year.

Health

- In 2007, 8% of youth ages 12–17 had a major depressive episode (MDE) in the past year, down from 9% in 2004. The percentage of youth with MDE receiving treatment for depression in the past year remained stable from 2004 to 2007 (40% in 2004 and 39% in 2007).

- In 2003–2004, on average, the quality of the diets of younger children was better when compared with that of older children with regard to fruit, milk, and extra calories. The quality of the diets of older children was better with regard to meat, oils, and saturated fat.

- In 2007, about 9% of children were reported to currently have asthma, and about 5% of children had one or more asthma attacks in the previous year. The prevalence of asthma was particularly high among Black, non-Hispanic children and Puerto Rican children (15% in each group).

Children with Special Health Care Needs

- In 2005–2006, an estimated 14% of children ages 0–17 had a special health care need, as measured by parents' reports that their child had a health problem expected to last at least 12 months and which required prescription medication, more services than most children, special therapies, or which limited his or her ability to do things most children can do.

Student Health and Academic Achievement

The academic success of America's youth is strongly linked with their health.

Health-related factors such as hunger, physical and emotional abuse, and chronic illness can lead to poor school performance. Health-risk behaviors such as substance use, violence, and physical inactivity are consistently linked to academic failure and often affect students' school attendance, grades, test scores, and ability to pay attention in class.

In turn, academic success is an excellent indicator for the overall well-being of youth and a primary predictor and determinant of adult health outcomes. Leading national education organizations recognize the close relationship between health and education, as well as the need to embed health into the educational environment for all students.

Health and Education Outcomes

Promoting academic achievement is one of the four fundamental outcomes of modern school health programs. Scientific reviews have documented that school health programs can have positive impacts on educational outcomes, as well as health-risk behaviors and health outcomes. Programs that are primarily designed to improve academic performance are increasingly being recognized as important public health interventions.

The Healthy People 2010 Objective 7-1 calls upon the nation to increase high school completion rates to 90% because "dropping out of school is associated with delayed employment opportunities, poverty, and multiple social and health problems, including substance abuse, delinquency, intentional and unintentional injury, and unintended pregnancy."

Educational interventions, such as reduced class size, are associated with improved health outcomes, as well as improved educational outcomes.

Data and Statistics

The Youth Risk Behavior Surveillance System (YRBSS) monitors behaviors that contribute markedly to the leading causes of death, disability, and social problems among youth and adults in the United States. Through the national Youth Risk Behavior Survey (YRBS), CDC monitors student health-risk behaviors and the extent to which these behaviors are associated with academic achievement.

There is a negative association between health-risk behaviors and academic achievement among high school students after controlling for sex, race/ethnicity, and grade level. This means that students with higher grades are less likely to engage in health-risk behaviors than their classmates with lower grades, and students who do not engage in health-risk behaviors receive higher grades than their classmates who do engage in health-risk behaviors. These associations do not prove causation. Further research is needed to determine whether low grades lead to health-risk behaviors, health-risk behaviors lead to low grades, or some other factors lead to both of these problems.

Science-Based Strategies

Student physical activity may help improve academic performance including academic achievement (e.g., grades, standardized test scores); academic behavior (e.g., on-task behavior, attendance); and factors that can positively influence academic achievement (e.g., concentration, attention, improved classroom behavior).

Physical activity is positively related to academic performance. Most importantly, adding time during the school day for physical activity does not appear to take away from academic performance. Schools should continue to offer and/or increase opportunities for student physical activity.

Students who feel connected to school believe that adults and peers in the school care about their learning as well as about them as individuals. When students feel connected to school, they are less likely to engage in a variety of risk behaviors, including tobacco use, alcohol and drug use, violence and gang involvement, and early sexual initiation.

Connected students are also more likely to have higher grades and test scores, have better school attendance, and stay in school longer.

Chapter 3

Physical and Emotional Changes in Teens

Early Adolescence (12–14 Years Old)

Developmental Milestones

Early adolescence is a time of many physical, mental, emotional, and social changes. Hormones change as puberty begins. Boys grow facial and pubic hair and their voices deepen. Girls grow pubic hair and breasts, and start menstruating. They might be worried about these changes and how they are looked at by others. This will also be a time when your teenager might face peer pressure to use alcohol, tobacco products, and drugs, and to have sex. Other challenges can be eating disorders, depression, and family problems.

At this age, teens make more of their own choices about friends, sports, studying, and school. They become more independent, with their own personality and interests.

Emotional/Social Changes

- More concern about body image, looks, and clothes

- Focus on self, going back and forth between high expectations and lack of confidence

From "Child Development," by the Centers for Disease Control and Prevention (CDC, www.cdc.gov), June 1, 2005. Reviewed by David A. Cooke, MD, FACP, March 16, 2010.

- Moodiness
- More interest in and influence by peer group
- Less affection shown toward parents
- May sometimes seem rude or short-tempered
- Anxiety from more challenging school work
- Eating problems sometimes start at this age

Mental/Cognitive Changes

- More ability for complex thought
- Better able to express feelings through talking
- A stronger sense of right and wrong

Many teens sometimes feel sad or depressed. Depression can lead to poor grades at school, alcohol or drug use, unsafe sex, and other problems.

Positive Parenting

- Trust is important for teenagers. Even as she develops independence, she will need to know she has your support. At the same time, she will need you to respect her need for privacy.
- Be honest and direct with your teenager when talking about sensitive subjects such as drugs, drinking, smoking, and sex.
- Encourage your teenager to get exercise. He or she might join a team or take up an individual sport. Helping with household tasks such as mowing the lawn, walking the dog, or washing the car also keeps your teen active.
- Meal time is very important for families. Eating together helps teenagers make better choices about the foods they eat, promotes healthy weight, and gives your family time to talk to each other.
- Meet and get to know your teenager's friends.
- Show an interest in your teenager's school life.
- Help your teenager make healthy choices while encouraging him to make his own decisions.
- Respect your teenager's opinions and take into account her thoughts and feelings. It is important that she knows you are listening to her.

Safety First

Motor vehicle crashes are the leading cause of death among 12- to 14-year-olds. Injuries from sports and other activities are also common.

- Make sure your teenager knows about the importance of wearing seatbelts. Visit the National Highway Traffic Safety Administration for more information.

- Encourage your teenager to wear a helmet when riding a bike, motorcycle, or all-terrain vehicle.

- Talk with your teenager about the dangers of drugs, drinking, smoking, and risky sexual activity. Ask him what he knows and thinks about these issues, and share your thoughts and feelings with him. Listen to what she says and answer her questions honestly and directly.

- Talk with your teenager about the importance of having friends who are interested in positive activities. Encourage him to avoid peers who pressure him to make unhealthy choices.

- Know where your teenager is and whether an adult is present. Make plans with her for when she will call you, where you can find her, and what time you expect her home.

- Set clear rules for your teenager when he is home alone. Talk about such issues as having friends at the house; how to handle unsafe situations (emergencies, fire, drugs, sex, etc.), and homework or household tasks to complete.

Middle Adolescence (15–17 Years Old)

Developmental Milestones

Middle adolescence is a time of physical, mental, cognitive, and sexual changes for your teenager. Most girls will be physically mature by now, and most will have completed puberty. Boys might still be maturing physically during this time. Your teenager might have concerns about her body size, shape, or weight. Eating disorders can also be common, especially among females. During this phase of development, your teenager is developing his unique personality and opinions. Peer relationships are still important, yet your teenager will have other interests as he develops a more clear sense of identity. Middle adolescence is also an important time to prepare for more independence and responsibility; many teenagers start working, and many will be leaving home soon after high school.

Emotional/Social Changes

- Increased interest in the opposite sex

- Decreased conflict with parents

- Increased independence from parents

- Deeper capacity for caring and sharing and the development of more intimate relationships

- Decreased time spent with parents and more time spent with peers

Mental/Cognitive Changes

- More defined work habits

- More concern about future educational and vocational plans

- Greater ability to sense right and wrong

- Sadness or depression, which can lead to poor grades at school, alcohol or drug use, unsafe sex, thoughts of suicide, and other problems (Note: Problems at school, alcohol and drug use, and other disorders can also lead to feelings of sadness or hopelessness.)

Positive Parenting Tips

- Talk to your teenager about her concerns and pay attention to any changes in her behavior. Ask her if she has had suicidal thoughts, particularly if she seems sad or depressed. Asking about suicidal thoughts will not cause her to have these thoughts, but it will let her know that you care about how she feels. Seek professional help if necessary.

- Show interest in your teenager's school and extracurricular interests and activities and encourage him to become involved in activities such as sports, music, theater, and art.

- Compliment your teenager and celebrate her efforts and accomplishments.

- Show affection for your teenager. Spend time together doing things you enjoy.

- Respect your teenager's opinion. Listen to him without playing down his concerns.

- Encourage your teenager to volunteer and become involved in civic activities in her community.

- Encourage your teenager to develop solutions to problems or conflicts. Help your teenager learn to make good decisions. Create opportunities for him to use his own judgment, and be available for advice and support.

- If your teenager engages in interactive Internet media such as games, chat rooms, and instant messaging, encourage him to be disciplined and respectful about the amount of time she is involved with it.

- If your teenager works, use the opportunity to talk about expectations, responsibility, and other aspects of behaving respectfully in a public setting.

- Talk with your teenager and help him plan ahead for difficult or uncomfortable situations. Discuss what he can do if he is in a group and someone is using drugs, under pressure to have sex, or offered a ride from someone who has been drinking.

- Respect your teenager's need for privacy.

- Encourage your teenager to get enough sleep and exercise, and to eat healthy, balanced meals.

- Encourage your teenager to have meals with the family. Eating together will help your teenager make better choices about the foods she eats, promote healthy weight, and give family members time to talk with each other. In addition, a teenager who eats meals with the family is more likely to have better grades and less likely to smoke, drink, or use drugs. She is also less likely to get into fights, think about suicide, or engage in sexual activity.

Safety First

Motor vehicle accidents are the leading cause of death from unintentional injury among teenagers, yet few teenagers take measures to reduce their risk of injury. Unintentional injuries resulting from participation in sports and other activities are also common.

- Talk with your teenager about the importance of wearing a seatbelt while driving. Insist that she obey speed limits and traffic lights, and strongly advise her not to drink and drive. Set clear rules for when and where she can use the car, and who can ride with her.

- Encourage your teenager to wear a helmet when riding a bike, motorcycle, or all-terrain vehicle.

- Suicide is the third leading cause of death among youth 15 through 24 years of age. Talk with your teenager about suicide and pay attention to warning signs.

- Talk with your teenager about the dangers of drugs, drinking, smoking, and risky sexual activity.

- Ask him what he knows and thinks about these issues, and share with him your feelings. Listen to what he says and answer his questions honestly and directly.

- Discuss with your teenager the importance of choosing friends who do not act in dangerous or unhealthy ways.

- Know where your teenager is and whether an adult is present. Make plans with her for when she will call you, where you can find her, and what time you expect her home.

Chapter 4

Understanding Adolescent Brain Development

Neuroscience, the scientific study of the biology of the brain, has made great strides over the past decade in revealing that remarkable changes occur in the brain during the second decade of life. Contrary to long-held ideas that the brain was mostly grown-up—"fully cooked"— by the end of childhood, it is now clear that adolescence is a time of profound brain growth and change. In fact, the brain of an early adolescent in comparison to that of a late adolescent differs measurably in anatomy, biochemistry, and physiology.

Between childhood and adulthood, the brain's "wiring diagram" becomes richer, more complex, and more efficient, especially in the brain's frontal lobe, or front outer mantle, which is the seat of such higher order functions as learning and socialization. An important part of the frontal lobes is the prefrontal cortex (PFC), which is often referred to as the "CEO" or executive of the brain and is responsible for such skills as setting priorities, organizing plans and ideas, forming strategies, controlling impulses, and allocating attention. New research suggests that the PFC is one of the last areas of the brain to fully mature.

The brain produces a large number of neural connections just before puberty—connections that diminish in number throughout adolescence through a "use-it-or-lose-it" pruning. Through this process, the brain

Excerpted from "The Adolescent Brain: A Work in Progress," by Daniel R. Weinberger, MD, Brita Elvevåg, PhD, and Jay N. Giedd, MD. © 2006 The National Campaign to Prevent Teen Pregnancy. Reprinted with permission. For additional information, visit www.thenationalcampaign.org. Reviewed by David A. Cooke, MD, FACP, April 4, 2010.

becomes leaner and more efficient. Like a sophisticated computer, the maturing brain also grows circuits that can perform several tasks simultaneously and with ever-greater efficiency. As circuits mature, they become coated with a layer of a white fatty substance, myelin, which speeds communication, much like the insulation on electric wire.

In addition, cells that use the chemical messenger dopamine—a neurotransmitter that, among other things, increases one's capacity to learn in response to reward—increase the density of their connections with the prefrontal cortex. Dopamine inputs to the prefrontal cortex grow dramatically during adolescence, probably representing one of the neuronal mechanisms that increase the capacity for more mature judgment and impulse control. Indeed, beginning in adolescence, the dopamine reward signal becomes especially important in the prefrontal cortex as ideas, per se, become increasingly reinforced and valued.

It is also apparent that regions of the cortex (i.e., the outer mantle layer of the brain) that handle abstract information and that are critical for learning and memory of such concepts as rules, laws, and codes of social conduct seem to become much more likely to share information in a parallel processing fashion as adulthood approaches. This increased information sharing is reflected in the patterns of connections between and among neurons in different regions of the cortex. For example, the branching of neurons in the prefrontal cortex becomes much more complex during adolescence, likely reflecting a more intricate web of information flow. It is as if the cells change their architecture in order to meet the increasingly difficult cognitive and emotional challenges that they are being asked to master. By the end of the twenties, the profile of cell-to-cell contacts reaches an adult pattern and the number of connections reaches a steady state that persists until old age.

Magnetic resonance imaging (MRI) is a medical imaging technique that safely provides exquisitely accurate pictures of the living, growing brain and has helped launch a new era of adolescent neuroscience. MRI studies show clearly that during adolescence, the brain is in a dynamic biologic state and that it exits this period in a different state from which it enters. Although it is not clear exactly what cellular processes account for the ebb and flow of the cortex's volume seen on MRI scans during adolescence, it is clear that changes are occurring. In healthy subjects, the cortical gray matter thickens throughout childhood as the brain cells grow an exuberance of connections to other brain cells—gray matter that is pruned in a back-to-front sequence through the teen years. MRI studies also show an opposite front-to-back wave of increases in white matter through childhood and adolescence. Like Michelangelo starting with a block of granite and eliminating rock to create the masterpiece David, certain connections are strengthened and others eliminated—in essence, brain functions are sculpted to reveal and allow increasing maturity in thought and action.

Scientists do not yet understand all of the forces that guide the building up or pruning down of connections between cells. Both are likely influenced by genetic and environmental factors. The roles of bacteria, viruses, nutrition, education, parenting, school, peers, drugs, video games, and many other factors are hotly debated. At present, the scientific jury is still out regarding how much of this process is automatic versus how much is susceptible to manipulation and intervention.

In addition to revealing more about the changing structure of the brain during adolescence, MRI can also be used to see the activity of the brain at work. For example, one key MRI study found that when identifying emotions expressed on faces, teens more often activated their amygdala—the brain area that experiences fear, threat, and danger—whereas adults more often activated their prefrontal cortex—the area of the brain linked more to reason and judgment—and performed better on the task. Behaviorally, the adult's responses were more intellectual, the teens' more from the gut. These findings and others suggest that although the plasticity and changeability of the adolescent brain are extremely well suited to meet the demands of teen life, guidance from parents and other adult institutions are essential while decision-making circuitry is being formed.

Impulse control, planning, and decision making are largely frontal cortex functions that are still maturing during adolescence. One way that the functions of the frontal lobes have been understood is by observing changes in the cognitive processes and behavior of adults who have suffered injury to this key area of the brain. For example, adults whose frontal lobes are damaged often tend to be more uninhibited and impulsive. Often unable to suppress irrelevant information, people with this kind of damage are often easily distracted and falter at even the simplest tasks requiring sustained attention and short-term memory. Such observations suggest that one reason adolescents may have difficulty inhibiting inappropriate impulses is that the circuitry needed for such control is not fully mature in early adolescence, thereby making such tasks relatively difficult.

Planning behavior is another case in point. Adults with damage to the prefrontal cortex tend to be inflexible in adapting to the environment. Studies show that the ability to plan improves with age until adulthood, since the process requires a temporary mental workspace—"working memory"—which is still developing throughout adolescence.

Similar parallels can be drawn with regard to decision making. Damage to the lower middle portion of the adult prefrontal cortex appears to impair the ability to imagine the future consequences of actions or to appropriately gauge their emotional significance. One needs to be able to estimate the probabilities of the possible outcomes of actions in order to make appropriate decisions and to appreciate the complex relationships of cause and effect. People with such damage tend to make decisions on the basis of immediate reward. And it has also been learned that teens are prone to certain types of flawed logic or to ignoring cues about how questions are framed in their decision making. Again, such observations suggest that one reason adolescents may have limited cognitive ability to simultaneously process information about antecedents and outcomes, hold it in working memory, and use it to make decisions is likely traceable, in part, to brain circuitry not fully developed and still under construction, particularly in the prefrontal cortex of the frontal lobes.

In sum, a large and compelling body of scientific research on the neurological development of teens confirms a long-held, common sense view: Teenagers are not the same as adults in a variety of key areas such as the ability to make sound judgments when confronted by complex situations, the capacity to control impulses, and the ability to plan effectively. Such limitations reflect, in part, the fact that key areas of the adolescent brain, especially the prefrontal cortex that controls many higher order skills, are not fully mature until the third decade of life. Teens are full of promise, often energetic and caring, capable of making many contributions to their communities, and able to make remarkable spurts in intellectual development and learning. But neurologically, they are not adults. They are, as we say in this paper often, a work in progress.

More research will be needed to fully understand the developing brain, of course, but in the interim, it seems prudent for adults to think carefully about this new evidence regarding teenage brain development. At a minimum, the data suggest that teens need to be surrounded by caring adults and institutions that help them learn specific skills and appropriate adult behavior. But within that fairly obvious suggestion are many more challenging and specific questions. For example, if teens are not the full neurological equivalent of adults, what specific systems and practices will best help them grow and mature in appropriate ways? What opportunities will be most effective in helping them develop the skills of judgment, planning, and impulse control? What styles of parenting and teaching can most help teens develop into solid adults? Under what circumstances should teens be allowed to make their own choices among many options, and under what circumstances should directed guidance be offered and options limited? Although such questions are often discussed and debated in schools, families, and communities, it is important that the answers arrived at take full note of teens' neurological development. Such biological underpinnings should not be the sole determinant of the answers, but they should clearly inform them.

Key Findings

What We Now Know

- Neuroscience—the study of brain development—has made great strides over the past decade. This progress is due, in large part, to the development and continued sophistication of magnetic resonance imaging (MRI) that safely provides detailed and accurate pictures of the living, growing brain and of molecular biology, which has allowed for the molecular characterization of changes in brain growth and development in biological model systems.

- Research has now determined that remarkable changes occur in the brain during the second decade of life.

- The understanding that adolescence is a time of profound brain growth and change is contrary to long-held ideas that the brain was mostly fully "formed" by the end of childhood.

How the Adolescent Brain Changes

- Between childhood and adulthood the brain's "wiring diagram" becomes more complex and more efficient, especially in the brain's prefrontal cortex or frontal outer mantle.

- An important part of the front lobes—and one of the last areas of the brain to fully mature—is the prefrontal cortex (PFC). The PFC is responsible for such skills as setting priorities, organizing plans and ideas, forming strategies, controlling impulses, and allocating attention.

How Such Changes Take Place

- Like a computer, the maturing brain grows "circuits"—neural connections—that can perform several tasks simultaneously and with ever-greater efficiency.

- Dopamine inputs to the PFC—a chemical messenger critical for focusing attention when necessary to choose between conflicting options—grow dramatically during adolescence.

Why Brain Changes during Adolescence Matter

- Impulse control, planning, and decision making are largely prefrontal cortex functions that are still maturing during adolescence.

- Adult response to stimuli tends to be more intellectual, while teens' is often more "from the gut." This suggests that while the changeability of the adolescent brain is well suited to meet the demands of teen life, guidance from adults are essential while this decision-making circuitry is being formed.

- The ability for the brain to plan, adapt to the social environment, and to imagine possible future consequences of action or to appropriately gauge their emotional significance, is still developing throughout adolescence.

- Brain functions that enhance teens' ability to connect gut feelings with their ability to help retrieve memories, to put situations into context, and to remember past details about a situation that might be important, are also under major construction during adolescence.

Implications

- Neurobiological factors should be one part of a wider universe of factors that are considered when trying to understand teen decision making and behavior, including pregnancy.

- Teens need to be surrounded by caring parents, adults, and institutions that help them learn specific skills and appropriate adult behavior.

- Teens themselves may be able to shape their own brain development. For example, neuroanatomical evidence suggests that learning and positive experiences help build complex, adaptive brains.

- More research is needed to fully understand the brain development, including the relative influence of genetic and environmental factors and how much of the brain's developing "wiring diagram" process is automatic versus how much is susceptible to manipulation and intervention.

Chapter 5

Adolescent Risk-Taking

Adolescent Risk-Taking: Healthy vs. Unhealthy

Healthy risk-taking is a positive tool in an adolescent's life for discovering, developing, and consolidating his or her identity. Adolescent risk-taking only becomes negative when the risks are dangerous. Healthy risks—often understood as "challenges"—can turn unhealthy risks in a more positive direction, or prevent them from ever taking place to begin with.

It is important to remember that learning how to assess risks is a process that we work on throughout our lives. Adolescents need both support and tools to be able to do this. Below are some suggestions for healthy alternatives to unhealthy risk-taking. In order to undertake healthy alternatives to dangerous risk-taking, adolescents need the active help and support of the adults in their lives, including parents and teachers. Any of the healthy risks in the right-hand column of Table 5.1 are excellent alternatives to any of the behaviors shown on the left.

This chapter includes text from "Adolescent Risk-Taking: Healthy vs. Unhealthy," "Guiding a Child or Teen in Risk Assessment," and "Ten Tips for Parents: Understanding Your Adolescent's Behavior," all adapted from *The Romance of Risk: Why Teenagers Do the Things They Do*, by Lynn E. Ponton, MD (Basic Books, 1997). © 1997 Lynn E. Ponton. Reprinted with permission. Additional information is available at http://lynnponton.com. Reviewed by David A. Cooke, MD, FACP, April 4, 2010.

Table 5.1. Risk Behaviors and Healthy Risk Alternatives

Unhealthy Risk Behavior	Healthy Risk Alternatives
Dangerous dieting, eating disorders	Physical activities such as sports teams, horseback riding, in-line skating, walking, or jogging
Using drugs or alcohol	Under the supervision of a trained expert, engaging in outlets for extreme physical and emotional thrills such as white-water rafting, rock climbing, camping, etc.; creative activity such as joining a band or the production of a play
Running away, staying out all night, living on the streets	Learning or practicing a creative art form such as photography, pottery, video, dance, or creative writing
Unprotected sexual activity	Learning to talk about sex and relationships, working on open communication with partners and parents
Gang violence, weapons, bullying, scapegoating	Seeking out new friends, volunteering in the community, participating in a student exchange program, transferring to a new school if necessary
Shoplifting, stealing	Getting a part-time job such as baby-sitting, camp or after-school counselor, retail clerk in clothing or music store, tutoring

Guiding a Child or Teen in Risk Assessment

Healthy risk-taking is a positive tool in an adolescent's life for discovering, developing, and consolidating his or her identity.

It is important to remember that learning how to assess risks is a process that we work on throughout our lives. Children and adolescents need support, tools, and practice in order to do this.

Young children give clues about how they do or don't take risks (e.g., how they ride a bike or skateboard, how they handle a new social situation). These clues contribute to styles or patterns of risk-taking.

Although there are many styles, certain patterns can be seen, such as the cautious risk-taker, the middle-of-the-roader, the adventurer or high-end risk-taker, the teen whose risk-taking increases when he or she is with friends.

Risk-taking can be accelerated in one area—social, physical, intellectual, artistic, or sexual, for example—and not in others.

Helping a child or teen understand or define his or her own risk-taking pattern is important.

This includes helping the child understand how and why he or she makes both healthy and unhealthy choices. Questions to ask:

- Do you feel pressured to make risky choices by friends?

- Do you rush into decisions?

- Do you think it is uncool to try things in a safe manner?

- Are dangerous risks more exciting? Do they feel more like you?

- Do you make dangerous choices to show others?

- Does it feel as though it's happening "in a dream" when you make dangerous choices?

Role-playing risk assessment with children and teens is crucial. Have them try out different roles.

Adults can share what we have learned about risk-taking. A nonjudgmental and nonbragging manner is most helpful. It is often most important to share feelings and mistakes.

Risk-taking can be practiced and learned in healthy, supportive situations.

10 Tips for Parents: Understanding Your Adolescent's Behavior

1. All teenagers take risks as a normal part of growing up. Risk-taking is the tool an adolescent uses to define and develop his or her identity, and healthy risk-taking is a valuable experience.

2. Healthy adolescent risk-taking behaviors which tend to have a positive impact on an adolescent's development can include participation in sports, the development of artistic and creative abilities, volunteer activities, travel, running for school office, making new friends, constructive contributions to the family or community, and others. Inherent in all of these activities is the possibility of failure. Parents must recognize and support their children with this.

3. Negative risk-taking behaviors which can be dangerous for adolescents include drinking, smoking, drug use, reckless driving, unsafe sexual activity, disordered eating, self-mutilation, running away, stealing, gang activity, and others.

4. Unhealthy adolescent risk-taking may appear to be "rebellion"—an angry gesture specifically directed at parents. However, risk-taking, whether healthy or unhealthy, is simply part of a teen's struggle to test out an identity by providing self-definition and separation from others, including parents.

5. Some adolescent behaviors are deceptive—a teen may genuinely try to take a healthy risk that evolves into more dangerous behavior. For example, many adolescent girls fail to recognize the trap of dieting and fall into a pattern of disordered eating, sometimes even developing a full eating disorder. Parents need to be well informed in order to help their adolescents with such struggles.

6. Red flags which help identify dangerous adolescent risk-taking can include psychological problems such as persistent depression or anxiety which goes beyond more typical adolescent "moodiness"; problems at school; engaging in illegal activities; and clusters of unhealthy risk-taking behaviors (e.g., smoking, drinking, and driving recklessly might be happening at the same time, as might disordered eating and self-mutilation, or running away and stealing).

7. Since adolescents need to take risks, parents need to help them find healthy opportunities to do so. Healthy risk-taking, not only important in itself, can help prevent unhealthy risk-taking.

8. Adolescents often offer subtle clues about their negative risk-taking behaviors through what they say about the behaviors of friends and family, including parents. Parents often stay silent about their own histories of risk-taking and experimenting, but it can be important to find ways to share this information with adolescents in order to serve as role models, to let teens know that mistakes are not fatal, and to encourage making healthier choices than those the parent may have made during his or her own adolescence.

9. Adolescents look to their parents for advice and modeling about how to assess positive and negative risks. Parents need to help their teens learn how to evaluate risks and anticipate the consequences of their choices, and develop strategies for diverting their energy into healthier activities when necessary.

10. Parents need to pay attention to their own current patterns of risk-taking as well. Teenagers are watching, and imitating, whether they acknowledge this or not.

Chapter 6

For Parents: Talking to Teens about Health Issues

Chapter Contents

Section 6.1

Communicating with Your Teen

"Parent-Teen Communication Tips," reprinted from http://www.solutions
.psu.edu, © 2006 Penn State Cooperative Extension.

If you're frustrated over an inability to communicate with your teenager, you are not alone. Take a look at how you are communicating with your teen. Ask yourself: "Do I talk *to* my teenager?" or, "Do I talk *with* my teenager?" The parent who talks to the teenager is very often reminding, threatening, blaming, questioning, ordering, or judging. Parents use this style to pressure teens into doing something parents want them to do, decreasing effective communication.

Parents who talk with teenagers listen. They make a point of listening to what the teen is thinking, feeling, or wanting. They respect their teen as a human being who is more than their child, and they try to understand and accept the teen's point of view. In addition, they are not afraid to express their own view or share feelings and concerns.

This can be done by using "I-messages" to get your point across without offending the other person. Start with the word "I," then add what you are thinking, feeling, needing, or wanting. For example, "I'm concerned when you stay out past 10:00 p.m. on weekends because our neighborhood isn't always safe in the evening."

Keep in mind that what you say while you're talking isn't the only thing that's getting communicated. Your tone of voice tells a lot about what you're thinking, especially if you're being sarcastic. You also communicate with your eyes and your body. Smiles, frowns, shrugs, clenched fists, hugs, and other body language say a lot. If you are the listener, remember that listening means concentrating on what the other person is saying rather than what you plan to say as soon as you get the chance. The focus needs to be on what the other person is trying to tell you, instead of what you are thinking about.

Both parents and teens can practice some of the following techniques to become more effective listeners:

- **Pay attention.** Look at the person who is talking to you. Make eye contact and don't interrupt. If it's a bad time to talk, tell the person you're interested in listening and set up a better time to talk, as soon as possible.

- **Don't interrupt while the other person is talking.** Avoid forming immediate judgments about the validity of what the other person is saying. Just listen. Make an effort to consider the issue from the other's point of view. If you have a habit of jumping in on the other's statement with comments of your own, listen with your chin in your hand and your fingers over your mouth until you break the habit. Listen and let the other person finish speaking before you begin thinking about what your response will be.

- **Listen for what is not said.** What a person hesitates to say is often the heart of the message. People also convey information with their tone of voice or body language. Listen with your eyes as well as your ears. Encourage the other person to keep talking.

- **Before you respond, be sure you understand the other's message.** Start out with the phrase "So, what you're saying is . . ." and then repeat what you've heard. It's an excellent technique and it works.

- Try very hard to keep your own emotions, such as anger, fear, and hurt under control while you listen.

Sometimes, old, ingrained, negative, or inefficient communication patterns make it impossible to change without getting help from outside the family. Sometimes it's hard for parents to recognize that their children are growing up and they have new needs and goals.

If you want to improve your communication with your teenager, but you can't seem to make it better, don't hesitate to ask for outside help. You and your teen will enjoy and appreciate each other more if you learn to talk with each other and listen with your hearts.

Section 6.2

Talking about Substance Abuse

Excerpted from "Talking to Teens about Drug and Alcohol Prevention: Parent's Resource Guide," © 2007 Newton Youth Commission (www .newtonma.gov/Youth/commission.htm). Reprinted with permission.

As children move from elementary-level schools into middle schools and then high schools, their world view opens up dramatically. Maturing children need a parents' help to safely navigate larger, more complex environments.

This text offers guidelines to help parents and children address the issues of alcohol and drug prevention. Taking time to talk to your teen is the first step you can take toward preventing drug and alcohol abuse.

Why Teens Take Risks

As your children grow, they rightfully demand a measure of independence in their life. They'll challenge you and disagree on things, and that's a healthy part of their efforts to mature and form a unique identity.

Stress

- Stress is the most cited concern by teens in survey after survey. Stress is compounded as teens move from middle school to high school and prepare for life after age 18.

- Students who are struggling for acceptance can fall prey to the influence of tobacco, alcohol, and illegal drug use to satisfy their curiosity, ease stress, win friends, and to appear cool.

- The need to fit in and striving for personal independence leads to the potential for making dangerous choices.

Behavior

- "Marijuana is not harmful because it is 'all natural' and comes from a plant," or "Everyone is doing it" may seem perfectly believable to a student. Talk to your kids about the illogical reasoning statements like this show.

- In today's society drinking and drug use is often portrayed as a normal part of adolescent development. Alcohol and drugs do not have to be part of a teen's rite of passage. Studies show that middle school binge drinking is growing and can lead to alcoholism later in life.

Celebrate Non-Use by Your Teen

- Teens who are involved in sports, theatre, and other activities are less likely to abuse drugs and alcohol. Encourage your child's involvement in extracurricular activities.

- Praise your teens and their friends when they demonstrate good judgment and make healthy decisions.

Prevention Really Works

Make Your Position Clear

- It's crucial for parents to clearly and consistently state their point of view when it comes to alcohol and illegal drug use.

- Engage your teens in a positive manner. As you listen carefully to what they have to say, you'll help them make appropriate choices on their own.

- Explain that there are serious health, social, and legal consequences for abusing of drugs and alcohol.

Set Expectations

- Agree on what is expected before an event happens. This is always preferable to disagreeing afterward.

- When your child goes out, ask: When will you be home? What will you be doing? Who will you be going with?

- If they're going to someone's house and you haven't met the parents, call to say hello and confirm your child's plans. Ask if they intend to be present and checking in on the event.

- Let your child know that you expect there to be adult supervision at all parties and events.

Be Involved

Stay Connected and Informed

- Teens are more likely to make good choices when they know you're looking after them.

- Attend your child's activities and events, when possible. Always discuss the event together if you are unable to attend.

- Try to eat several meals a week together without media distractions.

- Have conversations not associated with arguments or punishments.

Encourage Gatherings at Your Home

By having your child's friends in your home, you'll get to know their friends and you'll be able to see that they're enjoying themselves responsibly.

- If your house is the site for the party, remain in sight and be available.

- Make it clear no alcohol will be served to students or parents.

- Agree on a policy concerning uninvited guests. Never admit anyone whom no one knows.

- Promise a safe ride to all teens who attend a party. Do not allow anyone to get in a vehicle if they are under the influence.

- If the party will be large, it is courteous to inform the neighbors of the upcoming party and to assure them that there will be adults present.

- Teens gather informally at all times of the day, especially after school. Encourage your child to be involved in supervised activities.

Set Limits

Set Boundaries

- Establish cell phone protocol with your teen. Set a time when they need to call you or when they need to answer your phone call.

- Establish internet protocol with your child early on. There are many internet safety resources available.

- Oversee your teen's spending habits and discuss where their money is going. Talk about a budget plan together.

Guarantee a Safe Ride

- Know in advance who's transporting your teen and stress the importance of the driver staying sober or straight.

- Discuss the dangers and consequences of being in a car with a driver who is under the influence of drugs or alcohol.

- Assure your teen that they may call you to be picked up whenever they need to be, no questions asked.

- Discuss events later, preferably the next day.

Establish Reasonable Curfews

- Discuss reasonable and age appropriate curfews with your child.

- Be awake (or awakened) when young people come home at night.

- Establish communication to ensure that both parent and teen agree on any changes of plans.

Drug and Alcohol Abuse: Signs and Symptoms

Knowing the warning signs of drug or alcohol abuse may help avert a crisis.

Symptoms include [the following]:

- Withdrawn, depressed, tired; careless about dress and appearance

- Hostile and uncooperative; frequently breaks curfews

- Relationships with family members has deteriorated

- Appears stressed on a regular basis

- Hangs out with new friends; exhibiting secretive behavior

- Grades are slipping; school attendance is irregular

- Eating and sleeping patterns have changed

- Has a hard time concentrating on schoolwork and other activities

- Eyes are red and nose is runny in the absence of a cold

- Allowance or household money is disappearing

- Evidence of drug paraphernalia: Pipes, rolling papers, nail polish, aerosol cans, over-the-counter cold medicine, hair spray, correction fluid on body/clothes, rags/papers, use of incense, room deodorant, breath mints, mouthwash, eye drops

Prescription drugs: Kids are getting drugs from parent's medicine cabinets, friend's prescription medication, and over the internet. Be sure that you are in charge of dispensing all prescription medication to your kids.

Overdose Symptoms

If your child exhibits any signs of drug or alcohol overdose contact a professional immediately. These signs include:

- nausea and vomiting;
- trouble breathing;
- dizziness;
- drowsiness;
- confusion;
- unconsciousness;
- cold, clammy, hot reddish skin;
- coma.

Contact 911 immediately, if you suspect an overdose.

If You Suspect a Problem

Even in the best of school systems, and with the best of parenting, your children have the potential to fall prey to risky behaviors.

What to Do

- If you suspect a problem, be direct in your tone and approach. Tell your child that you are concerned and explain why.

- Remember that talking with your teen includes a lot of listening. Try to start the conversation by saying, "No matter what you tell me, I will continue to love you. I am concerned and I want to help you."

- If you feel that you are unable to "remove the emotion," ask your teen if he or she would be willing to speak with a counselor to better understand why he or she is using or misusing alcohol and/or other drugs.

- Check in with your teen's teachers or counselors to see how school is going. Consult with a professional counselor or therapist.

Section 6.3

Talking about Sex

From "Tips for Talking," by the U.S. Department of Health and Human Services (www.4parents.gov), 2009.

You don't want to talk about sex. Your kids don't want to talk about sex. Talking about sex is without a doubt one of the most important conversations you will ever have with your kids. It's also one of the most difficult. You need to talk with them early and often about why it's important for them to wait to have sex. But if you're like most parents, you're not sure how. Here are some tips.

- **Use teachable moments.** Many everyday occurrences offer a natural way to ease into the conversation. Maybe it's a scene from a movie or TV show. Perhaps a song lyric or news story. Use these, or anything else that seems appropriate, as conversation starters. And do it subtly.

- **Dole out bite-sized bits.** Don't try to cover the whole subject in one sitting. It's overwhelming and uncomfortable for your child and you. So toss out small bits of information and opinion at a time. Little by little, your kids will get the big picture and they'll appreciate not getting the big parental lecture.

- **Keep things light.** Talking about sex can be pretty heavy. So lighten up. Maybe use a little humor without underplaying the seriousness of the subject, but to disarm your child's anxiety (and yours). Don't feel you have to make direct eye contact either. That can increase the discomfort.

- **Don't preach. Share.** Let your children know how you felt when you were their age. So they know you understand what they're going through. And don't just talk, ask questions. This absolutely needs to be a two-way discussion. Because kids really respond better when they're talked with, not at. Believe it or not, your kids actually do want to know how you feel about sex and how you want them to behave. Of course they may never ask you about it. So you need to take the first step.

Chapter 7

For Teens: Talking to Your Parents or Other Adults

You probably talk to friends way more than you talk to your parents. That's natural as you get older. Even if you and your parents have a great relationship, you want to find your own path and make your own choices.

It still can feel good to talk with your parents, though. You probably want their help, advice, support, or just their company at times. But talking to parents can seem difficult or intimidating—especially when it comes to certain subjects. Here are some tips to make it easier.

Talk about Everyday Stuff—and Do It Every Day

The more you do something, the easier it gets. Talking to parents about everyday stuff builds a bond that can smooth the way for times you need to approach them with a topic that's more difficult.

Find something trivial to chat about each day. Talk about how your team did at the track meet. Share something one of your teachers said. Even small talk about what's for dinner can keep your relationship strong and comfortable.

It's never too late to start. If you feel your relationship with your parents is strained, try easing into conversations by mentioning that cute thing the dog or your little brother did. Talking to parents every day not only keeps an existing relationship strong, it also can help a frayed relationship get stronger.

When your parents feel connected to your daily life, they can be there for you when something really important comes up.

Raising Difficult Topics

Maybe you need to break bad news to a parent, like getting a speeding ticket or failing an exam. Perhaps you're feeling scared or stressed about something. Or maybe you just really, really want to tell your parents about your new boyfriend or girlfriend, but you don't know how they'll react, how it will feel to tell them, or how to find the words.

Here are three steps to help you prepare for that talk.

Step 1: Know What You Want from the Conversation

It takes maturity to figure out what you want to get out of a conversation. (Most adults aren't so good at this!)

What you hope to achieve can vary, but most often you'll probably want your parent to do one (or more) of these things:

- Simply listen and understand what you're going through without offering advice or commentary

- Offer you advice or help

- Give permission or support for something

- Guide you back on track if you're in trouble—in a way that's fair and without harsh criticism or put-downs

Why think about this before you begin talking? So you can tell mom or dad why you want to talk in a way that communicates what you need. For example:

- "Mom, I need to tell you about a problem I'm having, but I need you to just listen, OK? Don't give me advice—I just want you to know what's bothering me."

- "Dad, I need to get your permission to go on a class trip next week. Can I tell you about it?"

- "Mom, I need your advice about something. Can we talk?"

Step 2: Identify Your Feelings

Lots of people hesitate to bring up sensitive topics because talking about them can be so uncomfortable. Things like personal feelings or sex are awkward to discuss with anyone, let alone a parent.

It's natural to feel nervous before an important conversation. Recognize how you're feeling—for example, maybe you're worried that telling parents about a problem will make them disappointed or upset. But instead of letting those feelings stop you from talking, put them into words as part of the conversation. For example:

- "Mom, I need to talk to you—but I'm afraid I'll disappoint you."
- "Dad, I need to talk to you about something—but it's kind of embarrassing."

If you think a parent may be unsupportive, harsh, or critical, it can help to defuse things by beginning with a statement like, "Mom, I have something to tell you. I'm not proud of what I've done, and you might be mad. But I know I need to tell you. Can you hear me out?"

Step 3: Pick a Good Time to Talk

Approach your parent when he or she isn't busy with something else. Ask, "Can we talk? Is now a good time?" Driving in the car or going for a walk can be great opportunities to talk. If it's hard to find a good time, say, "I need to talk to you. When is a good time?"

Difficult conversations benefit from good planning. Think ahead about what you want to say or ask. Write down the most important ideas if you need to.

How to Talk So Parents Will Listen

As most of us know, talking and listening doesn't go smoothly every time. Emotions and past experiences can get in the way. Will parents take you seriously, believe what you say, listen to and respect your opinions, and hear you out without interrupting? A lot depends on your parent. Some parents are easy to talk to, some are great listeners, and some are harder to approach.

But some of what happens depends on you, too. Since communication is a two-way street, the way you talk can influence how well a parent listens and understands you.

So here are some guidelines to consider when talking to parents:

- **Be clear and direct.** Be as clear as you can about what you think, feel, and want. Give details that can help parents understand your situation. They can listen better or be more helpful if they understand what you mean and what's really going on.

- **Be honest.** If you're always honest, a parent will be likely to believe what you say. If you sometimes hide the truth or add too much drama to the truth, parents will have a harder time believing what you tell them. If you lie, they'll find it hard to trust you.

- **Try to understand their point of view.** If you have a disagreement, can you see your parents' side? If you can, say so. Telling parents you understand their views and feelings helps them be willing to see yours, too.

- **Try not to argue or whine.** Using a tone that's friendly and respectful makes it more likely parents will listen and take what you say seriously. It also makes it more likely that they'll talk to you in the same way. Of course, this is hard for any of us (adults included) when we're feeling heated about something. If you think your emotions might get the better of you, do something to blow off steam before talking: Go for a run. Cry. Hit your pillow. Do whatever it takes to sound calm when you need to.

What If Talking to Parents Doesn't Work?

Your parents won't always see things your way and they won't always say yes to what you ask. They might listen respectfully, understand your point of view, and do everything you need except say yes. It can be hard to take no for an answer. But gracefully accepting a no can help you get more yeses in the future.

But what if it's more than just saying no to something? What if you really need your parents to be there for you but they can't? Some parents have troubles of their own. Others just can't be available in the ways their kids need and deserve. Others have a hard time being flexible.

If you can't talk to your parent, seek out other adults you can trust. Find a relative, a teacher, or a counselor who will listen, understand, encourage, believe in you, and care. Then follow all the tips in this article to get the most from your conversation with that person.

Acting respectfully demonstrates maturity. Parents are more likely to think of their children as grown up (and, as a result, capable of making more important decisions) when they see them acting maturely. Give these tips a try and you'll come across that way—maybe even more mature than your parents!

Part Two

Staying Healthy
during Adolescence

Chapter 8

Medical Care and Your Teen

Chapter Contents

Section 8.1

What to Expect at the Doctor's Office

"Medical Care and Your 13- to 18-Year-Old," October 2008, reprinted with permission from www.kidshealth.org. Copyright © 2008 The Nemours Foundation. This information was provided by KidsHealth, one of the largest resources online for medically reviewed health information written for parents, kids, and teens. For more articles like this one, visit www.KidsHealth .org, or www.TeensHealth.org.

By meeting yearly with your teen, the doctor can keep track of changes in physical, mental, and social development and offer advice against unhealthy behaviors, such as smoking and drinking.

The doctor also can help your child understand the importance of choosing a healthy lifestyle that includes good nutrition, proper exercise, and safety measures. The more teens understand about their physical growth and sexual development, the more they will recognize the importance of active involvement in their own health care.

What to Expect at the Doctor's Office

Teens should visit their doctors annually. At least three of these visits should include a complete physical examination: one performed during early adolescence (ages 11 to 14), one during middle adolescence (ages 15 to 17), and one during late adolescence (ages 18 to 21). If your child has a chronic medical condition or if certain clinical signs or symptoms are present, more frequent exams may be needed.

Medical care should include screenings for high blood pressure, obesity, eating disorders, and, if indicated, hyperlipidemia (an excess of cholesterol and/or other fats in the blood). A tuberculin (PPD) test may be administered if your teen is at risk for tuberculosis.

Your teen's doctor will also check his or her teeth for tooth decay, abnormal tooth development, malocclusion (abnormal bite), dental injuries, and other problems. Your teen should also continue to have regular checkups with your dentist.

Vision and hearing will be checked. Teens are also checked for scoliosis (curvature of the spine).

Immunizations

Teens should receive a diphtheria and tetanus booster (Td) 10 years after their last childhood booster (usually at age 4 to 6 years) and every 10 years thereafter. They should have already completed their other immunizations, including varicella (if they have not had chickenpox); measles, mumps, and rubella (MMR); hepatitis B series (Hep B), and the HPV (human papillomavirus) vaccine. Before flu season each year, the flu vaccine (both seasonal and/or H1N1) is also recommended. And if your teen will be living in a group setting, such as a college dormitory, ask the doctor if the meningococcal meningitis vaccine also is required.

As kids go through puberty, issues of sexual health will be addressed. Your doctor will teach your daughter how to perform a monthly breast exam. The doctor also might perform (or refer her to a gynecologist for) a gynecologic exam and a Pap smear to check for cervical cancer. Males will be checked for hernias and testicular cancer and taught to perform a testicular self-exam.

Teens should be asked about behaviors or emotional problems that may indicate depression or the risk of suicide. The doctor also should provide counseling about risky behaviors and other issues, including:

- sexual activities that may result in unintended pregnancy and sexually transmitted diseases (STDs), including HIV [human immunodeficiency virus];

- emotional, physical, and sexual abuse;

- use of alcohol and other substances, including anabolic steroids;

- use of tobacco products, including cigarettes and smokeless tobacco;

- use of alcohol while driving;

- use of safety devices, including bicycle helmets, seat belts, and protective sports gear;

- how to resolve conflicts without violence, including how to avoid the use of weapons;

- learning problems or difficulties at school; and

- appropriate warm-ups before exercise and importance of regular physical activity.

If You Suspect a Medical Problem

Parents or other caregivers should receive health guidance at least once during early, middle, and late adolescence from their teen's doctor.

During these sessions, the doctor will provide information about normal development, including signs and symptoms of illness or emotional distress and methods to monitor and manage potentially harmful behaviors.

If you suspect that your teen has a physical disorder, a psychological problem, or a problem with drugs or alcohol, contact your doctor immediately.

Common Medical Problems

Issues involving puberty and sexual development are typical concerns for this age group. Doctors who establish a policy of confidentiality can serve as a valuable resource for a teen by answering questions and providing guidance during this period of physical and emotional changes. Teens should be reassured that anything they discuss with their doctor will be kept confidential, unless their health or the health of others is endangered by the situation.

Sports injuries are common concerns. Osgood-Schlatter disease, a painful inflammation of the area just below the front of the knee, is particularly common in the early teen years. Knee pain is also a frequent complaint. Your teen's doctor should evaluate any severe or persistent pain of the joints, muscles, or other areas of the body.

Section 8.2

Vaccines Teens Need

"Are you 11–19 years old?" © 2008 Immunization Action Coalition (www.immunize.org). Reprinted with permission.

Are you 11 to 19 years old? Then you need to be vaccinated against these serious diseases.

Many people between the ages of 11 and 19 think they are done with their vaccinations. They think vaccinations are just for little kids. But guess what? There are millions of people between the ages of 11 and 19 who need vaccinations to prevent whooping cough, tetanus, diphtheria, hepatitis B, hepatitis A, chickenpox, measles, mumps, rubella, polio, influenza, meningococcal disease, pneumococcal disease, and human papillomavirus infection. Are you one of them?

Getting immunized is a lifelong, life-protecting job. Make sure you and your healthcare provider keep your immunizations up-to-date. Check to be sure you've had all the vaccinations you need.

Hepatitis B (HepB)

You need a series of doses of hepatitis B vaccine if you have not already received them.

Measles, Mumps, Rubella (MMR)

Check with your healthcare provider to make sure you've had two doses of MMR.

Tetanus, Diphtheria, Pertussis (Whooping Cough) (Tdap, Td)

You need a booster dose of Tdap at age 11–12 years. If you're older and already had a Td booster, you should get a Tdap shot to get the extra protection against pertussis. After that you will need a Td booster dose every 10 years.

Polio (IPV)

If you haven't completed your series of polio vaccine doses and you are not yet 18, you should complete them now.

Varicella (Var) (Chickenpox Shot)

If you have not been previously vaccinated and have not had chickenpox, you should get vaccinated against this disease. The vaccine is given as a two-dose series. Any teenager who was vaccinated as a child with only one dose should get a second dose now.

Hepatitis A (HepA)

Anyone can get infected with hepatitis A. That is why many teens want to be protected by vaccine. Some teens, however, have an even greater chance of getting the disease. These risk factors include traveling outside the United States, babysitting or having household contact with a child who was adopted from a foreign country within the last 60 days, being a male who has sex with other males, using illegal drugs, or having a clotting factor disorder or chronic liver disease. Talk to your healthcare provider about this two-dose series of shots.

Human Papillomavirus (HPV)

All adolescent girls should get a series of three doses of HPV vaccine. One brand, Gardasil, prevents both cervical cancer and genital warts. Another brand of HPV vaccine, Cervarix, prevents cervical cancer. Adolescent boys, too, can get the Gardasil brand of the HPV vaccine to prevent genital warts.

Influenza

Every person, beginning at age 6 months and continuing throughout their lifetime, should receive annual vaccination against influenza every fall or winter. Vaccination is the most effective measure you can take to be protected from this serious disease.

Pneumococcal Disease (Pneumococcal Shot)

Do you have a chronic health problem? Talk to your healthcare provider about whether you should receive a pneumococcal shot.

Meningococcal Disease

This vaccine is recommended for all teens ages 11 through 18 years, college freshmen who will be or are living in dormitories, and those with certain special medical conditions.

Do You Travel outside the United States?

If so, you may need additional vaccines. The Centers for Disease Control and Prevention (CDC) operates an international traveler's health information line. Call 800-232-4636 or visit CDC's website at www.cdc.gov/travel for information about your destination. You may also consult a travel clinic or your healthcare professional.

Chapter 9

Nutrition Recommendations for Teens

Eating healthfully means getting the right balance of nutrients your body needs to perform every day. You can find out more about your nutritional needs by checking out the *Dietary Guidelines for Americans*. The guidelines suggest the number of calories you should eat daily based on your gender, age, and activity level.

According to the guidelines, a healthy eating plan includes the following:

- Fruits and vegetables

- Fat-free or low-fat milk and milk products

- Lean meats, poultry, fish, beans, eggs, and nuts

- Whole grains

In addition, a healthy diet is low in saturated and trans fats, cholesterol, salt, and added sugars.

When it comes to food portions, the Dietary Guidelines use the word "servings" to describe a standard amount of food. Serving sizes are measured as "ounce-" or "cup-equivalents." Here are some tips based on the guidelines that can help you develop healthy eating habits for a lifetime.

Excerpted from "Take Charge of Your Health!" by the Weight-control Information Network, National Institute of Diabetes and Digestive and Kidney Diseases (NIDDK, win.niddk.nih.gov), part of the National Institutes of Health, August 2009.

Eat fruits and vegetables every day.

When consumed as part of a well-balanced and nutritious eating plan, fruits and vegetables can help keep you healthy.

You may get your servings from fresh, frozen, dried, and canned fruits and vegetables. Teenagers who are consuming 2,000 calories per day should aim for 2 cups of fruit and 2½ cups of vegetables every day. You may need fewer or more servings depending on your individual calorie needs, which your health care provider can help you determine.

Power up with protein.

Protein builds and repairs body tissue like muscles and organs. Eating enough protein can help you grow strong and sustain your energy levels. Teens need five and one-half 1 ounce-equivalent of protein-rich foods each day.

Go whole grain.

Grain foods help give you energy. Whole-grain foods like whole-wheat bread, brown rice, and oatmeal usually have more nutrients than refined grain products. They give you a feeling of fullness and add bulk to your diet.

Try to get six 1 ounce-equivalents of grains every day, with at least three 1 ounce-equivalents coming from whole-grain sources.

Know your fats.

Fat is also an important nutrient. It helps your body grow and develop, and it is a source of energy as well—it even keeps your skin and hair healthy. But be aware that some fats are better for you than others. Limit your fat intake to 25% to 35% of your total calories each day.

Unsaturated fat can be part of a healthy diet—as long as you do not eat too much since it is still high in calories. Good sources include the following:

- Olive, canola, safflower, sunflower, corn, and soybean oils
- Fish like salmon, trout, tuna, and whitefish
- Nuts like walnuts, almonds, peanuts, and cashews

Limit saturated fat, which can clog your arteries and raise your risk for heart disease. Saturated fat is found primarily in animal products and in a few plant oils like:

- Butter
- Full-fat cheese
- Whole milk
- Fatty meats
- Coconut, palm, and palm kernel oils

Limit trans fat, which is also bad for your heart. Trans fat is often found in the following:

- Baked goods like cookies, muffins, and doughnuts
- Snack foods like crackers and chips
- Vegetable shortening
- Stick margarine
- Fried foods

Look for words like "shortening," "partially hydrogenated vegetable oil," or "hydrogenated vegetable oil" in the list of ingredients. These ingredients tell you that the food contains trans fat. Packaged food products are required to list trans fat on their Nutrition Facts labels.

Replenish your body with iron.

Teen boys need iron to support their rapid growth—most boys double their lean body mass between the ages of 10 and 17. Teen girls also need iron to support growth and replace blood lost during menstruation.

To get the iron you need, try eating these foods:

- Fish and shellfish
- Lean beef
- Iron-fortified cereals
- Enriched and whole-grain breads
- Cooked dried beans and peas like black beans, kidney beans, black-eyed peas, and chickpeas/garbanzo beans
- Spinach

Control your food portions.

The portion sizes that you get away from home at a restaurant, grocery store, or school event may contain more food than you need to eat in one sitting. Research shows that when people are served more food, they eat more food. So, how can you control your food portions?

When eating out, share your meal, order a half-portion, or order an appetizer as a main meal. Be aware that some appetizers are larger than others and can have as many calories as an entree.

Eat dinner with your family.

For many teens, dinner consists of eating on the run, snacking in front of the TV, or nonstop munching from after school to bedtime. Try to eat dinner as a family instead. Believe it or not, when you eat with your family you are more likely to get more fruits, vegetables, and other foods with the vitamins and minerals your body needs. Family meals also help you reconnect after a busy day. Talk to your family about fitting in at least a few meals together throughout the week.

Limit fast food and choose wisely.

Like many teens, you may eat at fast food restaurants often. If so, you are probably taking in a lot of extra calories from added sugar and fat. Just one value-sized fast food meal of a sandwich, fries, and sweetened soda can have more calories, fat, and added sugar than anyone needs.

The best approach is to limit the amount of fast food you eat. If you do order fast food, try these tips:

- Skip "value-sized" or "super-sized" meals.
- Choose a grilled chicken sandwich or a plain, small burger.
- Use mustard instead of mayonnaise.
- Limit fried foods or remove breading from fried chicken, which can cut half the fat.
- Order garden or grilled chicken salads with light or reduced-calorie dressings.
- Choose water, fat-free, or low-fat milk instead of sweetened soda.

Rethink your drinks.

Soda and other sugary drinks have replaced milk and water as the drinks of choice for teens and adults alike. Yet these drinks are actually more like desserts because they are high in added sugar and calories. In fact, soda and sugar-laden drinks may contribute to weight problems in kids and teens. Try sticking to water, low-fat milk, or fat-free milk.

Chapter 10

Talking with Your Teen about Healthy Food Choices

Parents who talk with their kids about food choices can help their children feel better today and stay healthy for tomorrow. As adults, we are encouraged to talk with kids about the birds and the bees and about alcohol and drugs. Talking about food choices combined with the Nutrition Facts label also makes sense. Nutrition influences growth and development.

What's a good food choice?

Lots of things. Fruits and vegetables. Low-fat dairy. Whole grain products. Lean meats. Fish. Poultry. Beans, eggs, and nuts. All have a place in a healthy diet.

Good food choices need to reflect balance and variety. Based on the latest scientific evidence, the *Dietary Guidelines for Americans* recommends choosing different fruits and vegetables from one day to the next. Varying selections within food groups is also suggested. For example, dark green and orange vegetables, legumes, starchy vegetables, and other vegetables should be eaten several times a week.

What's a good way to make food choices?

Everyone in the family can benefit from knowing how to use the Nutrition Facts label found on the side of packaged foods. Like a book's

"From Apples to Zucchini: Talk With Your Kids About Nutrition," by the Substance Abuse and Mental Health Services Administration (family.samhsa.gov), part of the U.S. Department of Health and Human Services, April 18, 2007.

table of contents, this label tells what nutrients are inside the food. Young people can use this information to make good food choices. They can make sure their bodies are getting the right combination of nutrients, such as vitamins, to work properly and be healthy.

The types and amounts of nutrients in a food aren't the only aspects of healthy eating. Counting calories matters—not only for individual foods like apple pie and broccoli but also for a person's total daily calorie intake. Consider the whole picture. Compare choices. Calculate daily needs.

The Nutrition Facts label gives calories per serving information. Be careful to check the portion size. For example, five small crackers or half a cup of canned green beans can constitute just one serving. Remember, fat free doesn't mean calorie free. Lower fat items may have as many calories as full-fat versions-as fat is reduced, sometimes more sugar is added.

Do fruits and vegetables require nutrition facts labels?

The Food and Drug Administration has voluntary guidelines for labeling of some raw fruits and vegetables but does not require nutrition labels on most fresh produce. Fresh fruits and vegetables are rich in nutrients and an important part of a healthy diet. Always follow safe handling and preparation practices.

How much is enough?

The *Dietary Guidelines for Americans* recommends four and one-half cups (nine servings) of fruits and vegetables (fresh, frozen, canned, or dried) daily for a 2,000-calorie diet, with higher or lower amounts depending on the individual calorie counts.

Unfortunately, most children and adults are simply not eating enough fruits and vegetables. In 2005, only one third of adults ate fruit two or more times a day.

The Centers for Disease Control and Prevention, Produce for Better Health Foundation, and other partners are collaborating through research, education, and environmental and policy strategies to encourage Americans to eat more fruits and vegetables. For cooking advice, nutrition information, and shopping tips, visit www.fruitsandveggiesmorematters.org.

What can parents do to ensure healthy eating?

First and foremost, be a good role model. The best way to encourage healthy habits in your children is to act healthfully. Youth watch what adults are doing. Parents' habits, both good and bad, have a strong influence on their children.

Provide regular meals and healthy snacks to ensure that your children get the energy and nutrients necessary for proper growth and development. Breakfast is especially important. Research shows that breakfast consumption may improve cognitive function related to memory, test grades, and school attendance.

Let your kids help plan the family menu. Take them to the grocery store with you. They can learn to read the food labels and make smart decisions about what they put in their bodies. By practicing good nutrition habits now, youth can protect their bodies and their health in the future.

What's all the talk about trans fat?

Fast food restaurants, manufacturers of potato chips and other snacks, even large cities like New York are making news about getting rid of trans fat. Trans fat has a "bad" reputation because it raises low-density lipoprotein (LDL) (or "bad") cholesterol levels in the blood, increasing the risk of heart disease. It's found in processed foods made with partially hydrogenated vegetable oils such as vegetable shortenings, some margarines (especially in stick form), and many crackers, candies, cookies, snack foods, fried foods, and baked goods.

Health experts recommend keeping intake of trans fat as well as saturated fat and cholesterol nutrients as low as possible while consuming a nutritionally adequate diet. Reducing trans fat does not mean cutting out fat entirely. Fats and oils are part of a healthful diet.

The *Dietary Guidelines for Americans* recommends keeping total fat intake between 20 to 35 percent of calories, with most fats coming from sources of polyunsaturated and monounsaturated fatty acids, such as fish, nuts, and vegetable oils.

Here are two tips on how you and your family can control trans fat intake:

- Use the Nutrition Facts label to compare foods. As of January 2006, trans fat must now be listed with saturated fat and cholesterol on the label.

- Substitute saturated and trans fats with mono- and polyunsaturated fats like olive, canola, soybean, sunflower, and corn oils.

Chapter 11

Calcium, Vitamin D, and Teens

Chapter Contents

Section 11.1

Facts about Calcium

Excerpted from "Milk Matters: For Strong Bones . . . For Lifelong Health," by the National Institute of Child Health and Human Development (NICHD, www.nichd.nih.gov), part of the National Institutes of Health, September 2005.

Growing tweens and teens have growing needs for milk. It takes calcium to build strong bones. And calcium is especially important during the tween and teen years, when bones are growing their fastest. Boys and girls in these age groups have calcium needs that they can't make up for later in life. Tweens and teens can get most of their daily calcium from 3 cups of low-fat or fat-free milk (900 mg of calcium), but they also need additional servings of calcium-rich foods to get the 1,300 mg of calcium necessary to build strong bones for life.

Low-fat or fat-free milk is a great source of calcium because it also has other important nutrients that are good for bones and teeth. One especially important nutrient is vitamin D, which helps the body absorb more calcium.

Starting around age 9, young people need almost twice as much calcium as younger kids to help during the critical bone-building time between the ages of 11 and 15. Unfortunately, fewer than one in 10 girls and only one in four boys ages 9 to 13 are at or above their adequate intake of calcium.

Building strong bones in the tween and teen years makes a lifelong difference. Having a calcium-rich diet when you're young makes a big difference in health, now and later. Drinking enough calcium will help with the following:

- It strengthens bones now. Our bodies continually remove and replace small amounts of calcium from our bones. If more calcium is removed than is replaced, bones will become weaker and have a greater chance of breaking. Some researchers suspect that the rise in forearm fractures in children is due to decreased bone mass, which may result because children are drinking less milk and more soda and are getting less physical activity.

- It helps prevent osteoporosis later in life. Osteoporosis is a condition that makes bones weak so they break more easily. Although the effects of osteoporosis might not show up until adulthood, tweens and teens can help prevent it by building strong bones when they are young.

Are there other reasons calcium is important?

Weight-bearing physical activity also builds strong bones. Bones are living tissue. Weight-bearing physical activity causes new bone tissue to form, which makes bones stronger. This kind of physical activity also makes muscles stronger. When muscles push and tug against bones during physical activity, bones and muscles become stronger. Weight-bearing activities are those that keep you active and on your feet so that your legs carry your body weight. Activities such as walking, running, dancing, climbing stairs, and playing team sports like basketball, soccer, and volleyball help make bones stronger. Older teenagers can build even more bone strength through weight training, but they should check with a health care provider before starting any type of training. Some activities, such as swimming, do not provide weight-bearing benefits. But they are good for cardiovascular fitness and overall good health.

Calcium is important for a healthy mouth, too. Even before they come in, baby teeth and adult teeth need calcium to develop fully. And after the teeth are in, calcium may also help protect them against decay. Calcium makes jawbones strong and healthy too! Besides making sure your children get enough calcium, there are other things you can do to keep their teeth healthy:

- Make sure your children brush with a fluoride toothpaste. Fluoride protects teeth from decay and helps heal early decay.

- Ask your child's dental care or health care provider if there is fluoride in your town or city's drinking water. If there is not, ask about fluoride tablets or drops for your child.

- Ask your child's dental care provider about proper brushing and flossing techniques and other ways your tween or teen can make sure teeth stay healthy.

What foods contain calcium?

There are lots of different calcium-rich foods to choose from, making it easy for tweens and teens to get the calcium they need every day. For example, just 1 cup of yogurt gives young people 25 percent of their daily calcium requirement. Low-fat and fat-free milk and milk products, such as low-fat or fat-free cheese and yogurt, are also excellent sources of calcium. Remember, tweens and teens can get most of their daily calcium from 3 cups of low-fat or fat-free milk (900 mg of calcium), but they also need additional servings of calcium-rich foods to get the 1,300 mg of calcium necessary.

Food labels can tell you how much calcium is in one serving of food. Look at the % Daily Value (% DV) next to the calcium number on the food label.

What if my teen doesn't like milk?

Even if your tweens or teens don't like the taste of plain milk, there are still plenty of ways to get calcium in the diet:

- Try a flavored low-fat or fat-free milk, such as chocolate, vanilla, or strawberry. Flavored milk has just as much calcium as plain.

- Serve foods that go with milk, such as fruit bars and fig bars.

- Drink milk or yogurt smoothies for breakfast or a snack. You can make these at home or try one of the ready-made versions now available at many grocery stores.

- Keep portable, calcium-rich foods on hand for snacks on the run, such as low-fat or fat-free string cheese or individual pudding cups with calcium added.

- In moderation, low-fat or fat-free ice cream and frozen yogurt are calcium-rich treats.

- Serve non-milk sources of calcium, such as calcium-fortified soy beverages or orange juice with added calcium.

- Try a spinach salad or have fresh or cooked broccoli.

Is one type of milk better than the other?

Today, tweens and teens have more milk choices than ever before. Most types of milk have approximately 300 mg of calcium per 8 fluid ounces (1 cup)—about 25 percent of the calcium that children and teenagers need every day. The best choices are low-fat or fat-free milk and milk products. Because these items contain little or no fat, it's easy to get enough calcium without adding extra fat to the diet.

Chocolate and other flavored milks have just as much calcium as plain milk, so it is fine for young people to drink these options if they prefer the taste. Remember to choose low-fat or fat-free.

Section 11.2

Low Vitamin D Levels Associated with Several Risk Factors in Teenagers

Study Highlights

- Low levels of vitamin D were associated with increased risk of high blood pressure, high blood sugar, and metabolic syndrome in teenagers.

- The highest levels of vitamin D were found in whites, the lowest levels in blacks, and intermediate levels in Mexican-Americans.

Low levels of vitamin D were associated with an increased risk of high blood pressure, high blood sugar, and metabolic syndrome in teenagers, researchers reported at the American Heart Association's 49th Annual Conference on Cardiovascular Disease Epidemiology and Prevention. In the study, researchers analyzed 3,577 adolescents, 12 to 19 years old (51 percent boys), who participated in the nationally representative National Health and Nutrition Examination Survey (NHANES) conducted from 2001–2004.

After adjusting for age, sex, race/ethnicity, body mass index, socioeconomic status, and physical activity, researchers found the adolescents with the lowest levels of vitamin D were:

- 2.36 times more likely to have high blood pressure;

- 2.54 times more likely to have high blood sugar; and

- 3.99 times more likely to have metabolic syndrome.

Metabolic syndrome is a cluster of cardiovascular disease and diabetes risk factors including elevated waist circumference, high blood pressure, elevated triglycerides, low levels of high-density lipoprotein (HDL or "good") cholesterol, and high fasting glucose levels. The presence of three or more of the factors increases a person's risk of developing diabetes and cardiovascular disease.

"We showed strong associations between low levels of vitamin D and higher risk of high blood pressure, hyperglycemia, and metabolic syndrome among adolescents, confirming the results of studies among adults," said Jared P. Reis, PhD, the study's lead author and postdoctoral research fellow at Johns Hopkins Bloomberg School of Public Health in Baltimore.

Researchers used a biomarker of vitamin D to measure levels in blood. The biomarker measures vitamin D obtained from food, vitamin supplementation, and exposure to sunlight.

The ethnic breakdown was similar to the general U.S. population: 64.7 percent non-Hispanic whites; 13.5 percent non-Hispanic blacks; and 11 percent Mexican Americans.

The study highlights the association between high levels of vitamin D and lower risk of heart disease. The highest levels of vitamin D were found in whites, the lowest levels in blacks, and intermediate levels in Mexican Americans. Whites had almost twice as high levels as blacks.

In whites, the average level of vitamin D was 28.0 nanograms per milliliter (ng/mL); in blacks, 15.5 ng/mL; and in Mexican Americans, 21.5 ng/mL.

"Although our study is important, we believe clinical trials designed to determine the effects of vitamin D supplementation on the risk of heart disease risk factors in adolescents should be conducted before recommendations can be made for vitamin D in the prevention of cardiovascular disease," Reis said.

The Institute of Medicine recommends a daily intake of vitamin D of 200 International Units (IU) for those less than 50 years, which includes children and adolescents. More recent recommendations, however, from the American Academy of Pediatrics suggests a daily intake of 400 IU daily. While these intakes have been shown to be important in the prevention of skeletal conditions such as rickets in children and osteoporosis in adults, some specialists have suggested intakes of at least 1,000 IU daily may be needed for overall health.

Low levels of vitamin D are strongly associated with overweight and abdominal obesity. Since vitamin D is a fat-soluble vitamin, it may be sequestered within adipose tissue. This may explain why those who are obese are more likely to be vitamin D deficient, Reis said.

Vitamin D plays a useful role in general human health, particularly in bone health. Other roles are emerging, Reis said. "This is an exciting time; since we are just now beginning to understand the role that vitamin D may play in cardiovascular health."

"These data on serum vitamin D levels in young people raise some concern about their food choices and even the amount of time they spend in the sunshine," said Robert H. Eckel, MD, American Heart Association past president. "The American Heart Association recommends an overall healthy diet and lifestyle, and that people get their nutrients primarily from food sources rather than supplements."

Co-authors are: Denise von Muhlen, MD, PhD; Edgar R. Miller III, MD, PhD; Erin D. Michos, MD, MHS; and Lawrence J. Appel, MD, MPH.

Chapter 12

Teens and Caffeine Use

Chapter Contents

Section 12.1

Energy Drinks: Power Boosts or Empty Boasts?

Excerpted from "Energy Drinks: Power Boosts or Empty Boasts?" by the Substance Abuse and Mental Health Services Administration (SAMHSA, family.samhsa.gov), part of the U.S. Department of Health and Human Services, April 30, 2007.

The energy drink market is hot. With names that suggest extreme power, a growing number of beverages are aimed at anyone who wants to improve athletic performance, study late, dance all night, or just counter a mid-afternoon slump.

These products are sold with claims that include boosting energy, raising alertness, lowering reaction time, improving concentration, speeding up metabolism, increasing stamina, and enhancing nutrition. Perhaps the most powerful energy drink is named after an illegal drug. Although this product does not contain the drug, it promises a high followed by a long-lasting energy buzz.

What's behind these claims? Although the makers of energy drinks tout mixtures of vitamins, minerals, and tropical extracts, the main ingredient is caffeine. The difference between the caffeine in energy drinks and other beverages is the amount—they have at least as much caffeine as coffee and much more than soft drinks.

Caffeine Concerns

Caffeine perks up the central nervous system and provides the lift that energy drinks are all about. The central nervous system, which includes the brain and the spinal cord, is the main "processing center" that controls all of the body's organs and systems.

However, the high levels of caffeine in energy drinks can cause problems. Because caffeine can send you to the bathroom more often, it can dehydrate your body—meaning that you do not have as much water and fluids as you should—when you are also sweating during exercise.

Caffeine also can speed up a person's heart and raise blood pressure. The amount of caffeine in energy drinks is not good for children. Caffeine may cause a child to become agitated, irritable, or nervous. In addition, caffeine is a concern for pregnant women as well as the children they carry.

What's in the Mix?

Other energy drink ingredients add to the possible problems. Guarana, or guarine, is a caffeine-like substance. Taurine is an amino acid that the body produces naturally, but exactly how it works or how much is too much is not known. Vitamins, minerals, and herbs added to energy drinks are not risky by themselves, but they could upset one's nutritional balance and could cause a bad reaction to medication.

Finally, energy drinks contain carbohydrates—carbs for short—that we need to fuel long exercise sessions. However, energy drinks provide more carbs than most people need for exercise. The result—excess calories—is just what we are trying to avoid or burn off. And because carbs make it harder for the body to absorb fluids, they can cause dehydration, especially in hot weather.

Choosing Wisely

While an energy drink every so often will not be a problem for most people, make sure that your child knows the real deal about these products. Talk with him about situations in which sports drinks could have unexpected effects. Remind him that many other products or just plain water can give him the lift he is looking for, often at a much lower cost than an energy drink. Making careful choices when he wants to kick it up a notch will pay off in safety and results. As a bonus, he'll end up with more money in his pocket.

Section 12.2

Caffeine and Teens' Sleep

"Caffeine and Teens' Sleep: An Eye-Opening Study," from the Substance Abuse and Mental Health Services Administration (SAMHSA, family.samhsa .gov), March 29, 2004. Reviewed by David A. Cooke, MD, FACP, March 16, 2010.

You may have spotted your teen staying up later than he used to. Activities that could be filling his late hours might include computer games, TV shows, phone calls, or music. Have you ever thought about caffeine intake as one of the reasons your teen is a night owl?

According to a recent study, eating foods, drinking beverages, or taking medications that have caffeine may lead to daytime sleepiness and breaks in sleep at night. Almost 200 high school students took part in this 14-day study. They reported on the time they went to bed and woke up, any caffeine intake, and any naps they took. At the end of the study, the researchers found that teens with higher caffeine intake slept fewer hours at night and took more naps during the day than those who had less caffeine.

What does this mean?

Broken sleep patterns can have many effects on a child. These include the following:

- Academic trouble
- Anxiety
- Decrease in cognitive development
- Depression (more common among females)
- Decreased immunity to illness
- Moodiness
- Reduced motivation

Caffeine can be found in many sodas, coffee, tea, and chocolate. It is also one of the most commonly used drugs in some pain medications and over-the-counter drugs. Caffeine stimulates the central nervous system and raises the heart rate, which can lead to nervous system disorders and heart problems.

Like many drugs, caffeine can be addictive. Once the body becomes used to the caffeine intake, it needs more to feel the same effect. This often causes a continued increase in caffeine intake.

What to do?

Now that you know some of the problems linked to loss of sleep and caffeine intake, you might be wondering how you can help your teen.

- Avoid caffeinated drinks and products in the evening. Offer juice, milk, and water instead of soft drinks or tea and coffee.

- Adjust plans to allow plenty of time for homework, studying, and writing reports and don't allow all-nighters. This will cut down on the desire to take coffee or drugs with caffeine.

- Talk with your teen and agree on a bedtime. Help your teen plan how to get enough sleep. Some activities may need to be cut out or cut down to keep with the bedtime.

- Urge your teen to stick to the plan as much as possible over the weekend.

These ideas can help reduce sleep deprivation. How do you help your teen kick the caffeine habit? Stopping caffeine intake cold turkey can cause withdrawal symptoms, including headaches, short-term depression or moodiness, and muscle aches. To avoid withdrawal, suggest slowly cutting back on caffeine. Cutting back may be hard at first, but after a few days your teen most likely will feel better rested and no longer suffer the effects of losing sleep.

Chapter 13

Physical Activity and Teens

Chapter Contents

Section 13.1

Tips to Help Teens Increase Physical Activity

Excerpted from "Take Charge of Your Health!" by the Weight-control Information Network, National Institute of Diabetes and Digestive and Kidney Diseases (NIDDK, win.niddk.nih.gov), part of the National Institutes of Health, August 2009.

Like eating well, physical activity may help you feel good. Being physically active may help you do the following:

- Help you control your weight, build lean muscle, and reduce your body fat
- Strengthen your bones
- Increase flexibility and balance
- Reduce your risk for chronic diseases like type 2 diabetes, heart disease, and high blood pressure

Physical activity also has possible emotional and social benefits, including the following:

- Improving your self-esteem and mood
- Decreasing feelings of anxiety and depression
- Helping you do better in school
- Improving your teamwork skills through sports

Be Active Every Day

Physical activity should be part of your daily life, whether you play sports, take physical education or other exercise classes, or even get from place to place by walking or bicycling. Teens should be physically active for 60 minutes or more on most, preferably all, days of the week.

Turn off the TV

Can too much TV contribute to weight problems? Several research studies say yes. In fact, one study noted that boys and girls who watched the most TV had more body fat than those who watched TV less than 2 hours a day.

Try to cut back on your TV, computer, and video game time and get moving instead. Here are some tips to help you break the TV habit.

- Tape your favorite shows and watch them later. This cuts down on TV time because you plan to watch specific shows instead of zoning out and flipping through the channels indefinitely.

- Replace after-school TV watching and video game use with physical activities.

- Get involved with activities at your school or in your community.

Making It Work

Look for chances to move more and eat better at home, at school, and in the community. It is not easy to maintain a healthy weight in today's environment. Fast food restaurants on every corner, vending machines at schools, and not enough safe places for physical activity can make it difficult to eat healthfully and be active. Busy schedules may also keep families from fixing and eating dinners together.

Old habits are hard to break and new ones, especially those related to eating and physical activity, can take months to develop and stick with. Here are some tips to help you in the process:

- Make changes slowly. Do not expect to change your eating or activity habits overnight. Changing too much too fast can hurt your chances of success.

- Look at your current eating and physical activity habits and at ways you can make them healthier. Use a food and activity journal for 4 or 5 days, and write down everything you eat, your activities, and your emotions. Review your journal to get a picture of your habits. Do you skip breakfast? Are you eating fruits and vegetables every day? Are you physically active most days of the week? Do you eat when you are stressed? Can you substitute physical activity for eating at these times? For tips on keeping a food and activity diary, check out the website of the American Academy of Family Physicians at www.familydoctor.org. You can also buy inexpensive journals at grocery stores, discount stores, or online bookstores.

- Set a few realistic goals for yourself. First, try cutting back the number of sweetened sodas you drink by replacing a couple of them with unsweetened beverages. Once you have reduced your sweetened soda intake, try eliminating these drinks from your diet. Then set a few more goals, like drinking low-fat or fat-free milk, eating more fruits, or getting more physical activity each day.

- Identify your barriers. Are there unhealthy snack foods at home that are too tempting? Is the food at your cafeteria too high in fat and added sugars? Do you find it hard to resist drinking several sweetened sodas a day because your friends do it? Use the tips above to identify changes you can make.

- Get a buddy at school or someone at home to support your new habits. Ask a friend, sibling, parent, or guardian to help you make changes and stick with your new habits.

- Know that you can do it! Stay positive and focused by remembering why you wanted to be healthier—to look, feel, move, and learn better. Accept relapses—if you fail at one of your nutrition or physical activity goals one day, do not give up. Just try again the next day. Also, share this information with your family. They can support you in adopting healthier behaviors.

Section 13.2

Strength Training in Adolescents

Reprinted with permission of the American College of Sports Medicine, "Strength Training in Children and Adolescents," September 2002. www .acsm.org. Reviewed by David A. Cooke, MD, FACP, March 16, 2010.

Benefits of Strength Training

Strength training in children and adolescents encourages a healthy lifestyle and builds confidence through successful completions of exercise and continued strength gains. Throughout the scientific literature, strength training has been shown to improve coordination by improving motor skills and sports performance. Especially in younger children, most strength gains are the result of improved technique, muscle fiber recruitment, and coordination as opposed to muscle enlargement. With childhood obesity on the increase nationwide, strength training has been shown to improve body composition by increasing lean body mass. Many studies looking at resistance training in children and adolescents reflect an improved cholesterol level, cardiorespiratory fitness, bone health, self-image, and self-esteem. A lower rate of sports-related injuries has been seen in adolescents who take part in a regular resistance training program. Children and adolescents who have experienced a sports-related injury often achieve more effective rehabilitation through strength training.

Safety Issues and Concerns

Severe injuries causing death or severe disability are exceedingly rare, but can occur while strength training in children and adolescents. These injuries are mostly due to the lack of appropriate adult supervision, instruction, or technique. Much controversy has surrounded the more explosive lifts involving children with open growth plates. A study involving 1109 children and adolescents lifting at national meets over a 4-year period showed not only no growth-plate injuries but no serious injuries requiring hospitalization or surgery. Minor injuries such as muscle strains are common among children and adolescents, as they are in their adult counterparts who do strength training. When compared to other sports in which children and adolescents participate—such as football, soccer, basketball and even baseball—the injuries due to all types of strength training are much lower. There is no current scientific evidence to support that early weight training can stunt a child's growth. Children and adolescents wishing to participate in intermediate and advanced strength training programs should consult with a certified or qualified strength specialist when developing individual programs.

Definitions

- **Strength training (a.k.a. resistance training, weight training):** Method of conditioning using resistance to increase muscular strength by various methods (i.e., free weights, weight machines, resistance bands).

- **Weightlifting:** Ballistic, explosive maneuvers involving a weighted barbell which is lifted from the ground to the overhead position. Weightlifting consists of two unique, complex lifts called the snatch and the clean and jerk.

- **Snatch:** One fluid motion, in which the barbell is pulled off the ground immediately into the overhead position. The lifter then stands upright with the barbell.

- **Clean and jerk:** A two-motion lift, in which the barbell is explosively lifted from the ground to the shoulder level. Then, after a brief pause, the lifter jerks the barbell overhead.

- **Powerlifting:** Non-ballistic maneuvers involving a weighted barbell, which is lifted in one of three methods: the bench press, the squat, or the deadlift.

- **Bench press:** A weighted barbell is lowered onto the lifter's chest with their arms while lying on a bench in a supine position. The barbell is then "pressed" or pushed off the chest until arms are fully extended.

- **Squat:** A weighted barbell is placed over the back of the shoulders on a standing lifter. The lifter then flexes at the knees and hips until thighs are parallel to the floor. Then the lifter attempts to stand upright with the barbell still on the shoulders.

- **Deadlift:** Lifter grasps weighted barbell on floor. The lifter then proceeds to raise the barbell to a position in front of the thighs by extending the legs, hips, and back.

- **Free weights:** Dumbbell, barbells, and other devices that are without external support and have independent motion.

- **Weight machine:** Devices which are used for resistance work through a certain, limited range of motion. May utilize weights, rubber bands, hydraulics, pulleys; are leveraged to create resistance.

- **Spotter:** A person with knowledge of strength training whose role is to assist the lifter and prevent injury.

- **Children:** Boys up to 13 years old; girls up to 11 years old

- **Adolescents:** Boys 14–18 years old; girls 12–18 years old

Guidelines

- Qualified adults should supervise and instruct youth at all times.

- Set realistic goals for the younger athlete.

- Focus on proper technique instead of amount lifted.

- Use a spotter when necessary.

- Each weight-training session should begin with a period of warm-up and stretching.

- Strength training should be part of a well-balanced exercise program.

- Increase the resistance gradually as technique, control, and strength improves.

Training Program

Basic (beginner) program (Example of a program): One should start with a basic program for 2 to 4 weeks that consists of one or two sets of each exercise.

- Warm-up (5 minutes)
- Leg extension (10–15 reps max)
- Leg press (10–15 repetitions max)
- Military press (10–15 reps max)
- Bench press (10–15 repetitions max)
- Reverse sit-up (10–15 reps max)
- Leg curls (10–15 repetitions max)

- Bent-leg sit-ups (10–15 reps max)
- Arm curls (10–15 repetitions max)
- Stretch (5 minutes)

Section 13.3

Sport Specialization: Advantages and Disadvantages

"Sports Specialization: Should children specialize in just one sport?" by Nima Zarrabi, January 2009, reprinted with permission from *Youth Fitness Magazine*, www.youthfitnessmag.com. © 2009 DHE, LLC. All rights reserved.

Why limit a child to a single athletic path? When people discuss the great athletes of the past century, the names that usually come to mind are not the players that are known for a single sport, but those who excelled in multiple sports. Athletes such as Bo Jackson, Deion Sanders, John Elway, Dave Winfield, Tony Gwynn, Marion Jones, and Lebron James, all starred in multiple sports before hitting the professional ranks.

Despite a history of splendid multi-sport athletes, youth sports have seen a rapid increase in its athletes specializing in one sport. Sports specialization is when a child picks a sport and trains in that sport year round. Rather than competing in a different sport each season, athletes who specialize, remain committed to improving in one sport. While sports specialization may seem like a good idea on the surface, there are several risks.

According to the American Academy of Pediatrics, early specialization has some distinct advantages, but may have negative physical, psychological, and social effects on a child. "Specialization leads to repetition and repetition leads to increased risk of injury," says Dr. Eric W. Edmonds, a Pediatric Orthopedic specialist at Rady Children's Hospital in San Diego, CA. "Injury leads to the inability to play that single sport that they have been training to participate. If they limit specialization, then they can be good at many sports, limit repetition by promoting cross-training, and decrease injury risk."

Parents also need to realize that when a child participates in different sports, certain skills carry over. The girl who plays basketball in the winter will likely have greater hand eye coordination for spring softball. The boy who runs track in the spring is likely to be faster on the gridiron when football season starts in the fall. There are tremendous benefits to challenging your body through various sports.

Dr. Edmonds isn't quite sure why so many parents have turned to sports specialization, although he cites convenience as a potential factor. "We all live very busy lives and sometimes feel like we can limit how many games and classes and events we have to drive to if our kids specialize in one sport," Dr. Edmonds says. "Also, a lot of parents are afraid that their child might not be a Jim Thorpe, so once they recognize a sport that their child likes or seems to be good at, then they actively push to have their child excel in that sport. Often times, people only know one way to get better at something, and that is to practice it over and over again—specialize. What you have to realize though, is that this is only one way to improve skills. The other is through cross-training, strength training, and diversifying activities."

By diversifying sports activities, parents can avoid one of the biggest pitfalls of sports specialization: burnout. Burnout happens when a highly committed athlete loses interest and motivation in their particular sport. It can occur in hard working, hard training athletes, who become emotionally, psychologically, or physically exhausted.

For Buffalo Bills quarterback Trent Edwards, playing multiple sports gave him an athletic edge. During high school, Edwards was a star football and basketball player. "The thing I liked about playing another sport outside of football was that it gave me another outlet," Edwards says. "To me, focusing on one sport for 12 months out of the year wasn't going to make me the best player. I needed another outlet so I didn't get burned out. If you look at most professional athletes, you will see that they played a variety of sports, which made them more athletic and helped build different muscles. I always enjoyed playing basketball. It gave me another opportunity to meet new people and work with different coaches. It also allowed me to get away from football for a bit, which was good as well."

By participating in numerous sports, a young athlete can develop other athletic skills that transfer to their primary activity. Quickness, balance, strength, and mental toughness are stressed differently in different sports.

For children that refuse to try any other sports, it is suggested that they take breaks from their primary sport to help the mind and body revitalize. To be competitive in one sport is fine, as long as it is not year round. "I don't know if children ever really know what they like," Dr. Edmonds says. "Their opinions can often be fickle and after 7 years of playing soccer because it was the greatest sport of all time, it may have just become the worst for no better reason then they didn't like their team name. I suggest that parents continually offer other activities and make sure that the athlete knows that she or he has the choice to do something different."

Dr. Edmonds believes a suitable age for young athletes to begin to specialize is 13 for girls and 15 for boys. "This is the average age at which girls and boys reach skeletal maturity," he explains. "At that time, bones are no longer growing, muscles and tendons have a chance to catch up, and focused training will be safer."

As sports specialization continues to grow in youth sports, it is important that parents are reminded that many of the professional athletes of today were two and three sport lettermen in high school. Once in a while a phenom comes around such as a Tiger Woods or Michael Jordan but that is less than 1 percent of high school athletes. According to the American Academy of Pediatrics, it is estimated that 98 percent of the athletes that specialize will never reach the highest levels of sport. Research has shown that early specialization does not ensure success in a particular sport. In fact, there is a better chance of injury or burnout. Sports specialization can be dangerous unless approached cautiously and in the right child.

Chapter 14

Weight Management in Teens

Chapter Contents

Section 14.1

Understanding Your Teen's Body Mass Index Measurement

Excerpted from "About BMI for Children and Teens," by the National Center for Chronic Disease Prevention and Health Promotion, Centers for Disease Control and Prevention (CDC, www.cdc.gov), January 27, 2009.

Body mass index (BMI) is a number calculated from a child's weight and height. BMI is a reliable indicator of body fatness for most children and teens. BMI does not measure body fat directly, but research has shown that BMI correlates to direct measures of body fat, such as underwater weighing and dual energy x-ray absorptiometry (DXA). BMI can be considered an alternative for direct measures of body fat. Additionally, BMI is an inexpensive and easy-to-perform method of screening for weight categories that may lead to health problems.

For children and teens, BMI is age- and sex-specific and is often referred to as BMI-for-age.

What is a BMI percentile?

After BMI is calculated for children and teens, the BMI number is plotted on the CDC BMI-for-age growth charts (for either girls or boys) to obtain a percentile ranking. Percentiles are the most commonly used indicator to assess the size and growth patterns of individual children in the United States. The percentile indicates the relative position of the child's BMI number among children of the same sex and age. The growth charts show the weight status categories used with children and teens (underweight, healthy weight, overweight, and obese). BMI-for-age weight status categories and the corresponding percentiles are shown in Table 14.1.

How is BMI used with children and teens?

BMI is used as a screening tool to identify possible weight problems for children. CDC and the American Academy of Pediatrics (AAP) recommend the use of BMI to screen for overweight and obesity in children beginning at 2 years old.

Table 14.1. Weight Status and BMI Percentiles

Weight Status Category	Percentile Range
Underweight	Less than the 5th percentile
Healthy weight	5th percentile to less than the 85th percentile
Overweight	85th to less than the 95th percentile
Obese	Equal to or greater than the 95th percentile

For children, BMI is used to screen for obesity, overweight, healthy weight, or underweight. However, BMI is not a diagnostic tool. For example, a child may have a high BMI for age and sex, but to determine if excess fat is a problem, a health care provider would need to perform further assessments. These assessments might include skinfold thickness measurements, evaluations of diet, physical activity, family history, and other appropriate health screenings.

How is BMI calculated and interpreted for children and teens?

Calculating and interpreting BMI using the BMI Percentile Calculator involves the following steps:

1. Before calculating BMI, obtain accurate height and weight measurements.

2. Calculate the BMI and percentile using the Child and Teen BMI Calculator [http://apps.nccd.cdc.gov/dnpabmi]. The BMI number is calculated using standard formulas.

3. Review the calculated BMI-for-age percentile and results. The BMI-for-age percentile is used to interpret the BMI number because BMI is both age-and sex-specific for children and teens. These criteria are different from those used to interpret BMI for adults—which do not take into account age or sex. Age and sex are considered for children and teens for two reasons:

    *   The amount of body fat changes with age. (BMI for children and teens is often referred to as BMI-for-age.)

    *   The amount of body fat differs between girls and boys.

    The CDC BMI-for-age growth charts for girls and boys take into account these differences and allow translation of a BMI number into a percentile for a child's or teen's sex and age.

4. Find the weight status category for the calculated BMI-for-age percentile as shown in Table 14.1. The CDC BMI-for-age growth charts are available at http://www.cdc.gov/growthcharts.

How can I tell if my child is overweight or obese?

CDC and the American Academy of Pediatrics (AAP) recommend the use of BMI to screen for overweight and obesity in children and teens aged 2 through 19 years. Although BMI is used to screen for overweight and obesity in children and teens, BMI is not a diagnostic tool.

For example, a child who is relatively heavy may have a high BMI for his or her age. To determine whether the child has excess fat, further assessment would be needed. Further assessment might include skinfold thickness measurements. To determine a counseling strategy, assessments of diet, health, and physical activity are needed.

Can I determine if my child or teen is obese by using an adult BMI calculator?

No. The adult calculator provides only the BMI number and not the BMI age- and sex-specific percentile that is used to interpret BMI and determine the weight category for children and teens. It is not appropriate to use the BMI categories for adults to interpret BMI numbers for children and teens.

Section 14.2

Helping Your Overweight Child

Excerpted from "Helping Your Overweight Child," by the Weight-control Information Network, National Institute of Diabetes and Digestive and Kidney Diseases (NIDDK, www.niddk.nih.gov), part of the National Institutes of Health, January 2008.

Healthy eating and physical activity habits are key to your child's well-being. Eating too much and exercising too little may lead to overweight and related health problems that may follow children into their adult years. You can take an active role to help your child—and your whole family—learn healthy eating and physical activity habits that last a lifetime.

Is my child overweight?

Children grow at different rates at different times, so it is not always easy to tell if a child is overweight. If you think that your child is overweight, talk to your health care provider. He or she can tell you if your child's weight and height are in a healthy range.

How can I help my overweight child?

Involve the whole family in building healthy eating and physical activity habits. This benefits everyone and does not single out the child who is overweight.

Do not put your child on a weight-loss diet unless your health care provider tells you to. If children do not eat enough, they may not grow and learn as well as they should.

How can I be supportive?

- Tell your child that he or she is loved, special, and important. Children's feelings about themselves are often based on how they think their parents feel about them.

- Accept your child at any weight. Children are more likely to accept and feel good about themselves when their parents accept them.

91

- Listen to your child's concerns about his or her weight. Over-weight children probably know better than anyone else that they have a weight problem. They need support, understanding, and encouragement from parents.

How can I encourage healthy eating habits?

- Buy and serve more fruits and vegetables (fresh, frozen, canned, or dried). Let your child choose them at the store.

- Buy fewer soft drinks and high-fat or high-calorie snack foods like chips, cookies, and candy. These snacks may be OK once in a while, but always keep healthy snack foods on hand. Offer the healthy snacks more often at snack times.

- Make sure your child eats breakfast every day. Breakfast may provide your child with the energy he or she needs to listen and learn in school. Skipping breakfast can leave your child hungry, tired, and looking for less healthy foods later in the day.

- Eat fast food less often. When you do visit a fast food restaurant, encourage your family to choose the healthier options, such as salads with low-fat dressing or small sandwiches without cheese or mayonnaise.

- Offer your child water or low-fat milk more often than fruit juice. Low-fat milk and milk products are important for your child's development. One hundred percent fruit juice is a healthy choice but is high in calories.

- Limit the amount of saturated and trans fats in your family's diet. Instead, obtain most of your fats from sources such as fish, vegetable oils, nuts, and seeds.

- Plan healthy meals and eat together as a family. Eating together at meal times helps children learn to enjoy a variety of foods.

- Do not get discouraged if your child will not eat a new food the first time it is served. Some kids will need to have a new food served to them 10 times or more before they will eat it.

- Try not to use food as a reward when encouraging kids to eat. Promising dessert to a child for eating vegetables, for example, sends the message that vegetables are less valuable than dessert. Kids learn to dislike foods they think are less valuable.

- Start with small servings and let your child ask for more if he or she is still hungry. It is up to you to provide your child with healthy meals and snacks, but your child should be allowed to choose how much food he or she will eat.

- Be aware that some high-fat or high-sugar foods and beverages may be strongly marketed to kids. Usually these products are associated with cartoon characters, offer free toys, and come in bright packages. Talk with your child about the importance of fruits, vegetables, whole grains, and other healthy foods—even if these foods are not often advertised on TV or in stores.

How do I encourage daily physical activity?

Like adults, kids need daily physical activity. Here are some ways to help your child move every day:

- Set a good example. If your child sees that you are physically active and that you have fun doing it, he or she is more likely to be active throughout life.

- Encourage your child to join a sports team or class, such as soccer, dance, basketball, or gymnastics at school or at your local community or recreation center.

- Be sensitive to your child's needs. If your child feels uncomfortable participating in activities like sports, help him or her find physical activities that are fun and not embarrassing, such as playing tag with friends or siblings, jumping rope, or dancing to his or her favorite music.

- Be active together as a family. Assign active chores such as making the beds, washing the car, or vacuuming. Plan active outings such as a trip to the zoo, a family bike ride, or a walk through a local park.

A preadolescent child's body is not ready for adult-style physical activity. Do not encourage your child to participate in activities such as long jogs, using an exercise bike or treadmill, or lifting heavy weights. FUN physical activities that kids choose to do on their own are often best.

Kids need about 60 minutes of physical activity a day, but this does not have to happen all at once. Several short 10- or even 5-minute periods of activity throughout the day are just as good. If your children are not used to being active, encourage them to start with what they can do and build up to 60 minutes a day.

How do I discourage inactive pastimes?

- Set limits on the amount of time your family spends watching TV, playing video games, and being on the computer.

- Help your child find fun things to do besides watching TV, like acting out favorite books or stories, or doing a family art project. Your child may find that creative play is more interesting than TV.

- Encourage your child to get up and move during commercials and discourage snacking when the TV is on.

How do I find more help?

Ask your health care provider for brochures, booklets, or other information about healthy eating, physical activity, and weight control. He or she may be able to refer you to other health care professionals who work with overweight children, such as registered dietitians, psychologists, and exercise physiologists.

You may want to think about a weight-control treatment program if the following are true:

- You have changed your family's eating and physical activity habits and your child has not reached a healthy weight.

- Your health care provider has told you that your child's health or emotional well-being is at risk because of his or her weight.

The overall goal of a treatment program should be to help your whole family adopt healthy eating and physical activity habits that you can keep up for the rest of your lives. Here are some other things a weight-control program should do:

- Include a variety of health care professionals on staff, including doctors, registered dietitians, psychiatrists or psychologists, and exercise physiologists

- Evaluate your child's weight, growth, and health before enrolling him or her in the program and monitor these factors while your child is enrolled

- Adapt to the specific age and abilities of your child

- Help your family keep up healthy eating and physical activity behaviors after the program ends

Chapter 15

Body Image in Youth

Chapter Contents

Section 15.1

For Teens: Developing Body Image and Self-Esteem

I'm fat. I'm too skinny. I'd be happy if I were taller, shorter, had curly hair, straight hair, a smaller nose, bigger muscles, longer legs.

Do any of these statements sound familiar? Are you used to putting yourself down? If so, you're not alone. As a teen, you're going through a ton of changes in your body. And as your body changes, so does your image of yourself. Lots of people have trouble adjusting, and this can affect their self-esteem.

Why Are Self-Esteem and Body Image Important?

Self-esteem is all about how much people value themselves, the pride they feel in themselves, and how worthwhile they feel. Self-esteem is important because feeling good about yourself can affect how you act. A person who has high self-esteem will make friends easily, is more in control of his or her behavior, and will enjoy life more.

Body image is how someone feels about his or her own physical appearance.

For many people, especially those in their early teens, body image can be closely linked to self-esteem. That's because as kids develop into teens, they care more about how others see them.

What Influences a Person's Self-Esteem?

Puberty

Some teens struggle with their self-esteem when they begin puberty because the body goes through many changes. These changes, combined with a natural desire to feel accepted, mean it can be tempting for people to compare themselves with others. They may compare themselves with the people around them or with actors and celebs they see on TV, in movies, or in magazines.

But it's impossible to measure ourselves against others because the changes that come with puberty are different for everyone. Some people start developing early; others are late bloomers. Some get a temporary layer of fat to prepare for a growth spurt, others fill out permanently, and others feel like they stay skinny no matter how much they eat. It all depends on how our genes have programmed our bodies to act.

The changes that come with puberty can affect how both girls and guys feel about themselves. Some girls may feel uncomfortable or embarrassed about their maturing bodies. Others may wish that they were developing faster. Girls may feel pressure to be thin but guys may feel like they don't look big or muscular enough.

Outside Influences

It's not just development that affects self-esteem, though. Many other factors (like media images of skinny girls and bulked-up guys) can affect a person's body image too.

Family life can sometimes influence self-esteem. Some parents spend more time criticizing their kids and the way they look than praising them, which can reduce kids' ability to develop good self-esteem.

People also may experience negative comments and hurtful teasing about the way they look from classmates and peers. Sometimes racial and ethnic prejudice is the source of such comments. Although these often come from ignorance, sometimes they can affect someone's body image and self-esteem.

Healthy Self-Esteem

If you have a positive body image, you probably like and accept yourself the way you are. This healthy attitude allows you to explore other aspects of growing up, such as developing good friendships, growing more independent from your parents, and challenging yourself physically and mentally. Developing these parts of yourself can help boost your self-esteem.

A positive, optimistic attitude can help people develop strong self-esteem—for example, saying, "Hey, I'm human" instead of "Wow, I'm such a loser" when you've made a mistake, or not blaming others when things don't go as expected.

Knowing what makes you happy and how to meet your goals can help you feel capable, strong, and in control of your life. A positive attitude and a healthy lifestyle (such as exercising and eating right) are a great combination for building good self-esteem.

Tips for Improving Your Body Image

Some people think they need to change how they look or act to feel good about themselves. But actually all you need to do is change the way you see your body and how you think about yourself.

The first thing to do is recognize that your body is your own, no matter what shape, size, or color it comes in. If you're very worried about your weight or size, check with your doctor to verify that things are OK. But it's no one's business but your own what your body is like—ultimately, you have to be happy with yourself.

Next, identify which aspects of your appearance you can realistically change and which you can't. Everyone (even the most perfect-seeming celeb) has things about themselves that they can't change and need to accept—like their height, for example, or their shoe size.

If there are things about yourself that you want to change and can (such as how fit you are), do this by making goals for yourself. For example, if you want to get fit, make a plan to exercise every day and eat nutritious foods. Then keep track of your progress until you reach your goal. Meeting a challenge you set for yourself is a great way to boost self-esteem!

When you hear negative comments coming from within yourself, tell yourself to stop. Try building your self-esteem by giving yourself three compliments every day. While you're at it, every evening list three things in your day that really gave you pleasure. It can be anything from the way the sun felt on your face, the sound of your favorite band, or the way someone laughed at your jokes. By focusing on the good things you do and the positive aspects of your life, you can change how you feel about yourself.

Where Can I Go If I Need Help?

Sometimes low self-esteem and body image problems are too much to handle alone. A few teens may become depressed, lose interest in activities or friends—and even hurt themselves or resort to alcohol or drug abuse.

If you're feeling this way, it can help to talk to a parent, coach, religious leader, guidance counselor, therapist, or an adult friend. A trusted adult—someone who supports you and doesn't bring you down—can help you put your body image in perspective and give you positive feedback about your body, your skills, and your abilities.

If you can't turn to anyone you know, call a teen crisis hotline (check the yellow pages under social services or search online). The most important thing is to get help if you feel like your body image and self-esteem are affecting your life.

Section 15.2

Why Do Teens Get Plastic Surgery?

"Plastic Surgery," December 2009, reprinted with permission from www .kidshealth.org. Copyright © 2009 The Nemours Foundation. This information was provided by KidsHealth, one of the largest resources online for medically reviewed health information written for parents, kids, and teens. For more articles like this one, visit www.KidsHealth.org, or www .TeensHealth.org.

When you hear of plastic surgery, what do you think of? A Hollywood star trying to delay the effects of aging? People who want to change the size of their stomachs, breasts, or other body parts because they see it done so easily on TV?

Those are common images of plastic surgery, but what about the 4-year-old boy who has his chin rebuilt after a dog bit him? Or the young woman who has the birthmark on her forehead lightened with a laser?

What Is Plastic Surgery?

Just because the name includes the word "plastic" doesn't mean patients who have this surgery end up with a face full of fake stuff. The name isn't taken from the synthetic substance but from the Greek word *plastikos*, which means to form or mold (and which gives the material plastic its name as well).

Plastic surgery is a special type of surgery that can involve both a person's appearance and ability to function. Plastic surgeons strive to improve patients' appearance and self-image through both reconstructive and cosmetic procedures.

- **Reconstructive procedures correct defects on the face or body.** These include physical birth defects like cleft lips and palates and ear deformities, traumatic injuries like those from dog bites or burns, or the aftermath of disease treatments like rebuilding a woman's breast after surgery for breast cancer.

- **Cosmetic (also called aesthetic) procedures alter a part of the body that the person is not satisfied with.** Common cosmetic procedures include making the breasts larger (augmentation mammoplasty) or smaller (reduction mammoplasty), reshaping the nose (rhinoplasty), and removing pockets of fat from specific spots on the body (liposuction). Some cosmetic procedures aren't even surgical in the way that most people think of surgery—that is, cutting and stitching. For example, the use of special lasers to remove unwanted hair and sanding skin to improve severe scarring are two such treatments.

Why Do Teens Get Plastic Surgery?

Most teens don't, of course. But some do. Interestingly, the American Society of Plastic Surgeons (ASPS) reports a difference in the reasons teens give for having plastic surgery and the reasons adults do: Teens view plastic surgery as a way to fit in and look acceptable to friends and peers. Adults, on the other hand, frequently see plastic surgery as a way to stand out from the crowd.

The number of teens who choose to get plastic surgery is on the rise. According to the ASPS, over 333,000 people 18 years and younger had plastic surgery in 2005, up from about 306,000 in 2000.

Some people turn to plastic surgery to correct a physical defect or to alter a part of the body that makes them feel uncomfortable. For example, guys with a condition called gynecomastia (excess breast tissue) that doesn't go away with time or weight loss may opt for reduction surgery. A girl or guy with a birthmark may turn to laser treatment to lessen its appearance.

Other people decide they want a cosmetic change because they're not happy about the way they look. Teens who have cosmetic procedures—such as otoplasty (surgery to pin back ears that stick out) or dermabrasion (a procedure that can help smooth or camouflage severe acne scars)—sometimes feel more comfortable with their appearance after the procedure.

The most common procedures teens choose include nose reshaping, ear surgery, acne and acne scar treatment, and breast reduction.

Is Plastic Surgery the Right Choice?

Reconstructive surgery helps repair significant defects or problems. But what about having cosmetic surgery just to change your appearance? Is it a good idea for teens? As with everything, there are right and wrong reasons to have surgery.

Cosmetic surgery is unlikely to change your life. Most board-certified plastic surgeons spend a lot of time interviewing teens who want plastic surgery to decide if they are good candidates for the surgery. Doctors want to know that teens are emotionally mature enough to handle the surgery and that they're doing it for the right reasons.

Many plastic surgery procedures are just that—surgery. They involve anesthesia, wound healing, and other serious risks. Doctors who perform these procedures want to know that their patients are capable of understanding and handling the stress of surgery.

Some doctors won't perform certain procedures (like rhinoplasty) on a teen until they are sure that person is old enough and has finished growing. For rhinoplasty, that means about 15 or 16 for girls and about a year older for guys.

Girls who want to enlarge their breasts for cosmetic reasons usually must be at least 18 because saline implants are only approved for women 18 and older. In some cases, though, such as when there's a tremendous size difference between the breasts or one breast has failed to grow at all, a plastic surgeon may get involved earlier.

Things to Consider

Here are a few things to think about if you're considering plastic surgery:

- Almost all teens (and many adults) are self-conscious about their bodies. Almost everyone wishes there were a thing or two that could be changed. A lot of this self-consciousness goes away with time. Ask yourself if you're considering plastic surgery because you want it for yourself or whether it's to please someone else.

- A person's body continues to change through the teen years. Body parts that might appear too large or too small now can become more proportionate over time. Sometimes, for example, what seems like a big nose looks more the right size as the rest of the person's face catches up during growth.

- Getting in good shape through appropriate weight control and exercise can do great things for a person's looks without surgery. It's never a good idea to choose plastic surgery as a first option for something like weight loss that can be corrected in a nonsurgical manner. Gastric bypass or liposuction may seem like quick and easy fixes compared with sticking to a diet. Both of these procedures, however, carry far greater risks than dieting, and doctors should reserve them for extreme cases when all other options have failed.

• Some people's emotions have a really big effect on how they think they look. People who are depressed, extremely self-critical, or have a distorted view of what they really look like sometimes think that changing their looks will solve their problems. In these cases, it won't. Working out the emotional problem with the help of a trained therapist is a better bet. In fact, many doctors won't perform plastic surgery on teens who are depressed or have other mental health problems until these problems are treated first.

What's Involved?

If you're considering plastic surgery, talk it over with your parents. If you're serious and your parents agree, the next step is meeting with a plastic surgeon to help you learn what to expect before, during, and after the procedure—as well as any possible complications or downsides to the surgery. Depending on the procedure, you may feel some pain as you recover, and temporary swelling or bruising can make you look less like yourself for a while.

Procedures and healing times vary, so you'll want to do your research into what's involved in your particular procedure and whether the surgery is reconstructive or cosmetic. It's a good idea to choose a doctor who is certified by the American Board of Plastic Surgery.

Cost will likely be a factor, too. Elective plastic surgery procedures can be expensive. Although medical insurance covers many reconstructive surgeries, the cost of cosmetic procedures almost always comes straight out of the patient's pocket.

Your parents can find out what your insurance plan will and won't cover. For example, breast enlargement surgery is considered a purely cosmetic procedure and is rarely covered by insurance. But breast reduction surgery may be covered by some plans because large breasts can cause physical discomfort and even pain for many girls.

Plastic surgery isn't something to rush into. If you're thinking about plastic surgery, find out as much as you can about the specific procedure you're considering and talk it over with doctors and your parents. Once you have the facts, you can decide whether the surgery is right for you.

Chapter 16

Sleep and Adolescents

Chapter Contents

Section 16.1

Is Your Teen Sleep Deprived?

High school teachers are all too familiar with the bleary eyes and giant yawns that often greet their lessons. But the responses might be less about teenage boredom and more about sleep deprivation, and the students' growing bodies themselves may be to blame.

As adolescents mature toward adulthood, nature seems to be preparing even their sleep cycles for the lifestyle change. Their bodies release the sleep-inducing hormone melatonin later in the evening than when the students were preteens, so they're not tired until later at night. Yet school bells still seem to ring at dawn.

Sleep Requirements

"Preteens can go to bed earlier, but for teens, the key lies in later school times, 8 to 8:30 in the morning," recommends Maninder Kalra, MD, a pediatric sleep specialist in the Sleep Disorders Center of Cincinnati Children's Hospital Medical Center. "Teenagers need that extra hour of sleep in the morning."

But what if the family's school district maintains an early start to the high school day? Preteens still need about 10 hours of sleep a night, and teens, 9. Yet surveys are showing that teens on average are sleeping 7.4 hours—"objective evidence that they're not getting enough sleep," says Dr. Kalra.

Students themselves feel the deficit. In a recent study, as many as 70 percent of American teens said they wished they got more sleep.

Less Sleep, More Problems

The effects of sleep deprivation are often swift and dramatic: Impaired alertness during the day and decreased cognitive ability, with the problems showing up "as soon as the next day," according to Dr.

Kalra. "We also see increased risk-taking behavior and depressed mood. The impaired alertness and increased risk-taking have serious implications when teens are driving."

In new studies, sleep deprivation is also proving to create serious medical complications. Lack of sleep affects the hormones that regulate how the body converts food to energy and decreases glucose tolerance. Sleep-starved children are then at risk for being overweight and developing cardiovascular problems.

To help counter sleep deprivation, Dr. Kalra recommends that "parents establish good sleep hygiene, with consistent bed and wake-up times. They can promote exposure to bright light in the morning, and avoid bright lights at night. This promotes the tendency to fall asleep earlier in the evening."

"Students should avoid caffeine in the late afternoon and evening, as well as exercise, TV, and video games right before bed."

When to Seek Help

In spite of all these efforts, some teens have trouble falling asleep, or feeling rested after sleep. But Dr. Kalra cautions against immediately reaching for an over-the-counter sleep aid: "That might mask the problem."

Instead, parents and children can seek help from their family doctor or a sleep specialist. "They will take a detailed sleep history, looking for mood disorders, psychosocial stressors or symptoms of medical problems, such as restless leg syndrome or sleep apnea."

Melatonin may be prescribed to help decrease the time it takes to fall asleep. A specialist might also set up a child's schedule of timed exposure to light, and work with chronotherapy—tapping into the body's natural biological rhythms—to shift sleep-time patterns. Occasionally, a sleeping pill will be recommended to help the teenager fall asleep.

"Once teens are evaluated, there are a variety of options to help them get the sleep they need," says Dr. Kalra.

Section 16.2

Sleep-Smart Tips for Parents and Teens

From "Sleepy Teens at School and Behind the Wheel," by the Substance Abuse and Mental Health Services Administration (SAMHSA, family.samhsa .gov), part of the U.S. Department of Health and Human Services, March 4, 2004. Reviewed by David A. Cooke, MD, FACP, March 16, 2010.

"Kids have so much energy!" is not true for many American teens, who actually require more sleep than they did as children. A poll by the National Sleep Foundation (NSF) shows that most teens are not getting the 9.25 hours of sleep they need each night. One reason is that a teen's biological clock changes during puberty and disrupts their normal sleep-wake cycle. Many teens find it is hard to fall asleep until late at night; then, they want to sleep later in the morning. However, many demands on teens, such as early school times, conflict with their new sleeping pattern. As a result, teens often do not get the sleep they need. They are sleepy when they most need to be alert. Teens can have trouble paying attention and learning in school, especially in the morning. In the NSF poll, 15 percent of teens said they fell asleep at school sometime during the year.

Teens who drive while sleepy are a danger to themselves and others. Driving drowsy can be like driving under the influence of drugs or alcohol. Sleepy teens are more likely to have breaks in attention, impaired memory and judgment, and slower reactions at critical times. Police report that drowsiness or fatigue causes at least 100,000 traffic crashes each year. These crashes kill more than 1,500 people and injure another 71,000. Drivers aged 25 and younger are involved in more than half of crashes in which the driver has fallen asleep.

Parents need to find ways to help their teens be well rested, ready to face the school day and the road. The tips below may help:

Sleep-Smart Tips for Parents and Teens

- **Set a bedtime routine.** A regular bedtime helps the body get used to a sleep schedule. Your teen's bedtime routine should include at least 15–30 minutes of low-key activities such as reading or taking a warm bath. He should avoid exercise, telephone use, and playing video games during this time. For a few hours before bedtime, your teen also should avoid caffeine, which is found in many beverages, in chocolate, and in other products.

- **Make sleep an important activity.** Help your teen set priorities for activities. Make sure that downtime and sleep are high on the list. Many teens lose sleep because they have too many demands on their time. Too many activities can lead to stress, poor health, and sleep problems.

- **Look for signs of lack of sleep.** Your teen may not be getting enough sleep if she finds it hard to wake up in the morning or falls asleep during quiet times of the day. Another sign is that your teen sleeps for extra long periods whenever she can. A teen who isn't getting enough sleep also may be cranky in the afternoon or may seem depressed.

- **Follow the light.** Use bright light and sunshine to help your teen wake up in the morning. Low light at night will help a teen's body get ready for sleep.

- **Be a good role model.** Create a home life that supports healthy sleep habits for the whole family. Set an example by making sure that you get enough sleep. You also need to be able to deal well with the challenges of your day, including being a good parent.

Part Three

Puberty, Sexuality, and Reproductive Health

Chapter 17

Overview of Reproductive and Sexual Health Trends in Teens

Sexual Activity

- Nearly half (46%) of all 15- to 19-year-olds in the United States have had sex at least once.[1]

- By age 15, only 13% of never-married teens have ever had sex. However, by the time they reach age 19, seven in 10 never-married teens have engaged in sexual intercourse.[1]

- Most young people have sex for the first time at about age 17, but they do not marry until their middle or late 20s. This means that young adults are at risk of unwanted pregnancy and sexually transmitted infections (STIs) for nearly a decade.[2]

- Teens are waiting longer to have sex than they did in the past. Some 13% of never-married females and 15% of never-married males aged 15–19 in 2002 had had sex before age 15, compared with 19% and 21%, respectively, in 1995.[1]

- The majority (59%) of sexually experienced teen females had a first sexual partner who was 1–3 years their senior. Only 8% had first partners who were 6 or more years older.[1]

Guttmacher Institute, Facts on American Teens' Sexual and Reproductive Health, In Brief. New York: Guttmacher, © 2006. http://www.guttmacher.org/pubs/fb_ATSRH.html, accessed May 12, 2010.

- More than three quarters of teen females report that their first sexual experience was with a steady boyfriend, a fiance, a husband, or a cohabiting partner.[1]

- Ten percent of young women aged 18–24 who have had sex before age 20 report that their first sex was involuntary. The younger they were at first intercourse, the higher the proportion.[1]

- Twelve percent of teen males and 10% of teen females have had heterosexual oral sex but not vaginal intercourse.[3]

- The proportion of teens who had ever had sex declined from 49% to 46% among females and from 55% to 46% among males between 1995 and 2002.[1]

Contraceptive Use

- A sexually active teen who does not use contraceptives has a 90% chance of becoming pregnant within a year.[4]

- The majority of sexually experienced teens (74% of females and 82% of males) used contraceptives the first time they had sex.[1]

- The condom is the most common contraceptive method used at first intercourse; it was used by 66% of sexually experienced females and 71% of males.[1]

- Nearly all sexually active females (98% in 2002) have used at least one method of birth control. The most common methods used are the condom (used at least once by 94%) and the pill (used at least once by 61%).[1]

- Nearly one quarter of teens who used contraceptives the last time they had sex combined two methods, primarily the condom and a hormonal method.[1]

- At most recent sex, 83% of teen females and 91% of teen males used contraceptives. These proportions represent a marked improvement since 1995, when only 71% of teen females and 82% of teen males had used a contraceptive method at last sex.[1]

Access to Contraceptive Services

- Twenty-one states and the District of Columbia explicitly allow all minors to consent to contraceptive services without a parent's involvement (as of January 2010). Two states (Texas and Utah) require parental consent for contraceptive services in state-funded family planning programs.[5]

- Ninety percent of publicly funded family planning clinics counsel clients younger than 18 about abstinence and the importance of communicating with parents about sex.[6]

- Sixty percent of teens younger than 18 who use a clinic for sexual health services say their parents know they are there.[7]

- Among those whose parents do not know, 70% would not use the clinic to obtain prescription contraceptives if the law required that their parents be notified.[7]

- One in five teens whose parents do not know they obtain contraceptive services would continue to have sex but would either rely on withdrawal or not use any contraceptives if the law required that their parents be notified of their visit.[7]

- Only 1% of all minor adolescents who use sexual health services indicate that their only reaction to a law requiring their parents' involvement in obtaining prescription contraceptives would be to stop having sex.[7]

STIs

- Of the 18.9 million new cases of STIs each year, 9.1 million (48%) occur among 15- to 24-year-olds.[8]

- Although 15- to 24-year-olds represent only one quarter of the sexually active population, they account for nearly half of all new STIs each year.[8]

- Human papillomavirus (HPV) infections account for about half of STIs diagnosed among 15- to 24-year-olds each year. HPV is extremely common, often asymptomatic, and generally harmless. However, certain types, if left undetected and untreated, can lead to cervical cancer.[8]

- In June 2006, the U.S. Food and Drug Administration approved the vaccine Gardasil as safe and effective for use among girls and women aged 9–26. The vaccine prevents infection with the types of HPV most likely to lead to cervical cancer.

Pregnancy

- Each year, almost 750,000 women aged 15–19 become pregnant. Overall, 71.5 pregnancies per 1,000 women aged 15–19 occurred in 2006; the rate declined 41% from its peak in 1990 to a low of 69.5 in 2005.[9]

- The majority of the decline in teen pregnancy rates is due to more consistent contraceptive use; the rest is due to higher proportions of teens choosing to delay sexual activity.[10]

- However, for the first time since the early 1990s, overall teen pregnancy rates increased in 2006, rising 3%. It is too soon to tell whether this reversal is simply a short-term fluctuation or the beginning of a long-term increase.[9]

- Black and Hispanic women have the highest teen pregnancy rates (126 and 127 per 1,000 women aged 15–19, respectively); non-Hispanic whites have the lowest rate (44 per 1,000).[9]

- The pregnancy rate among black teens decreased 45% between 1990 and 2005, more than the overall U.S. teen pregnancy rate declined during the same period (41%).[9]

- Eighty-two percent of teen pregnancies are unplanned; they account for about one fifth of all unintended pregnancies annually.[11]

- Two thirds of all teen pregnancies occur among 18- to 19-year-olds.[9]

Childbearing

- Ten percent of all U.S. births are to teens.[12]

- Fifty-nine percent of pregnancies among 15- to 19-year-olds ended in birth in 2006.[9]

- In 2006, there were 42 births per 1,000 women aged 15–19. The rate has dropped by 32% since 1991, when it was 62 per 1,000, but increased 4% between 2005 and 2006.[12]

- Seven percent of teen mothers receive late or no prenatal care. Babies born to teens are more likely to be low-birthweight than are those born to women in their 20s and 30s.[12]

- Teen mothers are now more likely than in the past to complete high school or obtain a GED [general educational development test], but they are still less likely than women who delay childbearing to go on to college.[13]

Abortion

- There were 200,420 abortions among 15- to 19-year-olds in 2006.[9]

- Twenty-seven percent of pregnancies among 15- to 19-year-olds ended in abortion in 2006.[9]

- The reasons teens give most frequently for having an abortion are concern about how having a baby would change their lives, inability to afford a baby now, and feeling insufficiently mature to raise a child.[14]

- As of January 2010, 34 states require that a minor seeking an abortion involve her parents in the decision.[15]

- Six in 10 minors who have abortions do so with at least one parent's knowledge. The great majority of parents support their daughter's decision to have an abortion.[16]

References

1. Abma JC et al., Teenagers in the United States: sexual activity, contraceptive use, and childbearing, 2002, *Vital and Health Statistics,* 2004, Series 23, No. 24.

2. The Alan Guttmacher Institute (AGI), *In Their Own Right: Addressing the Sexual and Reproductive Health Needs of American Men,* New York: AGI, 2002.

3. Mosher WD et al., Sexual behavior and selected health measures: men and women 15–44 years of age, United States, 2002, *Advance Data from Vital and Health Statistics,* 2005, No. 362.

4. Harlap S, Kost K and Forrest JD, *Preventing Pregnancy, Protecting Health: A New Look at Birth Control Choices in the United States,* New York: AGI, 1991.

5. Guttmacher Institute, Minors' access to contraceptive services, *State Policies in Brief,* updated Jan. 1, 2010, <http://www.guttmacher.org/statecenter/spibs/spib_MACS.pdf>, accessed Jan. 26, 2010.

6. Lindberg LD et al., Provision of contraceptive and related services by publicly funded family planning clinics, 2003, *Perspectives on Sexual and Reproductive Health,* 2006, 38(3):139–147.

7. Jones RK et al., Adolescents' reports of parental knowledge of adolescents' use of sexual health services and their reactions to mandated parental notification for prescription contraception, *Journal of the American Medical Association,* 2005, 293(3):340–348.

8. Weinstock H et al., Sexually transmitted diseases among American youth: incidence and prevalence estimates, 2000, *Perspectives on Sexual and Reproductive Health,* 2004, 36(1):6–10.

9. Guttmacher Institute, *U.S. Teenage Pregnancies, Births and Abortions: National and State Trends and Trends by Race and Ethnicity,* accessed Jan. 26, 2010.

10. Santelli JS et al., Explaining recent declines in adolescent pregnancy in the United States: the contribution of abstinence and improved contraceptive use, *American Journal of Public Health,* 2007, 97(1):150–156.

11. Finer LB et al., Disparities in rates of unintended pregnancy in the United States, 1994 and 2001, *Perspectives on Sexual and Reproductive Health,* 2006, 38(2):90–96.

12. Martin JA et al., Births: final data for 2002, *National Vital Statistics Reports,* 2003, Vol. 52, No. 10.

13. Hofferth SL et al., The effects of early childbearing on schooling over time, *Family Planning Perspectives,* 2001, 33(6):259–267.

14. Dauphinee LA, Guttmacher Institute, New York, personal communication, Mar. 23, 2006.

15. Guttmacher Institute, Parental involvement in minors' abortions, *State Policies in Brief,* updated Aug. 1, 2006, <http://www.guttmacher.org/statecenter/spibs/spib_PIMA.pdf>, accessed Aug. 8, 2006.

16. Henshaw SK and Kost K, Parental involvement in minors' abortion decisions, *Family Planning Perspectives,* 1992, 24(5):196–207 & 213.

Chapter 18

Puberty and Male Sexual Development

Adolescence is the time between childhood and adulthood. It lasts roughly from age 9 until adulthood. Adolescence includes puberty, physical changes, a change in thinking ability, and all the social and emotional changes that happen during this stage of life. Adolescence can be an exciting time and a tough time in a boy's life.

Puberty starts at the beginning of adolescence. It is when hormones change and a boy matures physically to become a young man. He experiences increases in height and weight, the size of his testicles and penis, and growth of pubic, facial, and body hair. He gains muscle mass and physical strength. His voice deepens. His brain is also maturing while his body is changing. It is during puberty that a boy's reproductive organs mature so that his body is ready for reproduction. He is then able to get a girl pregnant.

There is a master gland in males that controls all of this development called the pituitary gland. It is located in the brain and is about the size of a pea, and produces hormones that cause the testicles to produce male sex hormones. These hormones cause many of the physical changes that turn a boy's body into a young man's body.

Boys go through many physical and emotional changes during puberty.

Excerpted from "Boys and Puberty," by the U.S. Department of Health and Human Services (www.4parents.gov), August 6, 2008.

Physical Changes during Puberty for Boys

- Height and weight increase.

- Body hair grows in the pubic area, under the arms, and on the face, and becomes thicker on the legs.

- Muscles become stronger.

- Vocal cords get thicker and longer—boys' voices deepen.

- The body develops an increased number of red blood cells.

- Sweat and oil glands become more active, and body odor changes.

- Acne can develop.

- Some boys develop small and temporary breast tissue.

- Reproductive system begins to work.

Male Reproductive System

Men's reproductive organs are mostly on the outside of the body. Here is a list.

- **Cowper's glands:** These two glands provide a clear thick fluid that lubricates the urethra when the penis is erect so that sperm can pass through. The urethra is the tube in the penis that carries semen or urine.

- **Epididymis:** These coiled tubes are located at the back of the testes. Sperm move through these to be stored in the seminal vesicles.

- **Penis:** The penis is an external organ with a central tube called the urethra through which semen or urine leaves the body. The penis is made up of the shaft and the glans (head). The foreskin is a fold of skin that protects the glans (head) of the penis. The penis does not contain any bones or muscle but is made up of soft, spongy tissue that is full of blood vessels and lots of nerves. When a man is sexually excited, these vessels fill with blood. This causes the penis to enlarge and stiffen, which is called an erection. When semen comes out of the penis it is called ejaculation. Teenage boys often have erections even without sexual excitement. They also can release semen during the night (wet dreams). This is normal and common.

- **Prostate:** The prostate is a gland that produces a fluid that becomes part of semen.

- **Seminal vesicles:** These glands, located behind the bladder, produce a fluid that forms part of semen. They are also storage areas for sperm.

- **Scrotum:** The scrotum is the soft sac on the outside of the body that contains and protects the testicles. It is behind and underneath the penis. To protect sperm cells from temperature changes, muscles of the scrotum tighten when exposed to cold temperatures. This brings the testicles closer to the body. In warm weather, the scrotum hangs lower and the testicles seem larger—but there is actually no change in size of the testicles.

- **Sperm:** Under a microscope, these male reproductive cells look like a tadpole, with a head and a tail. Sperm are produced in the testicles when puberty begins. Sperm cells swim in semen, a whitish, sticky liquid. Once a boy's body begins to produce sperm, he will produce millions daily for the rest of his life.

- **Testes/Testicles:** In addition to sperm, these two glands also produce the male sex hormone testosterone. During puberty, the testicles become larger to allow the production of sperm. The testicles hang outside the body because sperm production requires a temperature slightly lower than body temperature. It is normal for the testicles to be slightly different sizes. New lumps or irregular areas on the testes should be checked by a doctor.

- **Urethra:** This narrow tube running from the bladder through the penis is the passage for urine and semen. Semen and urine do not mix. That is because urine is automatically cut off when semen is being released.

- **Vas deferens:** These narrow tubes carry sperm from the epididymis, past the seminal vesicles, and into the prostate gland.

Sexual Development of Boys

A boy goes through five stages of development during puberty. Boys usually start to show the physical changes of puberty between the ages of 11 and 14, which is slightly older than when girls start puberty. The male sex hormone called testosterone and other hormones cause the physical changes.

Here are the five stages and what happens.

119

Stage 1

- This stage may begin as early as age 9 and continue until 14.
- There is no sign of physical development but hormone production is beginning.

Stage 2

- This stage may begin anywhere from ages 11 to 13.
- Height and weight increase rapidly.
- Testicles become larger and scrotum hangs lower.
- Scrotum becomes darker in color.
- Fine hair growth begins at the base of the penis.
- Hair growth may begin on the legs and underarms.

Stage 3

- This stage may begin anywhere from ages 12 to 14.
- The penis, scrotum, and testicles grow.
- Pubic hair becomes darker, thicker, and curlier.
- Muscles become larger and shoulders become broader.
- Sweat and oil glands become more active, which can result in acne.
- Sperm production may begin.
- Temporary swelling and tenderness may occur around nipples.
- Height and weight continue to increase.
- Hair growth on the legs and underarms continues.

Stage 4

- This stage may begin anywhere from ages 13 to 16.
- Sperm production has usually begun.
- The larynx (Adam's apple) increases in size. Vocal chords become longer and thicker, and the voice begins to break or crack, then becomes low.
- Height and weight continue to increase.

- Penis and testicles continue to grow.

- Pubic hair increases in amount and becomes darker, coarser, and curly.

Stage 5

- This stage may begin anywhere from ages 14 to 18.

- Growth of facial hair begins.

- Chest hair growth may begin (not all males get much chest hair).

- Adult height is reached.

- Penis and testicles have reached full adult size.

- Pubic, underarm, and leg hair are adult color, texture, and distribution.

- Overall look is that of a young adult man.

Chapter 19

Male Reproductive Concerns

Chapter Contents

Section 19.1

How to Do a Testicular Self-Exam

For men over the age of 14, a monthly self-exam of the testicles is
an effective way of becoming familiar with this area of the body and
thus enabling the detection of testicular cancer at an early—and very
curable—stage. Why do you need to do it monthly? Because the point
of the self-exam is not to find something wrong today. The point is to
learn what everything feels like when things are normal, and to check
back every month to make sure that nothing has changed. If something
has changed, you will know it and you can do something about it.

The testicular self-exam is best performed after a warm bath or
shower. (Heat relaxes the scrotum, making it easier to spot anything
abnormal.)

Here is how to do the self-exam:

- If possible, stand in front of a mirror. Check for any swelling on
  the scrotal skin.

- Examine each testicle with both hands. Place the index and
  middle fingers under the testicle with the thumbs placed on
  top. Roll the testicle gently between the thumbs and fingers—
  you shouldn't feel any pain when doing the exam. Don't be
  alarmed if one testicle seems slightly larger than the other—
  that's normal.

- Find the epididymis, the soft, tubelike structure behind the testicle that collects and carries sperm. If you are familiar with this
  structure, you won't mistake it for a suspicious lump. Cancerous
  lumps usually are found on the sides of the testicle but can also
  show up on the front. Lumps on or attached to the epididymis
  are not cancerous.

- If you find a lump on your testicle or any of the other signs
  of testicular cancer listed in the following text, see a doctor,
  preferably a urologist, right away. The abnormality may not

be cancer, but if it is testicular cancer, it will spread if it is not stopped by treatment. Even if it is something else like an infection, you are still going to need to see a doctor. Waiting and hoping will not fix anything. Please note that free-floating lumps in the scrotum that are not attached in any way to a testicle are not testicular cancer. When in doubt, get it checked out—if only for peace of mind.

Other signs of testicular cancer to keep in mind are:

- any enlargement of a testicle;
- a significant loss of size in one of the testicles;
- a feeling of heaviness in the scrotum;
- a dull ache in the lower abdomen or in the groin;
- a sudden collection of fluid in the scrotum;
- pain or discomfort in a testicle or in the scrotum;
- enlargement or tenderness of the breasts.

Anything out of the ordinary down there should prompt a visit to the doctor, but you should be aware that the following symptoms are not normally signs of testicular cancer:

- A pimple, ingrown hair, or rash on the scrotal skin
- A free-floating lump in the scrotum, seemingly not attached to anything
- A lump on the epididymis or tubes coming from the testicle that kind of feels like a third testicle
- Pain or burning during urination
- Blood in the urine or semen

Remember, only a physician can make a positive diagnosis. For that matter, only a physician can make a negative diagnosis, too. If you think something feels strange, go see the doctor.

Finally, embarrassment is a poor excuse for not having any problem examined by a doctor. If you think there is something wrong or something has changed, please see your doctor.

Section 19.2

Disorders of the Testes

The testicles (also called testes) are part of the male reproductive system. The testicles are two oval organs about the size of large olives. They are located inside the scrotum, the loose sac of skin that hangs behind the penis. The testicles make the male hormones, including testosterone, and produce sperm, the male reproductive cells. Disorders of the testes can lead to serious complications, including hormonal imbalances, sexual dysfunction, and infertility.

What Disorders Affect the Testes?

Some of the more common disorders that affect the testes include the following:

Testicular Trauma

Because the testes are located within the scrotum, which hangs outside of the body, they do not have the protection of muscles and bones. This makes it easier for the testes to be struck, hit, kicked or crushed, which occurs most often during contact sports. Males can protect their testicles by wearing athletic cups during sports.

Trauma to the testes can cause severe pain, bruising, and/or swelling. In most cases, the testes—which are made of a spongy material—can absorb the shock of an injury without serious damage.

A rare type of testicular trauma, called testicular rupture, occurs when the testicle receives a direct blow or is squeezed against the hard surface of the pelvis. This injury can cause blood to leak into the scrotum. In severe cases, surgery to repair the rupture—and thus save the testicle—may be necessary.

Testicular Torsion

Within the scrotum, the testicles are secured at one end by a structure called the spermatic cord. Sometimes, this cord gets twisted, cutting off the testicle's blood supply. Symptoms of testicular torsion include sudden and severe pain, enlargement of the affected testicle, tenderness, and swelling.

This disorder, which occurs most often in young males between the ages of 12 and 18, can result from an injury to the testicles or from strenuous activity. It also can occur for no apparent reason.

Testicular torsion is an emergency. Treatment usually involves correction of the problem through surgery. Testicular function may be saved if the condition is diagnosed and corrected immediately. If the blood supply to the testicle is cut off for a long period of time, the testicle can become permanently damaged and may need to be removed.

Testicular Cancer

Testicular cancer occurs when abnormal cells in the testicles divide and grow uncontrolled. Testicular cancer can develop in one or both testicles in men or young boys. Symptoms of testicular cancer include a lump, irregularity or enlargement in either testicle; a pulling sensation or feeling of unusual heaviness in the scrotum; a dull ache in the groin or lower abdomen; and pain or discomfort (which may come and go) in a testicle or the scrotum.

The exact causes of testicular cancer are not known, but there are certain risk factors for the disease. A risk factor is anything that increases a person's chance of getting a disease. The risk factors for cancer of the testicles include:

- **Age:** Testicular cancer can occur at any age, but most often occurs in men between the ages of 15 and 40.

- **Undescended testicle (cryptorchidism):** This is a condition in which the testicles do not descend from the abdomen, where they are located during development, to the scrotum shortly before birth. This condition is a major risk factor for testicular cancer.

- **Family history:** A family history of testicular cancer increases the risk.

- **Race and ethnicity:** The risk for testicular cancer in Caucasian men is more than five times that of African-American men and more than double that of Asian-American men.

127

Testicular cancer is a rare form of cancer, and is highly treatable and usually curable. Surgery is the most common treatment for testicular cancer. Surgical treatment involves removing the cancerous testicle through an incision (cut) in the groin. In some cases, the doctor also may remove some of the lymph nodes in the abdomen. Radiation, which uses high-energy rays to attack cancer, and chemotherapy, which uses drugs to kill cancer, are other treatment options.

The success of treatment for testicular cancer depends on the stage of the disease when it is first detected and treated. If the cancer is found and treated before it spreads to the lymph nodes, the cure rate is excellent—greater than 98 percent. Even after testicular cancer has spread to the lymph nodes and other parts of the body, chemotherapy is highly effective, with a cure rate greater than 90 percent.

To prevent testicular cancer, all men should be familiar with the size and feel of their testicles, so they can detect any changes. The American Cancer Society recommends monthly testicular self-examinations (TSE) for men over age 15. A TSE is best performed after a warm bath or shower, when the skin of the scrotum is relaxed. After looking for any changes in appearance, carefully examine each testicle by rolling it between the fingers and thumbs of both hands to check for any lumps.

Epididymitis

Epididymitis is inflammation of the epididymis. The epididymis is the coiled tube that lies on and behind each testicle. It functions in the transport, storage, and maturation of sperm cells that are produced in the testicles. The epididymis connects the testicles with the vas deferens (the tubes that carry sperm).

Epididymitis often is caused by infection or by the sexually transmitted disease chlamydia. Symptoms of epididymitis include scrotal pain and swelling. In severe cases, the infection can spread to the adjacent testicle, causing fever and abscess (collection of pus).

Treatment for epididymitis includes antibiotics (drugs that kill the bacteria causing the infection), bed rest, ice to reduce swelling, the use of a scrotal supporter, and anti-inflammatory medicines (such as ibuprofen). The use of condoms during sex can help prevent epididymitis caused by chlamydia. If left untreated, epididymitis can produce scar tissue, which can block the sperm from leaving the testicle. This can cause problems with fertility, especially if both testicles are involved or if the man has recurring infections.

Hypogonadism

One function of the testes is to secrete the hormone testosterone. This hormone plays an important role in the development and maintenance of many male physical characteristics. These include muscle mass and strength, fat distribution, bone mass, sperm production, and sex drive.

Hypogonadism in men is a disorder that occurs when the testicles (gonads) do not produce enough testosterone. Primary hypogonadism occurs when there is a problem or abnormality in the testicles themselves. Secondary hypogonadism occurs when there is a problem with the pituitary gland in the brain, which sends chemical messages to the testicles to produce testosterone.

Hypogonadism can occur during fetal development, at puberty, or in adult men. When it occurs in adult men, hypogonadism may cause the following problems:

- Erectile dysfunction (the inability to achieve or maintain an erection)

- Infertility

- Decreased sex drive

- Decrease in beard and growth of body hair

- Decrease in size or firmness of the testicles

- Decrease in muscle mass and increase in body fat

- Enlarged male breast tissue

- Mental and emotional symptoms similar to those of menopause in women (hot flashes, mood swings, irritability, depression, fatigue)

There are various causes of hypogonadism, including:

- **Klinefelter's syndrome:** This syndrome involves the presence of abnormal sex chromosomes. A male normally has one X chromosome and one Y chromosome. The Y chromosome contains the genetic material with the codes that determine the male gender, and related masculine characteristics and development. Males with Klinefelter's syndrome have an extra X chromosome, which causes abnormal development of the testicles.

- **Undescended testicles:** The testicles develop inside the abdomen and usually move down into the scrotum before birth. Sometimes, this does not occur. However, in most cases, the testicles descend by the child's first birthday. An undescended testicle that remains outside the scrotum throughout childhood can result in abnormal testicular development.

- **Hemochromatosis:** Hemochromatosis, or too much iron in the blood, can cause the testicles or the pituitary gland to malfunction.

- **Testicular trauma:** Damage to the testicles can affect the production of testosterone.

- **Cancer treatment:** Chemotherapy or radiation therapy, common treatments for cancer, can interfere with testosterone and sperm production by the testicles.

- **Normal aging:** Older men generally have lower levels of testosterone, although the decline of the hormone varies greatly among men.

- **Pituitary disorders:** Problems affecting the pituitary gland—including a head injury or pituitary tumor—can interfere with the gland's signals to the testicles to produce testosterone.

- **Medications:** Certain drugs can affect testosterone production. Commonly used psychiatric drugs and some medicines used to treat gastroesophageal reflux disease (GERD) may cause hypogonadism.

Treatment for hypogonadism depends on the cause. Male hormone replacement (testosterone replacement therapy or TRT) often is used to treat disorders of the testicles. If the problem is related to the pituitary gland, pituitary hormones may help increase testosterone levels and sperm production.

Section 19.3

Gynecomastia (Male Breast Development)

"Gynecomastia," © 2010 A.D.A.M., Inc. Reprinted with permission.

Gynecomastia is the development of abnormally large breasts in males. It is related to the excess growth of breast tissue, rather than excess fat tissue.

Considerations

The condition may occur in one or both breasts and begins as a small lump beneath the nipple, which may be tender. The breasts often enlarge unevenly. Gynecomastia during puberty is not uncommon and usually goes away over a period of months.

In newborns, breast development may be associated with milk flow (galactorrhea). This condition usually lasts for a couple of weeks, but in rare cases may last until the child is 2 years old.

Causes

Androgens are hormones that create male characteristics, such as hair growth, muscle size, and a deep voice. Estrogens are hormones that create female characteristics. All men have both androgens and estrogens.

Changes in the levels of these hormones, or in how the body uses or responds to these hormones can cause enlarged breasts in men.

More than half of boys develop gynecomastia during puberty. Other causes include:

- aging;
- cancer chemotherapy;
- chronic liver disease;
- exposure to anabolic steroid hormones;
- exposure to estrogen hormone;
- kidney failure and dialysis;
- marijuana use;

- hormone treatment for prostate cancer;
- radiation treatment of the testicles;
- side effects of some medications (ketoconazole, spironolactone, metronidazole, cimetidine [Tagamet]); and
- testosterone (male hormone) deficiency.

Rare causes include:

- genetic defects;
- overactive thyroid; and
- tumors.

Breast cancer in men is rare. Signs that may suggest breast cancer include:

- one-sided breast growth;
- firm or hard breast lump that feels like it is attached to the tissue;
- skin ulcer over the breast; and
- bloody discharge from the nipple.

Home Care

Apply cold compresses and use analgesics as your health care provider recommends if swollen breasts are also tender.

Other tips include:

- stop taking all recreational drugs, such as marijuana; and
- stop taking all nutritional supplements or any drugs you are taking for bodybuilding.

When to Contact a Medical Professional

Call your health care provider if:

- you have recent swelling, pain, or enlargement in one or both breasts;
- there is dark or bloody discharge from the nipples;
- there is a skin sore or ulcer over the breast; or
- a breast lump feels hard or firm.

Note: Gynecomastia in children who have not yet reached puberty should always be checked by a health care provider.

What to Expect at Your Office Visit

Your health care provider will take a medical history and perform a physical examination.

Medical history questions may include:

- Is one or both breasts involved?

- What is the age and gender of the patient?

- What medications is the person taking?

- How long has gynecomastia been present?

- Is the gynecomastia staying the same, getting better, or getting worse?

- What other symptoms are present?

Testing may not be necessary, but the following tests may be done to rule out certain diseases:

- Blood hormone level tests

- Breast ultrasound

- Liver and kidney function studies

- Mammogram

Intervention

If an underlying condition is found, it is treated. Your physician should consider all medications that may be causing the problem. Gynecomastia during puberty usually goes away on its own.

Breast enlargement that is extreme, uneven, or does not go away may be embarrassing for an adolescent boy. Treatments that may be used in rare situations are:

- hormone treatment that blocks the effects of estrogens; and

- breast reduction surgery.

Chapter 20

Puberty and Female Sexual Development

Adolescence includes puberty, the physical changes, a change in thinking ability, and all the social and emotional changes that happen during this stage of life. It lasts roughly from age 9 until adulthood. Adolescence can be an exciting time and a tough time in a girl's life.

Puberty starts at the beginning of adolescence and is the time when hormones begin to change and a girl matures physically into a young woman. She develops breasts and her hips widen. Like boys, she experiences increases in height and weight, pubic and body hair, and she also begins menstruating. Her brain is also maturing while her body is changing. It is during puberty that the female reproductive organs mature and the body becomes ready for reproduction. Once a girl's reproductive organs begin maturing, she can get pregnant if she has sex.

There is a master gland in a female that controls all of this development. It's called the pituitary gland. It's located in the brain and is about the size of a pea. The pituitary gland produces hormones that cause the ovaries to produce the female sex hormone. These hormones cause some of the physical changes that turn a girl's body into a young woman's body.

Girls go through many physical and emotional changes during puberty. Both boys and girls begin to feel more and more independent.

Excerpted from "Girls and Puberty," by the U.S. Department of Health and Human Services (www.4parents.gov), October 5, 2009.

Physical Changes during Puberty for Girls

- Breasts develop.

- Height and weight increase.

- Hips and waist become more defined.

- Menstruation begins.

- Mood changes may occur.

- Body hair grows in the pubic area, under the arms, and becomes thicker on the arms and legs.

- Muscles become stronger.

- Fat tissue normally increases.

- Vocal cords get thicker and longer.

- Sweat and oil glands become more active, and body odor changes.

- Acne may develop.

- The reproductive system matures.

Female Reproductive System

A female's reproductive organs are mostly inside the body in the pelvis. The pelvic girdle, a ring of bone shaped like a basin, surrounds them. Here is a list of the female reproductive organs.

- **Cervix:** The cervix is the lower part of the uterus that opens into the vagina. The cervix is rounded and cone-shaped. It is about 1 inch in length. Menstrual fluid escapes through a small tube down the center of the cervix. The tube is small, about the size of the end of a pencil. The cervix can open (dilate) up to 10 centimeters during childbirth.

- **Clitoris:** A clitoris is a piece of body tissue with lots of nerve endings. The size and shape of a pencil eraser, the clitoris is located at the upper vulva, above the vaginal and bladder openings.

- **Egg (ovum):** The egg is the female reproductive cell released from an ovary each month. Upon release, a fully grown egg is a little smaller than the period at the end of this sentence.

- **Endometrium:** This lining provides oxygen and nutrition for an embryo during pregnancy. It leaves the body each month during a menstrual period if pregnancy does not happen.

- **Fallopian tubes:** The fallopian tubes are two tubes attached on either side of the uterus. Grown egg cells (ova) travel through these tubes toward the uterus. The inside contains hair-like projections called cilia. These cilia move the egg (ovum) from the ovary to the uterus.

- **Hymen:** This thin, flexible membrane partially covering the vaginal opening has an opening that allows menstrual fluid to leave the body.

- **Ovaries:** The ovaries are two glands that produce hormones and reproductive cells called eggs or ova. The ovaries are the size of a small bird's egg and the shape of an almond. They are located on either side of the uterus. The ovaries contain thousands of undeveloped egg cells (ova). Only a few hundred of these will mature and be released during a female's reproductive years.

- **Uterus:** It is in the uterus where a baby develops. The uterus is about the size and shape of an upside-down pear. It can stretch up to 20 times its normal size during pregnancy. The muscle contracts to help push the baby through the birth canal at delivery and can also contract and cause cramps during menstruation.

- **Vagina:** The vulva is the passageway leading from the uterus to the outside of the body. The vagina is 4 to 5 inches in length. At the top it is connected to the cervix and at the bottom it opens between the inner thighs. It is often called the birth canal. The opening to the vagina is protected by flexible folds of skin called the labia.

- **Vulva:** The vulva is the name for the external female genitalia. The two pairs of fleshy folds between the upper thighs are called the labia, and they surround and cover the vaginal opening.

Sexual Development of Girls

Girls go through five stages of development during puberty.

Girls usually start to show the physical changes of puberty between the ages of 9 and 13, which is slightly sooner than boys. The female sex hormone called estrogen and other hormones cause the physical changes. Many girls are fully developed by the age of 16. Some girls will continue to develop through age 18.

Here are the five stages and what happens.

137

Stage 1

- This stage occurs between ages 8 to 12.

- There are no visible signs of physical development but the ovaries are enlarging and hormone production is beginning.

Stage 2

- This stage may begin anywhere from ages 8 to 14.

- Height and weight increase rapidly.

- Fine hair growth begins close to the pubic area and underarms.

- Breast buds appear; nipples become raised and this area may be tender.

- Sweat and oil glands become more active, which can result in acne.

Stage 3

- This stage may begin anywhere from ages 9 to 15.

- Breasts become rounder and fuller.

- Hips may start to widen in relation to waist.

- The vagina begins secreting a clear or whitish fluid.

- Pubic hair becomes darker, thicker, and curlier.

- Height and weight continue to increase.

- For some girls, ovulation and menstruation (periods) begin, but may be irregular.

Stage 4

- This stage may begin anywhere from ages 10 to 16.

- Underarm hair becomes darker.

- Pubic hair starts to form a triangular patch in front and around the sides of the genital area.

- The nipple and the dark area around the breast (areola) may stick out from the rest of the breast.

- For many girls, ovulation and menstruation (periods) begin, but may be irregular.

Stage 5

- This stage may begin anywhere from ages 12 to 19.
- Adult height is probably reached.
- Breast development is complete.
- Pubic hair forms a thick, curly, triangular patch.
- Ovulation and menstruation (periods) usually occur regularly.
- The overall look is that of a young adult woman.

Chapter 21

Menstruation and the Menstrual Cycle

Menstruation is a woman's monthly bleeding. When you menstruate, your body sheds the lining of the uterus (womb). Menstrual blood flows from the uterus through the small opening in the cervix and passes out of the body through the vagina. Most menstrual periods last from 3 to 5 days.

What is the menstrual cycle?

When periods (menstruations) come regularly, this is called the menstrual cycle. Having regular menstrual cycles is a sign that important parts of your body are working normally. The menstrual cycle provides important body chemicals, called hormones, to keep you healthy. It also prepares your body for pregnancy each month. A cycle is counted from the first day of one period to the first day of the next period. The average menstrual cycle is 28 days long. Cycles can range anywhere from 21 to 35 days in adults and from 21 to 45 days in young teens.

The rise and fall of levels of hormones during the month control the menstrual cycle.

What happens during the menstrual cycle?

In the first half of the cycle, levels of estrogen (the "female hormone") start to rise. Estrogen plays an important role in keeping you

From "Frequently Asked Questions about Menstruation and the Menstrual Cycle," by the Office on Women's Health (www.womenshealth.gov), part of the U.S. Department of Health and Human Services, October 21, 2009.

healthy, especially by helping you to build strong bones and to help keep them strong as you get older. Estrogen also makes the lining of the uterus (womb) grow and thicken. This lining of the womb is a place that will nourish the embryo if a pregnancy occurs.

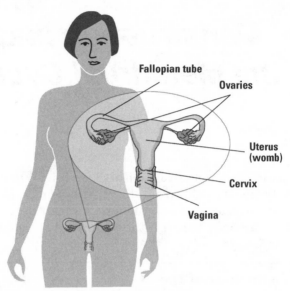

Figure 21.1. *The female reproductive system.*

At the same time the lining of the womb is growing, an egg, or ovum, in one of the ovaries starts to mature. At about day 14 of an average 28-day cycle, the egg leaves the ovary. This is called ovulation.

After the egg has left the ovary, it travels through the fallopian tube to the uterus. Hormone levels rise and help prepare the uterine lining for pregnancy. A woman is most likely to get pregnant during the 3 days before or on the day of ovulation. Keep in mind, women with cycles that are shorter or longer than average may ovulate before or after day 14.

A woman becomes pregnant if the egg is fertilized by a man's sperm cell and attaches to the uterine wall. If the egg is not fertilized, it will break apart. Then, hormone levels drop, and the thickened lining of the uterus is shed during the menstrual period.

What is a typical menstrual period like?

During your period, you shed the thickened uterine lining and extra blood through the vagina. Your period may not be the same every month. It may also be different than other women's periods. Periods can be light, moderate, or heavy in terms of how much blood comes out of the vagina. This is called menstrual flow. The length of the period also varies. Most periods last from 3 to 5 days, but anything from 2 to 7 days is normal.

For the first few years after menstruation begins, longer cycles are common. A woman's cycle tends to shorten and become more regular with age. Most of the time, periods will be in the range of 21 to 35 days apart.

What kinds of problems do women have with their periods?

Women can have a range of problems with their periods, including pain, heavy bleeding, and skipped periods.

Some women may experience amenorrhea—the lack of a menstrual period. This term is used to describe the absence of a period in young women who haven't started menstruating by age 15 and women and girls who haven't had a period for 90 days, even if they haven't been menstruating for long. Causes can include pregnancy, breastfeeding, extreme weight loss, eating disorders, excessive exercising, stress, and serious medical conditions in need of treatment.

When your menstrual cycles come regularly, this means that important parts of your body are working normally. In some cases, not having menstrual periods can mean that your ovaries have stopped producing normal amounts of estrogen. Missing these hormones can have important effects on your overall health. Hormonal problems, such as those caused by polycystic ovarian syndrome (PCOS) or serious problems with the reproductive organs, may be involved. It's important to talk to a doctor if you have this problem.

Dysmenorrhea is a term for painful periods, including severe cramps. Menstrual cramps in teens are caused by too much of a chemical called prostaglandin. Most teens with dysmenorrhea do not have a serious disease, even though the cramps can be severe. In older women, the pain is sometimes caused by a disease or condition such as uterine fibroids or endometriosis.

For some women, using a heating pad or taking a warm bath helps ease their cramps. Some over-the-counter pain medicines can also help with these symptoms. They include ibuprofen (for instance, Advil, Motrin, Midol Cramp); ketoprofen (for instance, Orudis KT); and naproxen (for instance, Aleve).

If these medicines don't relieve your pain or the pain interferes with work or school, you should see a doctor. Treatment depends on what's causing the problem and how severe it is.

Abnormal uterine bleeding—vaginal bleeding that's different from normal menstrual periods—is another period problem. It includes the following:

- Bleeding between periods
- Bleeding after sex
- Spotting anytime in the menstrual cycle
- Bleeding heavier or for more days than normal
- Bleeding after menopause

Abnormal bleeding can have many causes. Your doctor may start by checking for problems that are most common in your age group. Some of them are not serious and are easy to treat. Others can be more serious. Treatment for abnormal bleeding depends on the cause.

In both teens and women nearing menopause, hormonal changes can cause long periods along with irregular cycles. Even if the cause is hormonal changes, you may be able to get treatment. You should keep in mind that these changes can occur with other serious health problems, such as uterine fibroids, polyps, or even cancer. See your doctor if you have any abnormal bleeding.

When does a girl usually get her first period?

In the United States, the average age for a girl to get her first period is 12. This does not mean that all girls start at the same age. A girl can start her period anytime between the ages of 8 and 15. Most of the time, the first period starts about 2 years after breasts first start to develop. If a girl has not had her first period by age 15, or if it has been more than 2 to 3 years since breast growth started, she should see a doctor.

How long does a woman have periods?

Women usually have periods until menopause. Menopause occurs between the ages of 45 and 55, usually around age 50. Menopause means that a woman is no longer ovulating (producing eggs) or having periods and can no longer get pregnant. Like menstruation, menopause can vary from woman to woman and these changes may occur over several years.

The time when your body begins its move into menopause is called the menopausal transition. This can last anywhere from 2 to 8 years. Some women have early menopause because of surgery or other treatment, illness, or other reasons. If you don't have a period for 90 days, you should see your doctor. He or she will check for pregnancy, early menopause, or other health problems that can cause periods to stop or become irregular.

When should I see a doctor about my period?

See your doctor about your period if the following occur:

- You have not started menstruating by the age of 15.

- You have not started menstruating within 3 years after breast growth began, or if breasts haven't started to grow by age 13.

- Your period suddenly stops for more than 90 days.

- Your periods become very irregular after having had regular, monthly cycles.

- Your period occurs more often than every 21 days or less often than every 35 days.

- You are bleeding for more than seven days.

- You are bleeding more heavily than usual or using more than one pad or tampon every one to two hours.

- You bleed between periods.

- You have severe pain during your period.

- You suddenly get a fever and feel sick after using tampons.

How often should I change my pad and/or tampon?

You should change a pad before it becomes soaked with blood. Each woman decides for herself what works best. You should change a tampon at least every 4 to 8 hours. Make sure to use the lowest absorbency tampon needed for your flow. For example, use junior or regular tampons on the lightest day of your period. Using a super absorbency tampon on your lightest days increases your risk for toxic shock syndrome (TSS). TSS is a rare but sometimes deadly disease. TSS is caused by bacteria that can produce toxins. If your body can't fight the toxins, your immune (body defense) system reacts and causes the symptoms of TSS.

Young women may be more likely to get TSS. Using any kind of tampon puts you at greater risk for TSS than using pads. The Food and Drug Administration (FDA) recommends the following tips to help avoid tampon problems:

- Follow package directions for insertion.
- Choose the lowest absorbency for your flow.
- Change your tampon at least every four to eight hours.
- Consider switching between pads and tampons.
- Know the warning signs of TSS.
- Don't use tampons between periods.

If you have any of these symptoms of TSS while using tampons, take the tampon out, and contact your doctor right away:

- Sudden high fever (over 102 degrees Fahrenheit)
- Muscle aches
- Diarrhea
- Vomiting
- Dizziness and/or fainting
- Sunburn-like rash
- Sore throat
- Bloodshot eyes

Chapter 22

Female Reproductive Health Concerns

Chapter Contents

Section 22.1

Breast and Pelvic Exams

Why You Need These Exams

The American College of Obstetricians and Gynecologists recommends that a girl make her first visit to a gynecologist when she is between the ages of 13 and 15. Not all girls will need a pelvic exam during this initial visit, though. Many gynecologists will just do a regular health exam and talk to the girl about her development.

Yearly gyn visits are important for a number of reasons, including:

- **as a routine check.** You'll want to be sure you're developing normally.

- **to deal with a problem.** There may be a number of concerns that lead to a pelvic exam. For example, if you have problems with your periods, missed periods, pain, signs of infection, and worries about development, it's a good idea to see a doctor.

Also, if you have ever had sex, you are probably going to need a pelvic exam.

Choosing the Right Doctor

If you're going to be involved in deciding who you'll see for your pelvic exam, you have a few choices. These experts can prescribe birth control and provide education about reproductive health, STD [sexually transmitted disease] prevention, and birth control:

Family doctors and pediatricians: If your family doctor or and pediatrician does pelvic and breast exams and advises teens on sexual health, it means you can see a doctor you already know and feel comfortable with for your first pelvic exam.

Specialists: A number of different kinds of doctors and nurses have special training in women's reproductive health:

- Gynecologists are doctors who have been specially trained in women's health issues.

- Adolescent medicine doctors have been trained in the health and management of teen issues. They are familiar with the concerns most young women have about their reproductive systems and can advise them on birth control and STD prevention.

- Nurse practitioners who specialize in gynecology have advanced training that allows them to pay special attention to women's reproductive health, including giving breast and pelvic exams.

Whether you want to see a male or female health care professional is up to you. Some women say that they prefer being examined by a female doctor or nurse because it puts them more at ease and they feel like they can talk more openly about women's health problems and sexuality issues. Other women feel comfortable being examined by a male doctor or nurse. If the doctor or nurse is male, he will usually have a female assistant in the room with him during all parts of the exam.

Making the Appointment

It's best to involve your parents in your health care. If you want to go to a doctor's office for your exam, you may need to involve an adult for insurance purposes (it may be expensive otherwise).

If for some reason you can't involve your parents, you can take advantage of health clinics like Planned Parenthood or your local teen clinic. These clinics have fully trained staff who often can care for you at a lower cost and respect your need for confidentiality. Each state has different guidelines on which medical issues teens can get confidential care for. Your doctor should be able to explain these issues to you.

The most important thing is that you feel comfortable with the person who is examining you. You want to be able to talk with him or her about important personal health and relationship issues, including birth control.

What Happens When You Go for Your Gyn Exam

You don't need to do anything special before going for your exam. When you make the appointment, try to schedule the exam for a time when you won't have your period. For many young women, that can be hard to predict, though—lots of girls have irregular periods at first. Ask the doctor's office or clinic when you make the appointment what you should do if you get your period. Some doctors say it's OK to come for an exam if your period is just beginning or just ending and it's very light, but everyone has a different policy.

When you arrive for your appointment, you may be asked to fill out some forms while you wait. These forms ask questions about any illnesses or conditions you have, your health habits (like whether you drink or smoke), any family illnesses that you know of, and your history regarding sexual activity, pregnancy, and birth control. You might also be asked for the date of your last period (or a doctor or nurse will ask during your exam).

When you first go into the exam room, a nurse or medical assistant will do a few things that your doctor has probably done a million times before, such as recording your weight and taking your blood pressure. You'll then be left alone to change out of your clothes. It may feel weird taking off even your underwear because you may not have had to undress completely for a medical exam before. The nurse or medical assistant will leave you a paper sheet or gown—or maybe both—to cover you. If you're cold, most doctors and nurses won't mind if you keep your socks on.

After a few minutes, the doctor (or nurse practitioner, if that is who you choose to see) will knock on the door to make sure you're in your gown. If you're ready, he or she will come in and start the exam. The doctor may start by going over anything you wrote down on your forms, or you may talk about these things later.

If this is your first gynecologic exam, let the doctor know. That way, he or she will know to go slowly and explain everything that's going on. Now is also the time to ask about birth control or sexuality if you need to. Some doctors like to discuss these things before the exam, and some like to do it after. Your aim is to make sure you get your questions answered.

The Breast Exam

During the physical part of the gynecologic exam, you'll be asked to lie on your back on the table. You'll have the paper sheet or gown covering you, and the doctor will only uncover the parts of your body being examined.

The doctor will give you a breast exam by lightly pressing on different parts of your breasts. After finishing, he or she may show you how to examine your own breasts. This helps you become familiar with how your breasts feel so you know which lumps are normal and which may be the result of a change.

The Pelvic Exam

During the pelvic part of the exam, the doctor or nurse practitioner will ask you to move down so your behind is at the end of the table. You'll bend your knees and rest your feet in two stirrups, which are metal triangular loops that stick out from the end of the table. These might look a little scary, but they're just there to rest your feet in and keep you more comfortable. The doctor will ask you to relax your knees out to the sides as far as they will go. It might feel a little funny to be lying with your legs opened like this, but everyone feels that way at first.

The doctor will put on gloves and examine the outside of your vagina to make sure that there are no sores or swelling and that everything looks OK on the outside.

The Internal Exam

Next, the doctor will want to look at the inside of your vagina and will do so with the help of a speculum (pronounced: speh-kyuh-lum). A speculum is a thin piece of plastic or metal with a hinged piece on one end that allows it to open and close. The doctor or nurse will warm the speculum with water (some offices keep the speculum warmed in a drawer with a heating pad). The doctor or nurse will then slide the speculum into your vagina. Usually the doctor will tell you when he or she is about to place the speculum inside you so it doesn't come as a surprise.

Once the speculum is in the vagina, it can be opened to allow the doctor to see inside. Putting in and opening the speculum should not be painful, although some women say that it can cause a bit of pressure and discomfort. Naturally, if this is your first exam, you might feel a little tense. Because the vagina is surrounded by muscles that can contract or relax, the exam can be more comfortable if you try to stay calm and relax the muscles in that area.

If you feel like you're tensing up the muscles in your vagina, try breathing deeply or doing some breathing exercises to help you stay relaxed. Sometimes humming your favorite song or making small talk can distract you and allow you to feel more relaxed.

After the speculum is in place, the doctor will shine a light inside the vagina to look for anything unusual, like redness, swelling, discharge, or sores.

Because the ovaries and uterus are so far inside a girl's body that they can't be seen at all, even with the speculum, the doctor will need to feel them to be sure they're healthy. While your feet are still in the stirrups, and after the speculum is removed from the vagina, the doctor will put lubricant on two fingers (while still wearing the gloves) and slide them inside your vagina. Using the other hand, he or she will press on the outside of your lower abdomen (the area between your vagina and your stomach). With two hands, one on the outside and one on the inside, the doctor can make sure that the ovaries and uterus are the right size and free of cysts or other growths.

During this part of the exam, you may feel a little pressure or discomfort. Again, it's important to relax your muscles and take slow, deep breaths if you feel nervous.

Pap Smears

A Pap smear may be part of the pelvic exam, although not all teens need to get a pap smear. Pap smears are used to check for abnormal cells. The American College of Obstetricians and Gynecologists recommends that girls should get a Pap smear about 3 years after first having sex and then every year after that. All women should have a Pap smear by age 21.

To do a Pap smear, the doctor will gently touch the cervix to pick up cells from that area.

The Pap smear shouldn't hurt, but it might be uncomfortable, especially if this is your first pelvic exam. The good news is this part of the exam is over quickly.

The cells that have been collected are sent to a laboratory where they are studied for any abnormal cells, which might indicate infection or warning signs of cervical cancer. (Like breast cancer, cervical cancer is very unusual in teen girls.)

STD Tests

If you have had sex, the doctor or nurse practitioner may test for STDs. He or she will swab the inside of the cervix with what looks like a cotton swab. The speculum is then slid out of the vagina. As with the Pap smear, the sample is sent out to a laboratory where it is tested for various STDs.

Talk to your doctor or a nurse about how you want to be contacted with results, and what they should do if they are unable to reach you. Again, doctors and nurses will do their best to maintain confidentiality, but they need to be able to reach you.

After the Exam

Although reading this article may make it seem long, the entire pelvic exam (the parts involving your vagina, cervix, uterus, and ovaries) really only takes about 3 to 5 minutes.

Afterward, you'll be left alone to get dressed. Some women say that they bleed a tiny bit from the Pap smear after the exam, so they like to put a pantiliner in their underwear as they get dressed. If you bleed a tiny bit, it's no big deal—it's nothing like a period and it won't last.

If you haven't discussed your questions before the exam, now's the time. Don't be afraid of questions that sound stupid or silly—no question about your body is stupid, and this is the best time to get answers.

The Pap smear is almost always normal in teen girls. But if for any reason the doctor or nurse practitioner needs to see you again, the office or clinic will let you know. Unless you notice any health problems, you won't need to go for an exam for another 6 months to a year.

It's very important to go for pelvic exams on a yearly basis—even when you're feeling good—because they help detect any problems early on. If you don't want to return for another exam because you didn't like the doctor or nurse practitioner, look into finding a new doctor or clinic.

And if the physical discomfort of the exam left you not wanting another, remember that each time it gets easier and easier to relax. Naturally, no one loves getting an exam, but having a doctor or nurse practitioner you trust can really help.

Section 22.2

Premenstrual Syndrome

From "Frequently Asked Questions about Premenstrual Syndrome," by the Office on Women's Health (www.womenshealth.gov), part of the U.S. Department of Health and Human Services, April 1, 2007.

What is premenstrual syndrome (PMS)?

Premenstrual syndrome (PMS) is a group of symptoms linked to the menstrual cycle. PMS symptoms occur in the week or 2 weeks before your period (menstruation or monthly bleeding). The symptoms usually go away after your period starts. PMS can affect menstruating women of any age. It is also different for each woman. PMS may be just a monthly bother or it may be so severe that it makes it hard to even get through the day. Monthly periods stop during menopause, bringing an end to PMS.

What causes PMS?

The causes of PMS are not clear. It is linked to the changing hormones during the menstrual cycle. Some women may be affected more than others by changing hormone levels during the menstrual cycle. Stress and emotional problems do not seem to cause PMS, but they may make it worse.

Diagnosis of PMS is usually based on your symptoms, when they occur, and how much they affect your life.

What are the symptoms of PMS?

PMS often includes both physical and emotional symptoms. Common symptoms include the following:

- Acne
- Breast swelling and tenderness
- Feeling tired
- Having trouble sleeping

- Upset stomach, bloating, constipation, or diarrhea

- Headache or backache

- Appetite changes or food cravings

- Joint or muscle pain

- Trouble concentrating or remembering

- Tension, irritability, mood swings, or crying spells

- Anxiety or depression

Symptoms vary from one woman to another. If you think you have PMS, keep track of which symptoms you have and how severe they are for a few months. You can use a calendar to write down the symptoms you have each day or you can use a form to track your symptoms. If you go to the doctor for your PMS, take this form with you.

What is the treatment for PMS?

Many things have been tried to ease the symptoms of PMS. No treatment works for every woman, so you may need to try different ones to see what works. If your PMS is not so bad that you need to see a doctor, some lifestyle changes may help you feel better. The following are some lifestyle changes that may help ease your symptoms.

- Take a multivitamin every day that includes 400 micrograms of folic acid. A calcium supplement with vitamin D can help keep bones strong and may help ease some PMS symptoms.

- Exercise regularly.

- Eat healthy foods, including fruits, vegetables, and whole grains.

- Avoid salt, sugary foods, caffeine, and alcohol, especially when you are having PMS symptoms.

- Get enough sleep. Try to get 8 hours of sleep each night.

- Find healthy ways to cope with stress. Talk to your friends, exercise, or write in a journal.

- Don't smoke.

- Over-the-counter pain relievers such as ibuprofen, aspirin, or naproxen may help ease cramps, headaches, backaches, and breast tenderness.

In more severe cases of PMS, prescription medicines may be used to ease symptoms. One approach has been to use drugs such as birth control pills to stop ovulation from occurring. Women on the pill report fewer PMS symptoms, such as cramps and headaches, as well as lighter periods.

What is premenstrual dysphoric disorder (PMDD)?

There is evidence that a brain chemical called serotonin plays a role in a severe form of PMS, called premenstrual dysphoric disorder (PMDD). The main symptoms, which can be disabling, include the following:

- Feelings of sadness or despair, or possibly suicidal thoughts
- Feelings of tension or anxiety
- Panic attacks
- Mood swings, crying
- Lasting irritability or anger that affects other people
- Disinterest in daily activities and relationships
- Trouble thinking or focusing
- Tiredness or low energy
- Food cravings or binge eating
- Having trouble sleeping
- Feeling out of control
- Physical symptoms, such as bloating, breast tenderness, headaches, and joint or muscle pain

You must have five or more of these symptoms to be diagnosed with PMDD. Symptoms occur during the week before your period and go away after bleeding starts.

Making some lifestyle changes may help ease PMDD symptoms.

Antidepressants called selective serotonin reuptake inhibitors (SS-RIs) that change serotonin levels in the brain have also been shown to help some women with PMDD. The Food and Drug Administration (FDA) has approved three medications for the treatment of PMDD:

- Sertraline (Zoloft®)
- Fluoxetine (Sarafem®)
- Paroxetine HCI (Paxil CR®)

Individual counseling, group counseling, and stress management may also help relieve symptoms.

Section 22.3

Menstrual Irregularities

From "Menstrual Irregularities," by the National Institute of Child
Health and Human Development (NICHD, www.nichd.nih.gov), part of
the National Institutes of Health, May 24, 2007.

What are menstruation and the menstrual cycle?

The menstrual cycle is the process by which a woman's body gets
ready for the chance of a pregnancy each month.

Menstruation is the part of a woman's monthly menstrual cycle in
which blood and tissue are discharged from the vagina. It is also commonly called a period or menstrual period.

What are menstrual irregularities?

Sometimes women have problems in their menstrual cycle—called
menstrual irregularities or menstrual problems. They may not get periods, get periods too frequently, have unpredictable menstrual bleeding,
or they may have painful periods.

When not caused by pregnancy, menstrual irregularities are usually
a sign of a larger condition or problem. There are many conditions that
can cause menstrual irregularities.

Amenorrhea: Amenorrhea occurs when a woman does not get her
period by age 16, or when she stops getting her period for at least 3
months and is not pregnant.

Amenorrhea is not a disease. Instead, it is a symptom of another
condition. Possible causes can include moderate or excessive exercising,
eating disorders (such as anorexia nervosa), physical or psychological
stress, tumors, and hormonal problems. Women with polycystic ovary
syndrome (PCOS) may also experience amenorrhea.

It is important for you to see your health care provider to determine
the cause of amenorrhea. Treatment for amenorrhea depends on the
underlying cause. Sometimes lifestyle changes can help if weight,
stress, or extreme physical activity is causing the amenorrhea. Other
times, medications and oral contraceptives can help the problem.

Oligomenorrhea: This term refers to infrequent menstrual periods, or having a period only now and then. Like amenorrhea, oligomenorrhea is not a disease itself, but is a symptom of a larger condition. For example, many women with polycystic ovary syndrome (PCOS) have oligomenorrhea.

Premature ovarian failure (POF): POF describes a stop in the normal functioning of the ovaries in a woman younger than age 40. Women with POF may not have periods or may get them irregularly. Although getting pregnant is difficult for women with POF, it may still be possible.

There is no proven treatment to make a woman's ovaries work normally again. However, estrogen replacement therapy (ERT) gives women the estrogen and other hormones their bodies are not making and can help women have regular periods and lower their risk for osteoporosis.

Uterine fibroids: Uterine fibroids are the most common, noncancerous tumors in women of childbearing age. Most women with fibroids do not have problems with fertility and can get pregnant. But some women with fibroids may not be able to get pregnant naturally.

Women who have uterine fibroids but show no symptoms may not need any treatment. Some women with fibroids have heavy menstrual periods, and some may bleed in between periods. Medications can often offer relief from many of the symptoms of fibroids, such as pain, and can even slow or stop their growth. There are also several types of surgery that can remove the fibroids.

Endometriosis: Endometriosis occurs when tissues that usually grow inside a woman's uterus grow on the outside instead. Endometriosis may cause pain before and during the first few days of the menstrual period. About 30 percent to 50 percent of women with endometriosis are infertile, making it one of the top three causes for female infertility. Women with endometriosis may also have very heavy periods.

There are several ways to treat pain, including pain medication, hormone therapy, and surgery.

There are also some treatments for infertility associated with endometriosis. In vitro fertilization often works to improve fertility in women with the condition. Hormone treatments and surgery offer other infertility treatment options.

Dysmenorrhea: Dysmenorrhea refers to painful periods, including severe menstrual cramps. The condition is usually not serious, although it can sometimes be caused by infection, endometriosis, or ovarian cysts.

158

Painful periods can sometimes be eased by using heating pads or taking a warm bath. Over-the-counter pain relievers can also help with the pain. Your health care provider might recommend birth control pills or a birth control shot to make periods less painful.

Section 22.4

Vaginal Discharge Concerns

Excerpted from "Douching," by the Office on Women's Health (www.womenshealth.gov), part of the U.S. Department of Health and Human Services, December 1, 2005.

What is douching?

The word "douche" means to wash or soak in French. Douching is washing or cleaning out the vagina (also called the birth canal) with water or other mixtures of fluids. Usually douches are prepackaged mixes of water and vinegar, baking soda, or iodine. Women can buy these products at drug and grocery stores. The mixtures usually come in a bottle and can be squirted into the vagina through a tube or nozzle.

Why do women douche?

Women douche because they mistakenly believe it gives many benefits. In reality, douching may do more harm than good. Common reasons women give for using douches include the following:

- To clean the vagina
- To rinse away blood after monthly periods
- To get rid of odors from the vagina
- To avoid sexually transmitted infections (STIs)
- To prevent pregnancy

Is douching safe?

Most doctors and the American College of Obstetricians and Gynecologists (ACOG) suggest that women steer clear of douching. All healthy vaginas contain some bacteria and other organisms called vaginal flora. The normal acidity of the vagina keeps the amount of bacteria down. But douching can change this delicate balance. This may make a woman more prone to vaginal infections. Plus, douching can spread existing vaginal infections up into the uterus, fallopian tubes, and ovaries.

Should I douche to clean inside my vagina?

No. Doctors and the ACOG suggest women avoid douching completely. Most experts believe that douching increases a woman's chances of infection. The only time a woman should douche is when her doctor recommends it.

What is the best way to clean my vagina?

Most doctors say that it is best to let your vagina clean itself. The vagina cleans itself naturally by producing mucus. Women do not need to douche to wash away blood, semen, or vaginal discharge. The vagina gets rid of it alone. Also, it is important to note that even healthy, clean vaginas may have a mild odor.

Regular washing with warm water and mild soap during baths and showers will keep the outside of the vagina clean and healthy. Doctors suggest women avoid scented tampons, pads, powders, and sprays. These products may increase a woman's chances of getting vaginal infections.

My vagina has a terrible odor. Can douching help?

No. Douching will only cover up the smell. It will not make it go away. If your vagina has a bad odor, you should call your doctor right away. It could be a sign of a bacterial infection, urinary tract infection, STI, or a more serious problem.

Should I douche to get rid of vaginal discharge, pain, itching, or burning?

No. Douching may even make these problems worse. It is very important to call your doctor right away if you have the following:

- Vaginal discharge with a bad smell

- Thick, white or yellowish-green discharge with or without a smell

- Burning, redness, and swelling of the vagina or the area around it

- Pain when urinating

- Pain or discomfort during sex

These may be signs of a bacterial infection, yeast infection, urinary tract infection, or STI. Do not douche before seeing your doctor. This can make it hard for the doctor to figure out what is wrong.

Section 22.5

Vaginal Yeast Infections

Excerpted from "Frequently Asked Questions about Vaginal Yeast Infections," by the Office on Women's Health (www.womenshealth.gov), part of the U.S. Department of Health and Human Services, September 23, 2008.

What is a vaginal yeast infection?

A vaginal yeast infection is irritation of the vagina and the area around it called the vulva.

Yeast is a type of fungus. Yeast infections are caused by overgrowth of the fungus *Candida albicans*. Small amounts of yeast are always in the vagina. But when too much yeast grows, you can get an infection.

Yeast infections are very common. About 75 percent of women have one during their lives. And almost half of women have two or more vaginal yeast infections.

What are the signs of a vaginal yeast infection?

The most common symptom of a yeast infection is extreme itchiness in and around the vagina.

Other symptoms include the following:

- Burning, redness, and swelling of the vagina and the vulva

- Pain when passing urine

- Pain during sex

- Soreness

- A thick, white vaginal discharge that looks like cottage cheese and does not have a bad smell

- A rash on the vagina

You may only have a few of these symptoms. They may be mild or severe.

Should I call my doctor if I think I have a yeast infection?

Yes, you need to see your doctor to find out for sure if you have a yeast infection. The signs of a yeast infection are much like those of sexually transmitted infections (STIs) like *Chlamydia* and gonorrhea. So, it's hard to be sure you have a yeast infection and not something more serious.

If you've had vaginal yeast infections before, talk to your doctor about using over-the-counter medicines.

How are yeast infections treated?

Yeast infections can be cured with antifungal medicines that come as creams, tablets, or ointments or suppositories that are inserted into the vagina.

These products can be bought over the counter at the drug store or grocery store. Your doctor can also prescribe you a single dose of oral fluconazole. But do not use this drug if you are pregnant.

Infections that don't respond to these medicines are starting to be more common. Using antifungal medicines when you don't really have a yeast infection can raise your risk of getting a hard-to-treat infection in the future.

Is it safe to use over-the-counter medicines for yeast infections?

Yes, but always talk with your doctor before treating yourself for a vaginal yeast infection if the following are true:

- You are pregnant.

- You have never been diagnosed with a yeast infection.

- You keep getting yeast infections.

Studies show that two thirds of women who buy these products don't really have a yeast infection. Using these medicines the wrong way may lead to a hard-to-treat infection. Plus, treating yourself for a yeast infection when you really have something else may worsen the problem. Certain STIs that go untreated can cause cancer, infertility, pregnancy problems, and other health problems.

If you decide to use these over-the-counter medicines, read and follow the directions carefully. Some creams and inserts may weaken condoms and diaphragms.

Chapter 23

Precocious and Delayed Puberty

Chapter Contents

Section 23.1

Precocious Puberty

From "Precocious Puberty," by the National Institute of Child Health and Human Development (NICHD, www.nichd.nih.gov), part of the National Institutes of Health, January 15, 2007.

What is precocious puberty?

Precocious puberty is puberty that begins before age 8 years for girls and before age 9 years for boys. The word "precocious" means developing unusually early.

What are the signs of precocious puberty?

The signs of precocious puberty are the same as those for regular puberty. The difference is that they start to occur at a younger age than normal.

- For females, signs include development of breasts, pubic hair, and underarm hair; increased growth rate; and menstrual bleeding.

- In boys, signs include growth of the penis and testicles, development of pubic and underarm hair, muscle growth, voice changes, and increased growth rate.

What causes precocious puberty?

Sometimes precocious puberty is the result of a structural problem in the brain that triggers puberty to begin too early. There are many conditions that may lead to precocious puberty, such as the following:

- Congenital adrenal hyperplasia

- McCune-Albright syndrome

- Gonadal (testicles or ovaries) or adrenal gland disorders or tumors

- hCG [human chorionic gonadotropin]-secreting tumors

- Hypothalamic hamartoma

But in many cases, there is no identifiable cause for the precocious puberty. Puberty just starts earlier than normal. If you think your child is beginning puberty early, talk to your child's health care provider.

What is the treatment for precocious puberty?

Treatment for precocious puberty can help stop puberty until the child is closer to the normal time for sexual development. One reason to consider treating precocious puberty is that rapid growth and bone maturation can prevent a child from reaching his or her full height potential.

Children grow rapidly in height during puberty and reach their final adult height after puberty. Children who go through puberty too early may not reach their full adult height potential because their growth stops too soon.

Another reason to consider treating precocious puberty is that a young child may not be psychologically ready for the physical and hormonal changes that occur in puberty.

If precocious puberty is caused by a specific medical problem, treating the underlying problem can often stop the puberty. In addition, precocious puberty can often be stopped by medical treatment to block the hormones that cause puberty.

Section 23.2

Delayed Puberty

Jeff hates gym class. It's not that he minds playing soccer or basketball or any of the other activities. But he does dread going into the
locker room at the end of class and showering in front of his friends.
Although the other guys' bodies are growing and changing, his body
seems to be stuck at a younger age. He's shorter than most of the other
guys in his grade, and his voice hasn't deepened at all. It's embarrassing to still look like a little kid.

Abby knows what it's like to feel different, too. The bikini tops that
her friends fill out lie flat on her. Most of them have their periods, too,
and she hasn't had even a sign of one.

Both Jeff and Abby wonder if there's anything wrong.

What Is Delayed Puberty?

Puberty is the time when your body grows from a child's to an
adult's. You'll know that you are going through puberty by the way
that your body changes.

If you're a girl, you'll notice that your breasts develop and your pubic
hair grows, that you have a growth spurt, and that you get your period
(menstruation). The overall shape of your body will probably change,
too—your hips will widen and your body will become curvier.

If you're a guy, you'll start growing pubic and facial hair, have a
growth spurt, and your testicles and penis will get larger. Your body
shape will also begin to change—your shoulders will widen and your
body will become more muscular.

These changes are caused by the sex hormones (testosterone in
guys and estrogen in girls) that your body begins producing in much
larger amounts than before.

Puberty takes place over a number of years, and the age at which it starts and ends varies widely. It generally begins somewhere between the ages of 7 and 13 for girls, and somewhere between the ages of 9 and 15 for guys, although it can be earlier or later for some people. This wide range in age is normal, and it's why you may develop several years earlier (or later) than most of your friends.

Sometimes, though, people pass this normal age range for puberty without showing any signs of body changes. This is called delayed puberty.

What Causes Delayed Puberty?

Puberty can be delayed for several reasons. Most often, it's simply a pattern of growth and development in a family. A guy or girl may find that his or her parent, uncle, aunt, brothers, sisters, or cousins developed later than usual, too. This is called constitutional delay (or being a late bloomer), and it usually doesn't require any kind of treatment. These teens will eventually develop normally, just later than most of their peers.

Medical problems also can cause delays in puberty. Some people with chronic illnesses like diabetes, cystic fibrosis, kidney disease, or even asthma may go through puberty at an older age because their illnesses can make it harder for their bodies to grow and develop. Proper treatment and better control of many of these conditions can help make delayed puberty less likely to occur.

A person who's malnourished—without enough food to eat or without the proper nutrients—may also develop later than peers who eat a healthy, balanced diet. For example, teens with the eating disorder anorexia nervosa often lose so much weight that their bodies can't develop properly. Girls who are extremely active in sports may be late developers because their level of exercise keeps them so lean. Girls' bodies require a certain amount of fat before they can go through puberty or get their periods.

Delayed puberty can also happen because of problems in the pituitary or thyroid glands. These glands produce hormones important for body growth and development.

Some people who don't go through puberty at the normal time have problems with their chromosomes (pronounced: kro-muh-soamz), which are made up of DNA [deoxyribonucleic acid] that contain our body's construction plans. Problems with the chromosomes can interfere with normal growth processes.

Turner syndrome is an example of a chromosome disorder. It happens when one of a female's two X chromosomes is abnormal or missing.

This causes problems with how a girl grows and with the development of her ovaries and production of sex hormones. Women who have untreated Turner syndrome are shorter than normal, are usually infertile, and may have other medical problems.

Males with Klinefelter syndrome are born with an extra X chromosome (XXY instead of XY). This condition can slow sexual development.

What Do Doctors Do?

The good news is that if there is a problem, doctors usually can help teens with delayed puberty to develop more normally. So if you are worried that you're not developing as you should, you should ask your parents to make an appointment with your doctor.

In addition to doing a physical examination, the doctor will take your medical history by asking you about any concerns and symptoms you have, your past health, your family's health, any medications you're taking, any allergies you may have, and other issues like growth patterns of your family members. He or she will chart your growth to see if your growth pattern points to a problem and also may order blood tests to check for thyroid, pituitary, chromosomal, or other problems. You may also have a "bone age" x-ray, which allows the doctor to see whether your bones are maturing normally.

In many cases, the doctor will be able to reassure you that there's no underlying physical problem; you're just a bit later than average in developing. If the doctor does find a problem, though, he or she might refer you to a pediatric endocrinologist (pronounced: en-doh-krih-nah-leh-jist), a doctor who specializes in treating kids and teens who have growth problems, or to another specialist for further tests or treatment.

Some teens who are late developers may have a difficult time waiting for the changes of puberty to finally get going—even after a doctor has reassured them that they are normal. In some cases, doctors may offer teens a short course (usually a few months) of treatment with hormone medications to get the changes of puberty started. Usually, when the treatment is stopped a few months later, the teen's own hormones will take over from there to complete the process of puberty.

Dealing with Delayed Puberty

It can be really hard to watch your friends grow and develop when the same thing's not happening to you. You may feel like you're never going to catch up. People at school may joke about your small size or your flat chest. Even when the doctor or your parents reassure you that things will be OK eventually—and even when you believe they're right—it's difficult to wait for something that can affect how you feel about yourself.

If you're feeling depressed or having school or other problems related to delays in your growth and development, talk to your mom or dad, your doctor, or another trusted adult about finding a counselor or therapist you can talk to. This person can help you sort out your feelings and suggest ways to cope with them.

Delayed puberty can be difficult for anyone to accept and deal with—but it's a problem that usually gets solved. Ask for help if you have any concerns about your development. And remember that in most cases kids will eventually catch up with their peers.

Chapter 24

Teaching Teens about Sexual Activity

Chapter Contents

Section 24.1

Making Healthy Sexual Decisions

As a teenage girl or young woman, you may be thinking about what it means to be involved in a sexual relationship. Deciding to have a sexual relationship is a big deal, since it involves both your body and your emotions. You need to make sure that it is the right decision for you. There are many things that you need to think about before you decide to have sex, including whether this is the right person, the right time in your life, and how you will feel if the relationship breaks up. If you do decide to have sex, you definitely need to first think about how to prevent getting pregnant, and how to protect yourself from getting a sexually transmitted disease (STD).

You should talk to your parents, guardian, a trusted adult, or your health care provider if you are thinking about having a sexual relationship. It is a good idea to discuss all of your choices and all of the concerns and worries you may have so that you can make good decisions. This can be a very confusing time for you, and it is always good to have someone to talk to.

What do I need to know if I am sexually active or I'm thinking about becoming sexually active?

Young people have to make lots of decisions about their sexuality, including whether to abstain from sexual intercourse (not have sex) or become, or continue being, sexually active. Other sexuality issues that teens need to make decisions about are the gender of partners, the type of contraception to use, and the intensity of the relationship. You should never let others pressure you into having sex if you don't want to. The decision as to when you want to have sex for the first time (and every time after the first time) is yours, not anyone else's! Remember that it's completely okay to wait until you're older to have sex. You are young and there are risks involved, like STDs and pregnancy. Many young people just don't want to even deal with the possibility of getting an STD or getting pregnant, so they choose to wait.

Before you decide to have a sexual relationship, talk to your partner about whether this is the right decision. Ask about his or her sexual history, including if he or she has had any sexually transmitted diseases (STDs). Talk about whether you or your partner has been, or will be sexually involved with other people. Remember, the risk of getting a sexually transmitted disease or a virus that can cause cancer or AIDS [acquired immunodeficiency syndrome] is increased if you or your partner are having sexual intercourse with other people. The more partners, the greater the risk. The only way to absolutely prevent getting a sexually transmitted disease is to not have sex. If you do decide to have sex, the best way to avoid getting any sexually transmitted diseases is to have sex with only one person who has never been exposed to an STD. You should use a latex condom every time you have sex, from start to finish.

If you are in a heterosexual relationship (you are a female dating a male), talk about birth control (latex condom, birth control pill, injection hormones) and what you would do if it failed. If you feel that you cannot talk to your partner about these issues, then you should rethink whether or not you should be having a sexual relationship with him. Talk to your primary care provider about what methods of birth control are right for you. If you are in a serious relationship, it is equally important to talk about how to prevent sexually transmitted infections (STIs).

How do I find a health care provider to discuss birth control and STD protection?

Many teens and young women can talk to their moms, dads, or guardians about these issues, while others need confidential services. You can talk to your primary care provider about birth control or STD protection. You also have the options of talking to a gynecologist, a health care provider (HCP) at a family planning clinic, or an HCP at a student health center or school clinic. You should feel comfortable with your HCP, since it is important to share personal information and any health problems with her/him. You need to find a provider who will listen to your concerns, answer your questions, and take the time to explain things clearly to you.

Make sure you know how to receive confidential, non-judgmental services when talking about your sexual choices and health. Practice these questions to ask:

- What happens to the bills from my visits here or to a gynecologist in the community?

- If I'm covered by my parents' insurance, will they find out about examinations and tests that are done on me?

- What if I need birth control?

- Can you tell me what happens to my lab test results? Who do you call?

- What if I want to be tested for STDs or HIV [human immunodeficiency virus]?

- What if you find out that I have a STD?

- What if you find out that I am pregnant?

- Is there any information that you are obligated to tell my parents?

- What happens if I have a big problem and need help telling my parents?

- What should I know about emergency contraception?

If your birth control method fails, you do have an option called emergency contraception, also known as the "morning-after pill." Emergency contraception can prevent pregnancy after unprotected sex. Emergency contraception pills are taken in two doses. The first dose should be taken within the first 72 hours after unprotected sex, and the second dose should be taken 12 hours later. The sooner you start the medicine after unprotected sex, the more effective the treatment is. You can usually get emergency contraception from your health care provider or family planning clinics, through Planned Parenthood, at: 800-230-PLAN, or by calling 800-NOT2LATE.

What if I'm not sure whether I'm gay, straight, or bisexual?

Many young people may also be trying to figure out their sexual orientation. If you feel like you need to talk to someone or you need more support, your HCP can help you find a counselor or support group for gay, lesbian, bisexual, and transgender teens. If you don't feel comfortable talking to your provider, you can call any of the following to talk to someone and get advice on where you can find a counselor or support group.

- BAGLY (Boston Alliance of Gay, Lesbian, Bisexual, and Transgendered Youth): 617-227-4313

- Massachusetts Gay and Lesbian Youth Peer Listening Line: 800-399-7337
- Gay and Lesbian National Hotline: 800-843-4564
- LGBT HelpLine: 888-340-4528

Quiz: Are you ready for sex?

Ask yourself the following questions to see if you are ready to have a sexual relationship:

- Is your decision to have sex completely your own (you feel no pressure from others, including your partner)?
- Is your decision to have sex based on the right reasons? (It shouldn't be based on peer pressure, a need to fit in or make your partner happy, or a belief that sex will make your relationship with your partner better, or closer. If you decide to have sex, it should be because you feel emotionally and physically ready and your partner should be someone you love, trust, and respect.)
- Do you feel your partner would respect any decision you made about whether to have sex or not?
- Do you trust and respect your partner?
- Are you able to comfortably talk to your partner about sex, and your partner's sexual history?
- Have you and your partner talked about what both of you would do if you became pregnant or got an STD?
- Do you know how to prevent pregnancy and STDs?
- Are you and your partner willing to use contraception to prevent pregnancy and STDs?
- Look inside yourself. Do you really feel ready and completely comfortable with yourself and your partner to have sex?

If you answered **no** to any of these questions, you are not really ready for sex.

If you think you should have sexual intercourse because others want you to or you feel like you should since everyone else is doing it, these are not the right reasons. You should only decide to have sex because you trust and respect your partner, you know the possible risks, you know how to protect yourself against the risks, and most importantly, because you really know that you are ready!

Section 24.2

Facts on Sex Education in the United States

Guttmacher Institute, "Facts on Sex Education in the United States, In Brief." New York: Guttmacher, © 2006. http://www.guttmacher.org/pubs/ fb_sexEd2006.html, accessed May 24, 2010.

Sex and Pregnancy among Teens

- By their 18th birthday, six in 10 teenage women and more than five in 10 teenage men have had sexual intercourse.[1]

- Between 1995 and 2002, the number of teens aged 15–17 who had ever engaged in sexual intercourse declined 10%.[2]

- Of the approximately 750,000 teen pregnancies that occur each year, 82% are unintended. More than one-quarter end in abortion.[3]

- The pregnancy rate among U.S. women aged 15–19 has declined steadily—from 117 pregnancies per 1,000 women in 1990 to 75 per 1,000 women in 2002.[4]

- Approximately 14% of the decline in teen pregnancy between 1995 and 2002 was due to teens' delaying sex or having sex less often, while 86% was due to an increase in sexually experienced teens' contraceptive use.[5]

- Despite the decline, the United States continues to have one of the highest teen pregnancy rates in the developed world—almost twice as high as those of England, Wales, and Canada, and eight times as high as those of the Netherlands and Japan.[6]

- Every year, roughly nine million new sexually transmitted infections (STIs) occur among teens and young adults in the United States. Compared with rates among teens in Canada and Western Europe, rates of gonorrhea and chlamydia among U.S. teens are extremely high.[7]

- Though teens in the United States have levels of sexual activity similar to levels among their Canadian, English, French and Swedish peers, they are more likely to have shorter and more sporadic sexual relationships and are less likely to use contraceptives.[8]

Sex Education: Teens' Perspectives

- By 2002, one-third of teens had not received any formal instruction about contraception.[9]

- More than one in five adolescents (21% of females and 24% of males) received abstinence education without receiving instruction about birth control in 2002, compared with 8–9% in 1995.[10]

- In 2002, only 62% of sexually experienced female teens had received instruction about contraception before they first had sex, compared with 72% in 1995.[11]

- Only one out of three sexually experienced black males and fewer than half of sexually experienced black females had received instruction about contraception before the first time they had sex.[12]

- One-quarter of sexually experienced teens had not received instruction about abstinence before first sex.[13]

Sex Education: Teachers' Perspectives

- Sex education teachers were more likely to focus on abstinence and less likely to provide students with information on birth control, how to obtain contraceptive services, sexual orientation, and abortion in 1999 than they were in 1988.[14]

- In 1999, one in four sex education teachers taught abstinence as the only way to prevent pregnancy and STIs—a huge increase from 1988, when the fraction was just one in 50.[15]

- The majority of teachers believe that topics such as birth control methods and how to obtain them, the correct way to use a condom, sexual orientation, and factual and ethical information about abortion should also be taught by the end of the 12th grade. These topics are currently being taught less often and later than teachers think they should be.[16]

- More than nine in 10 teachers believe that students should be taught about contraception, but one in four are prohibited from doing so.[17]

- One in five teachers believe that restrictions on sex education are preventing them from meeting their students' needs.[18]

- Eighty-two percent of adults support comprehensive sex education that teaches students about both abstinence and other methods of preventing pregnancy and STIs.[19]

- Only one-third of adults surveyed support abstinence-only education, while half oppose the abstinence-only approach.[20]

Sex Education Policy

- Currently, 35 states mandate either sex education or education about HIV/AIDS [human immunodeficiency virus and acquired immunodeficiency syndrome] and other STIs, but their laws tend to be very general. Policies specifying the content of sex education are typically set at the local level.[21]

- More than two out of three public school districts have a policy to teach sex education. The remaining one-third of districts leave policy decisions up to individual schools or teachers.[22]

- Eighty-six percent of the public school districts that have a policy to teach sex education require that abstinence be promoted. Some 35% require abstinence to be taught as the only option for unmarried people and either prohibit the discussion of contraception altogether or limit discussion to its ineffectiveness. The other 51% have a policy to teach abstinence as the preferred option for teens and permit discussion of contraception as an effective means of preventing pregnancy and STIs.[23]

- More than half of the districts in the South with a policy to teach sex education have an abstinence-only policy, compared with one in five of such districts in the Northeast.[24]

Government Support of Abstinence-Only Education

- There are three federal programs dedicated to funding restrictive abstinence-only education: Section 510 of the Social Security Act, the Adolescent Family Life Act's teen pregnancy prevention component, and Community-Based Abstinence Education (CBAE). The total funding for these programs is $176 million for FY 2006.[25]

- Federal law establishes a stringent eight-point definition of "abstinence-only education"—that requires programs to teach that sexual activity outside of marriage is wrong and harmful—for people of any age. The law also prohibits programs from advocating contraceptive use or discussing contraceptive methods except to emphasize their failure rates.[26]

- Federal guidelines now define sexual activity to include any behavior between two people that may be sexually stimulating, which could be interpreted as including even kissing or hand-holding.[27]

- New federal restrictions have been expanded to target adolescents and young adults between the ages of 12 and 29.[28]

- There is currently no federal program dedicated to supporting comprehensive sex education that teaches young people about both abstinence and contraception.[29]

- Despite years of evaluation in this area, there is no evidence to date that abstinence-only education delays teen sexual activity. Moreover, recent research shows that abstinence-only strategies may deter contraceptive use among sexually active teens, increasing their risk of unintended pregnancy and STIs.[30]

- Evidence shows that comprehensive sex education programs that provide information about both abstinence and contraception can help delay the onset of sexual activity among teens, reduce their number of sexual partners, and increase contraceptive use when they become sexually active. These findings were underscored in "Call to Action to Promote Sexual Health and Responsible Sexual Behavior," issued by former Surgeon General David Satcher in June 2001.[31]

Sources

1. Abma JC et al., Teenagers in the United States: sexual activity, contraceptive use, and childbearing, 2002, *Vital and Health Statistics,* 2004, Series 23, No. 24.

2. Ibid.

3. Guttmacher Institute, U.S. Teenage Pregnancy Statistics: National and State Trends and Trends by Race and Ethnicity, 2006, <http://www.guttmacher.org/pubs/2006/09/11/USTPstats.pdf>, accessed Nov. 28, 2006; Finer LB et al., Disparities in rates of unintended pregnancy in the United States, 1994 and 2001, *Perspectives on Sexual and Reproductive Health,* 2006, 38(2):90–96.

4. Guttmacher Institute, 2006, op. cit. (see reference 3).

5. Santelli JS et al., Explaining recent declines in adolescent pregnancy in the United States: the contribution of abstinence and improved contraceptive use, *American Journal of Public Health,* 2007, 97(1):1–7.

6. Singh S and Darroch JE, Adolescent pregnancy and childbearing: levels and trends in developed countries, *Family Planning Perspectives,* 1998, 32(1):14–23.

7. Weinstock H et al., Sexually transmitted diseases among American youth: incidence and prevalence estimates, 2000, *Perspectives on Sexual and Reproductive Health,* 2004, 36(1): 6–10.; Darroch JE, Frost JJ and Singh S, Teenage Sexual and Reproductive Behavior in Developed Countries: Can More Progress Be Made?, *Occasional Report,* New York: The Alan Guttmacher Institute, 2001, No. 3.

8. Ibid.

9. Lindberg LD, Changes in formal sex education: 1995–2002, *Perspectives on Sexual and Reproductive Health,* 2006, 38(4):182–189.

10. Ibid.

11. Ibid.

12. Ibid.

13. Ibid.

14. Darroch JE et al, Changing emphases in sexuality education in U.S. public secondary schools, 1988–1999, *Family Planning Perspectives,* 2000, 32(5):204–211 & 265.

15. Ibid.

16. Ibid.

17. Ibid.

18. Ibid.

19. Bleakley A et al., Public opinion on sex education in U.S. schools, *Archives of Pediatrics and Adolescent Medicine, 2006,* 160(11):1151–1156.

20. Ibid.

21. Guttmacher Institute, Sex and STD/HIV education, *State Policies in Brief,* November 2006, <http://www.guttmacher.org/statecenter/spibs/spib_SE.pdf>, accessed Nov. 28, 2006.

22. Landry DJ et al, Abstinence promotion and the provision of information about contraception in public school district

sexuality education policies, *Family Planning Perspectives,* 1999, 31(6):280–286.

23. Ibid.

24. Ibid.

25. Unpublished tabulations based on annual federal government appropriations for abstinence-only sex education.

26. Dailard C, Abstinence promotion and teen family planning: the misguided drive for equal funding, *The Guttmacher Report on Public Policy,* 2002, 5(1):1–3; and Dailard C, Fueled by campaign promises, drive intensifies to boost abstinence-only education funds, *The Guttmacher Report on Public Policy,* 2000, 3(2):1–2 & 12.

27. Dailard C, Legislating against arousal: the growing divide between federal policy and teenage sexual behavior, *Guttmacher Policy Review,* 2006, 9(3):12–16.

28. Dailard C, New Bush Administration policy promotes abstinence until marriage among people in their 20s, *Guttmacher Policy Review,* 2006, 9(4):23.

29. Dailard C, 2002, op. cit. (see reference 26); and Dailard C, Sex education: politicians, parents, teachers and teens, *The Guttmacher Report on Public Policy,* 2001, 4(1):9–12.

30. Kirby D, Emerging Answers: *Research Findings on Programs to Reduce Teen Pregnancy,* Washington, DC: National Campaign to Prevent Teen Pregnancy, 2001; Bearman PS and Bruckner H, Promising the future: virginity pledges and first intercourse, *American Journal of Sociology, 2001,* 106(4):859–912; Bruckner H and Bearman PS, After the promise: the STI consequences of adolescent virginity pledges, *Journal of Adolescent Health,* 2005, 36(4):271–278.

31. Dailard C, 2002, op. cit. (see reference 26); and Kirby D, 2001, op. cit. (see reference 30).

Chapter 25

Sexually Transmitted Diseases (STDs) and Their Prevention

Chapter Contents

Section 25.1

Frequently Asked Questions about STDs

From "Teen Talk: Commonly Asked Questions about Sexually Transmitted Diseases (STDs)," by the Office of Public Health and Science–Office of Population Affairs (opaclearinhouse.org), U.S. Department of Health and Human Services, March 2003. Reviewed and revised by David A. Cooke, MD, FACP, March 16, 2010.

What is an STD?

STD stands for sexually transmitted disease. These infections are passed from person to person during sexual activity (vaginal, oral, or anal intercourse). Some infections are curable, while others are not. It is estimated that more than 19 million new cases of STDs occur in the United States each year. Approximately one half of the new cases occur among young people aged 15–24 years old.

Who can get an STD?

Anyone who engages in sexual activity.

How do I know if I have an STD?

Since many STDs do not have any obvious symptoms, the only sure way to know is by having a medical exam and lab tests.

Do latex condoms protect you from getting an STD?

For sexually active people, the most effective strategy for reducing the risk of STDs and preventing HIV/AIDS is correct and consistent use of latex condoms. However, research shows that condoms may not provide as much protection against some STDs such as HPV (human papillomavirus/genital warts). Abstinence—not having sex—is the only 100% sure way to avoid an STD.

Who can I talk to?

A parent, teacher, school nurse, family doctor, clergyman, or other responsible adult.

Here are some common myths about STDs.

Myth: If I don't have symptoms, that means I don't have an STD.

Fact: You can be infected with an STD and not know it. The only sure way to know if you have an STD is by having a medical exam and lab tests.

Myth: HIV/AIDS is the only STD that can't be cured.

Fact: STDs caused by viruses—genital herpes, genital warts, and HIV/AIDS—cannot be cured, although some medications may reduce the severity and/or delay the appearance of symptoms.

STDs caused by bacteria (like chlamydia, gonorrhea, and syphilis) can usually be cured with antibiotics. If they are not treated early, serious long-term problems, like pain and infertility, can develop.

What should I do if I think I have an STD?

If you think you have been exposed to an STD, you should go to a clinic or doctor as soon as possible to be tested and treated. Health departments, which diagnose and treat STDs, are located in almost every county and city. They provide confidential information and will help answer any questions you may have about STDs.

When should I have a checkup?

All sexually active teens should be seen by a health provider to be screened for STDs. Teens who have had sex with more than one person are at greater risk of getting an STD or HIV/AIDS. Many experts recommend that testing for gonorrhea and chlamydia be performed routinely during Pap smears and that all teens should be tested annually for HIV.

Section 25.2

STD Testing

STD Testing at a Glance

- You must ask for an STD test if you want to be tested.
- STD tests are easy to get.
- Consider testing if you have had unprotected sex, even if you don't have symptoms.
- There are different tests for different STDs.

You might be wondering if you need a test for sexually transmitted diseases (STDs). You might be wondering if your partner needs one. Or you may simply be interested in learning more about STD testing. Whatever the reason, the more information you have, the better you can protect your sexual health.

If you think you may have been exposed to an infection, getting tested for STDs is a great way to protect your sexual health. It's also a great way to protect the health of your sex partners.

Should I get tested for STDs?

If you have symptoms of an STD, it's important to be tested. Some common symptoms of STDs include sores on the genitals, discharge from the penis or vagina, itching, and burning during urination.

But remember, many infections often do not cause any symptoms. Many people have sexually transmitted infections and never know it. Many people get or spread infections without ever having symptoms.

If you've had sex play with another person and did not use a condom, female condom, dental dam, or other barrier, it's a good idea to talk to your health care provider about STD testing. Getting tested can put your mind at ease or get you (and your partner) needed treatment. It's also important to learn about ways you and your partner can protect yourselves in the future through safer sex.

How do I get tested for STDs?

You must ask your health care provider to give you an STD test.

Some people assume they will be tested for STDs when they have an exam for another reason, such as when a woman has a Pap test or when a man has a physical. This is not true—you will not automatically be tested for STDs.

If you are seeing your health care provider for another reason, and are not sure if you need an STD test, just ask. Your provider can help you decide if you need any tests, and which one(s) you may need.

Where can I get an STD test?

Your local Planned Parenthood health center, many other clinics, private health care providers, and health departments offer STD tests.

Which STD tests do I need?

There is no single test for every sexually transmitted disease—tests are specific to each infection. And some infections can be found using different kinds of tests.

You and your health care provider will decide what STD tests make the most sense for you. In most cases, your provider will first ask you questions about:

- your sexual practices—such as how many partners you have, whether you use condoms or other barrier methods, and what body parts are used during sex play;

- whether you have symptoms—and to describe the symptoms if you do have any;

- whether you have had symptoms in the past;

- whether you've ever had any STDs;

- whether you have used over-the-counter medications to treat your symptoms;

- whether your partner(s) have any STDs or symptoms of STDs;

- any drug allergies you may have;

- your last period, if you're a woman—to see if you could you be pregnant.

It is important to be honest with your health care provider. Your provider will be helping you make important decisions about what test(s) you may need.

Table 25.1. STD Testing Quick Reference Guide

Which STD is being tested?	What's the test?
HIV/AIDS	Blood test; Oral swab test—a special tool is used to test cells from inside the mouth; Urine test (rarely used)
Bacterial vaginosis (BV; affects only women)	Pelvic exam; Test of vaginal discharge
Chlamydia	Physical exam; Test of discharge from the anus, urethra, or vagina; Test of a cell sample—cells from the cervix, penis, vagina, or anus; Urine test
Cytomegalovirus	Blood test
Genital warts	Physical exam—some warts can be seen by the naked eye during a pelvic exam. A special tool called a colposcope may be used to detect warts that are too small to be seen by the naked eye.
Gonorrhea	Test of discharge from the anus, urethra, or vagina; Test of a cell sample—cells from the cervix, penis, anus, or throat; Urine test
Hepatitis B blood test	Herpes blood test; Test of fluid taken from a herpes sore
High-risk HPV	No HPV test for men; Test of cell samples from the cervix
Intestinal parasites	Test of a stool (feces) sample; Proctoscopy may be needed—a test that involves a health care provider inserting a thin lighted tube into the rectum
Molluscum contagiosum	Physical exam; Test of a cell sample
Pelvic inflammatory disease (affects only women)	Pelvic exam; Blood test; Test of discharge from the cervix or vagina; Laparoscopy—a special instrument is inserted through a small cut in the navel to look at the reproductive organs
Pubic lice	Physical exam; May be self-diagnosed based on symptoms
Scabies	Physical exam; May be self-diagnosed based on symptoms; Test of a cell sample; Biopsy may be necessary
Syphilis	Blood test; Test of fluid taken from a syphilis sore
Trichomoniasis	Test of discharge from the vagina or urethra

How are STD tests done?

It depends on which infection you may have. And some infections can be tested for in more than one way. Your test may include a:

- **Physical exam:** Your health care provider may look at your genitals and/or your anus for any signs of an infection, such as a rash, discharge, sores, or warts. For women, this exam can be similar to a pelvic exam.

- **Blood sample:** Your provider may take a blood sample, either with a needle or by pricking the skin to draw drops of blood.

- **Urine sample:** You may be asked to urinate into a special cup.

- **Discharge, tissue, cell, or saliva sample:** Your provider will use a swab to collect samples that will be looked at under a microscope.

Sometimes a diagnosis can be made based on your symptoms and/or a physical exam. Treatment could be prescribed right away. Other times, your health care provider may need to send a sample to a lab to be tested. In that case, the results may not be available for several days or weeks.

Section 25.3

Vaccine to Prevent Human Papillomavirus

This section includes text from "HPV Vaccine Information for Young Women," by the Centers for Disease Control and Prevention (CDC, www.cdc.gov), June 26, 2008, and "FDA Approves New Indication for Gardasil to Prevent Genital Warts in Men and Boys," by the U.S. Food and Drug Administration (FDA, www.fda.gov), October 16, 2009.

Human Papillomavirus Vaccine Information for Young Women

There is now a vaccine that prevents the types of genital human papillomavirus (HPV) that cause most cases of cervical cancer and genital warts. The vaccine, Gardasil®, is given in three shots over 6 months. The vaccine is routinely recommended for 11 and 12-year-old girls. It is also recommended for girls and women age 13 through 26 who have not yet been vaccinated or completed the vaccine series.

Why the HPV Vaccine Is Important

Genital HPV is a common virus that is passed on through genital contact, most often during sex. Most sexually active people will get HPV at some time in their lives, though most will never even know it. It is most common in people in their late teens and early 20s.

There are about 40 types of HPV that can infect the genital areas of men and women. Most HPV types cause no symptoms and go away on their own. But some types can cause cervical cancer in women and other less common genital cancers—like cancers of the anus, vagina, and vulva (area around the opening of the vagina). Other types of HPV can cause warts in the genital areas of men and women, called genital warts. Genital warts are not a life-threatening disease. But they can cause emotional stress and their treatment can be very uncomfortable.

Every year, about 12,000 women are diagnosed with cervical cancer and almost 4,000 women die from this disease in the United States.

About 1% of sexually active adults in the United States (or 1 million people) have visible genital warts at any point in time.

Who Should Get the HPV Vaccine

The HPV vaccine is recommended for 11- and 12-year-old girls. It is also recommended for girls and women age 13 through 26 years of age who have not yet been vaccinated or completed the vaccine series. The vaccine can also be given to girls 9 or 10 years of age.

Ideally females should get the vaccine before they become sexually active, when they may be exposed to HPV. Females who are sexually active may also benefit from the vaccine, but they may get less benefit from it. This is because they may have already gotten an HPV type targeted by the vaccine. Few sexually active young women are infected with all HPV types covered by the vaccine so they would still get protection from those types they have not yet gotten. Currently, there is no test available to tell if a girl/woman has had HPV in the past or which types.

The vaccine is not recommended for pregnant women. There has been limited research looking at vaccine safety for pregnant women and their unborn babies. So far, studies suggest that the vaccine does not cause health problems for pregnant women or their developing children. But more research is still needed. For now, pregnant women should wait until their pregnancy is over before getting the vaccine. If a woman finds out she is pregnant after she has started getting the vaccine series, she should wait until her pregnancy is over before finishing the three-dose series.

Girls/women do not need to get an HPV test or Pap test to find out if they should get the vaccine. Neither of these tests can tell the specific HPV type(s) that a woman has (or has had in the past), so there's no way to know if she has already had the HPV types covered by the vaccine.

The vaccine has been widely tested in girls/women 9 through 26 years of age. New research is being done on the vaccine's safety and efficacy in women older than 26 years of age. The U.S. Food and Drug Administration (FDA) will consider licensing the vaccine for these women when there is enough research to show that it is safe and effective for them.

Effectiveness of the HPV Vaccine

This vaccine targets the types of HPV that most commonly cause cervical cancer and genital warts. The vaccine is highly effective in preventing those types of HPV and related diseases in young women.

The vaccine is less effective in preventing HPV-related disease in young women who have already been exposed to one or more HPV types. That is because the vaccine does not treat existing HPV infections or the diseases they may cause. It can only prevent HPV before a person gets it.

Research suggests that vaccine protection will last a long time. More research is being done to find out if women will need a booster vaccine many years after getting vaccinated to boost protection.

The vaccine does not protect against all types of HPV—so it will not prevent all cases of cervical cancer. About 30% of cervical cancers will not be prevented by the vaccine, so it will be important for women to continue getting screened for cervical cancer (regular Pap tests). Also, the vaccine does not prevent other sexually transmitted infections (STIs). So it will still be important for sexually active persons to lower their risk for other STIs.

It is not yet known how much protection girls/women would get from receiving only one or two doses of the vaccine. For this reason, it is very important that girls/women get all three doses of the vaccine.

Safety of the HPV Vaccine

This vaccine has been licensed by the FDA and approved by CDC as safe and effective. It was studied in thousands of females (ages 9 through 26 years) around the world and its safety continues to be monitored by CDC and the FDA. Studies have found no serious side effects. The most common side effect is soreness in the arm (where the shot is given). There have recently been some reports of fainting in teens after they got the vaccine. For this reason, it is recommended that patients wait in their doctor's office for 15 minutes after getting the vaccine.

Cost and Paying for the HPV Vaccine

The retail price of the vaccine is about $125 per dose ($375 for full series).

While some insurance companies may cover the vaccine, others may not. Most large insurance plans usually cover the costs of recommended vaccines.

Children age 18 and younger may be eligible to get vaccines, including the HPV vaccine, for free through the Vaccines for Children (VFC) program if they are: Medicaid eligible; uninsured; or American Indian or Alaska Native. Doctors may charge a small fee to give each shot. However, VFC vaccines cannot be denied to an eligible child if the family cannot afford the fee.

Some states also provide free or low-cost vaccines at public health department clinics to people without health insurance coverage for vaccines. Contact your State Health Department to see if your state has such a program.

What Vaccinated Girls/Women Need to Know

Women will still need regular cervical cancer screening (Pap tests) because the vaccine will **not** protect against all HPV types that cause cervical cancer. Also, women who got the vaccine after becoming sexually active may not get the full benefit of the vaccine if they had already acquired HPV.

Another HPV vaccine is now being considered for licensure by the FDA. This vaccine would protect against the types of HPV that cause most cervical cancers, but it would not protect against genital warts.

Regular cervical cancer screening and follow-up can prevent most cases of cervical cancer. The Pap test can detect cell changes in the cervix before they turn into cancer. Pap tests can also detect most, but not all, cervical cancers at an early, treatable stage. Most women diagnosed with cervical cancer in the United States have either never had a Pap test, or have not had a Pap test in the last 5 years. The HPV test can tell if a woman has HPV on her cervix. This test can be used with the Pap test to help your doctor determine next steps in cervical cancer screening.

The only sure way to prevent HPV is to abstain from all sexual activity. For those who are sexually active, condoms may lower the chances of getting HPV, if used all the time and the right way. Condoms may also lower the risk of developing HPV-related diseases (genital warts and cervical cancer). But HPV can infect areas that are not covered by a condom—so condoms may not fully protect against HPV.

Sexually active adults can also lower their risk of HPV by being in a mutually faithful relationship with someone who has had no or few sex partners, or by limiting their number of sex partners. The fewer partners a person has had—the less likely he or she is to have HPV. But even persons with only one lifetime sex partner can get HPV, if their partner has had previous partners.

Gardasil Vaccine for Boys

The U.S. Food and Drug Administration (FDA) approved use of the vaccine Gardasil for the prevention of genital warts (condyloma acuminata) due to human papillomavirus (HPV) types 6 and 11 in boys and men, ages 9 through 26.

Each year, about two out of every 1,000 men in the United States are newly diagnosed with genital warts.

Gardasil currently is approved for use in girls and women ages 9 through 26 for the prevention of cervical, vulvar, and vaginal cancer caused by HPV types 16 and 18; precancerous lesions caused by types 6, 11, 16, and 18; and genital warts caused by types 6 and 11.

HPV is the most common sexually transmitted infection in the United States and most genital warts are caused by HPV infection.

"This vaccine is the first preventive therapy against genital warts in boys and men ages 9 through 26, and, as a result, fewer men will need to undergo treatment for genital warts," said Karen Midthun, MD, acting director of the FDA's Center for Biologics Evaluation and Research.

Gardasil's effectiveness was studied in a randomized trial of 4,055 males ages 16 through 26 years old. The results showed that in men who were not infected by HPV types 6 and 11 at the start of the study, Gardasil was nearly 90 percent effective in preventing genital warts caused by infection with HPV types 6 and 11.

Studies were conducted to measure the immune response to the vaccine in boys ages 9 through 15. The results showed that the immune response was as good as that found in the 16 through 26 years age group, indicating that the vaccine should have similar effectiveness.

The manufacturer will conduct postmarketing studies to obtain additional information on the safety and effectiveness of Gardasil in boys and men.

Gardasil is given as three injections over a 6-month period. Headache, fever, and pain at the injection site, itching, redness, swelling, and bruising were the most common side effects observed.

Gardasil is manufactured by Merck and Company Inc. of Whitehouse Station, NJ. Gardasil product information is available at www .fda.gov/cber/products/gardasil.htm.

Section 25.4

Practicing Safer Sex: What It Means

We all care about protecting ourselves and the ones we love. For sexually active people that means practicing safer sex. We can use it to reduce our risk of getting sexually transmitted diseases (STDs). It lets us protect ourselves—and our partners—while we enjoy sex play with them. Safer sex is for responsible people who care about their and their partners' pleasure and health.

What is safer sex?

Safer sex is anything we do during sex play to reduce our risk of getting an infection. Even though a lot of people say "safe sex" instead of "safer sex," there is no kind of skin-to-skin sex play with a partner that is totally risk-free. But being "safer" is something all of us can do.

These are the most important ways to practice safer sex:

- Understand and be honest about the risks we take.

- Keep our blood, pre-cum, semen, or vaginal fluids out of each other's bodies.

- Always use latex or female condoms for anal or vaginal intercourse.

- Don't have sex play when we have a sore caused by a sexually transmitted disease.

- Find ways to make safer sex as pleasurable as possible.

How can I lower my risk using safer sex?

One way to have safer sex is to only have one partner who has no sexually transmitted infections and no other partners than you.

But, this isn't always the safest kind of safer sex. That's because most people don't know when they have infections. They are very likely to pass them on without knowing it.

Another other reason is that some people aren't as honest as they should be. In fact, about one out of three people will say they don't have an infection when they know they do, just to have sex. So most of us have to find other ways to practice safer sex.

Another way to practice safer sex is to only have sex play that has no risk—or a lower risk—of passing STDs. This means no vaginal or anal intercourse. Many of us find that great sex is about a lot more than a penis going in a vagina or anus. It is about exploring the many other ways you and your partner can turn each other on. Not only is it a way to discover new sexual pleasures, it's also safer.

No-risk safer sex play includes:

• masturbation;

• mutual masturbation;

• cybersex;

• phone sex; and

• sharing fantasies.

Low-risk safer sex play includes:

• kissing;

• fondling—manual stimulation of one another;

• body-to-body rubbing—frottage, grinding, or dry humping;

• oral sex (even safer with a condom or other barrier); and

• playing with sex toys—alone or with a partner.

The highest risk kinds of sex play are:

• vaginal intercourse; and

• anal intercourse.

How do different sexually transmitted infections get passed along?

Infections are passed in different ways. Here are the basics:

Vaginal or anal intercourse without a condom (high risk for passing):

• chancroid;

• chlamydia;

• cytomegalovirus (CMV);

- genital warts;
- gonorrhea;
- hepatitis B;
- herpes;
- human immunodeficiency virus (HIV);
- human papillomavirus (HPV);
- pelvic inflammatory disease (PID);
- pubic lice;
- scabies;
- syphilis; and
- trichomoniasis.

Oral sex without a condom (high risk for passing CMV):

- gonorrhea;
- hepatitis B;
- herpes; and
- syphilis.

Skin-to-skin sex play without sexual intercourse (risky for passing CMV):

- herpes;
- HPV;
- pubic lice; and
- scabies.

Lots of other infections, from the flu to mononucleosis, can also be passed during sex play. Luckily, we can use condoms during vaginal and anal intercourse to make them safer.

How do condoms make sex safer?

Condoms work by forming a barrier between the penis and anus, vagina, or mouth. The barrier keeps one partner's fluids from getting into or on the other. And condoms reduce the amount of skin-to-skin contact. There are two main kinds of condoms—latex condoms and female condoms.

- Latex condoms are great safer sex tools for anal or vaginal intercourse. They are easy to get at a pharmacy, grocery store, or at a Planned Parenthood health center. They are cheap. And they come in a variety of shapes, sizes, and textures.

- People with latex allergies can use condoms made of non-latex rubber or plastic. They also make sex safer, but they are not as widely available as latex condoms.

- Female condoms reduce your risk of infection, too. Female condoms aren't quite as easy to find as latex condoms, but they are available in some drugstores and many Planned Parenthood health centers. You can also order them online if you can't find them in your neighborhood. Follow the instructions on the package for using female condoms correctly.

Is oral sex safer sex?

When it comes to HIV, oral sex is safer sex than vaginal or anal intercourse. But other infections, like herpes, syphilis, and hepatitis B, can be passed by oral sex. Condoms or other barriers can also be used to make oral sex even safer.

How can I use Sheer Glyde or dental dams to make oral sex safer?

Dental dams are small, thin, square pieces of latex used to protect the throat during certain kinds of dental work. They can also be placed on the vulva or the anus when the mouth, lips, or tongue are used to sexually arouse a partner. Like the condom, dams keep partners' body fluids out of each other's bodies. They also prevent skin-to-skin contact. A special kind of dam, the Sheer Glyde dam, has been approved by the FDA especially for safer sex. Like dental dams, Sheer Glyde dams are available online, in some drugstores, and at many Planned Parenthood health centers.

If Sheer Glyde dams or dental dams aren't handy, you can use plastic wrap or a cut-open condom.

How can I have safer sex with my sex toys?

Many people like to spice up sex play with sex toys—dildos, vibrators, strap-ons, butt plugs, and more. These toys need special care, too, when used alone or with partners. Unless they are kept clean between uses, they can build up bacteria, which can cause an infection. And if they are shared between partners, they can pass along sexually transmitted diseases.

The best way to keep sex toys clean and safe is to protect them with a latex condom. The condom should be changed whenever the toy is passed from partner to partner or from one body opening to another—mouth, anus, or vagina.

If you don't use condoms to keep a sex toy clean, it's important to clean it before and after every use. Sex toys are made of many different materials—silicone, jelly rubber, vinyl, stainless steel, acrylic, etc. They all may have to be cleaned different ways. Some toys can be soaked in water—and some cannot. Please read the instructions on the package carefully. Never use breakable household objects, like glass bottles, as sex toys.

Keeping your sex toys clean will help them last longer, and they'll give you pleasure instead of infections.

How can I use lubricant for safer sex?

A good lubricant can go a long way in making sure that safer sex is pleasurable and fun. Lubricant is important in safer sex because it also makes condoms and dams slippery and less likely to break. Lubricants make safer sex feel better by cutting down on the dry kind of friction that a lot of people find irritating.

When buying lube, it's important to find the right kind—one that works for you and for your condom. Never use oil-based lube with a latex or non-latex rubber condom. Use only water or silicone-based lube with latex and non-latex rubber condoms. Read the package insert if you have any questions about what you can use.

What about safer sex and drugs and alcohol?

Alcohol and other drugs can make you forget you promised yourself to have safer sex. The use of too much alcohol or any amount of drugs often leads to high-risk sex.

How does safer sex make sex feel better?

Worrying about sexually transmitted infections can make sex less satisfying. Safer sex can reduce that worry. Practicing safer sex can also help you and your partner:

- add variety to sexual pleasure;
- make sex play last longer by postponing orgasms;
- increase intimacy and trust;

- strengthen relationships; and

- improve communication—verbal and nonverbal.

The bottom line is that safer sex can be fun. It is a great way to explore who we are sexually, express our feelings, bond with others, and have a good time. Practicing safer sex can enhance our pleasure—and who doesn't want more pleasure?

Am I ready for safer sex?

Which of the following statements are true for you?

- I am ready to let my partner know where and how I like to be touched.

- I am ready to buy condoms, even if it's embarrassing.

- If I decide I want to use sex toys, I'm ready to keep them clean.

- I am ready to let my partner know my limits when it comes to taking risks.

- I am ready to say no to sex when I don't want to have it.

- I am ready to have regular physical exams and tests for sexually transmitted infections.

- I am ready to talk with my health care provider about my sex life.

- I am ready to enjoy sex without having to get high.

Section 25.5

Talking to Your Partner about Condoms

It's much smarter to talk about condoms before having sex, but that doesn't make it easy. Some people—even those who are already having sex—are embarrassed by the topic of condoms. But not talking about condoms affects a person's safety. Using condoms properly every time is the best protection against sexually transmitted disease (STDs)—even if you're using another form of birth control like the Pill.

So how can you overcome your embarrassment about talking about condoms? Well, for starters it can help to know what a condom looks like, how it works, and what it's like to handle one. Buy a box of condoms so you can familiarize yourself.

The next thing to get comfortable with is bringing up the topic of condoms with a partner. Practice opening lines. If you think your partner will object, work out your response ahead of time. Here are some possibilities:

Your partner says: "It's uncomfortable." You might answer this by suggesting a different brand or size. Wearing a condom also may take some getting used to.

Your partner says: "It puts me right out of the mood." Say that having unsafe sex puts you right out of the mood. Permanently.

Your partner says: "If we really love each other, we should trust each other." Say that it's because you love each other so much that you want to be sure you're both safe and protect each other.

Your partner says: "Are you nervous about catching something?" The natural response: "Sometimes people don't even know when they have infections, so it's better to be safe."

Your partner says: "I won't enjoy sex if we use a condom." Say you can't enjoy sex unless it's safe.

Your partner says: "I don't know how to put it on." This one's easy: "Here, let me show you."

Timing

After you've familiarized yourself with condoms and practiced your routine, you'll want to pick the right time to bring up the subject with your partner. A good time to do this is long before you're in a situation where you might need a condom. When people are caught up in the heat of the moment, they may find they're more likely to be pressured into doing something they regret later.

Try bringing up the topic in a matter-of-fact way. You might mention that you've bought some condoms and checked them out. Offer to bring the unopened condoms along. Or suggest that your partner buy his or her favorite brand (and then bring some of yours with you, just to be on the safe side). Offer to try different types of condoms to find which works best for both of you.

Make it clear that you won't have sex without a condom. If someone threatens you or says they'd rather break up than wear a condom, it's time for you to say good-bye. Tell the person you won't have sex with someone who doesn't respect you or themselves enough to use protection.

Here are some tips for using condoms:

- Check the expiration date (condoms can dry and crack if they're old). Don't use a condom if it seems brittle or sticky—throw it away and get another one.

- Choose condoms made of latex, which is thought to be more effective in preventing STDs. (If one of you has an allergy to latex, use polyurethane condoms instead.)

- If you use lubricants with condoms, always use water-based ones. Shortening, lotion, petroleum jelly, or baby oil can break down the condom.

- Open the condom packet with your hands, not your teeth, and open it carefully so you don't tear the condom.

- Choose a condom with a reservoir tip to catch semen after ejaculation. Lightly pinch the top of the condom and place it at the top of your (or your partner's) penis. This gets rid of trapped air, which can cause a condom to burst.

- Roll the condom down until it's completely rolled out—if it's inside out, throw it away and start over with a new condom.

- Remove the condom immediately after ejaculation, before the penis softens. You or your partner should hold the condom at the base of the penis (the part nearest the guy's body) while he withdraws to prevent the condom from slipping off.

- Slide the condom off the penis, keeping the semen inside. Since condoms can clog the toilet if they are flushed, tie it off or put in a plastic bag (so it's not a health risk for others) and throw it out.

These aren't the only tips on discussing and using condoms. If you want more advice, talk to your friends, siblings, or parents. Yes, parents. Not everyone feels comfortable talking about sex with their parents, but lots of teens do. Parents often have the best tips.

Health professionals are also great sources of advice on sex and sexuality. A doctor or nurse practitioner or someone at a local health or family planning clinic can offer you advice—confidentially if necessary.

Of course, the only way to be 100% protected from pregnancy and STDs is abstinence (not having sex). But if you do decide to have sex, using a condom allows you to protect yourself.

Chapter 26

Understanding Abstinence

Is abstinence right for me?

People are abstinent for many reasons, including to prevent pregnancy. Here are some of the most common questions we hear people ask about abstinence. We hope the answers help you decide if it is right for you.

What is abstinence?

You may have heard people talk about abstinence in different ways. Some people think of abstinence as not having vaginal intercourse. They may enjoy other kinds of sex play that don't lead to pregnancy. This is better described as outercourse.

Some people define abstinence as not having vaginal intercourse when a woman might get pregnant. This is better described as periodic abstinence, which is one of the fertility awareness-based methods of birth control.

And some people define abstinence as not having any kind of sex play with a partner. This is the definition used in this text.

Being continuously abstinent is the only way to be absolutely sure that you won't have an unintended pregnancy or get a sexually transmitted disease (STD).

How does abstinence prevent pregnancy?

Abstinence prevents pregnancy by keeping sperm out of the vagina.

How effective is abstinence?

Used continuously, abstinence is 100 percent effective in preventing pregnancy. It also prevents STDs.

How safe is abstinence?

Abstinence is one of the safest ways to prevent pregnancy—there are no side effects.

What are the benefits of abstinence?

Abstinence:

- has no medical or hormonal side effects; and
- is free.

Women and men abstain from sex play for many reasons—even after they've been sexually active. A couple may even choose to be abstinent after having had sex play with each other. The reasons people choose to be abstinent may change throughout life.

People choose abstinence to:

- prevent pregnancy;
- prevent STDs;
- wait until they're ready for a sexual relationship;
- wait to find the right partner;
- have fun with romantic partners without sexual involvement;
- focus on school, career, or extracurricular activities;
- support personal, moral, or religious beliefs and values;
- get over a breakup;
- heal from the death of a partner; or
- follow medical advice during an illness or infection.

Any woman or man can abstain from sex play. Many do so at various times in their lives. Some choose to abstain from sex play for long periods in their lives.

Sexual relationships present risks. Abstinence is a very good way to postpone taking those risks until you are better able to handle them. Women who abstain until their 20s—and who have fewer partners in their lifetimes—may have certain health advantages over women who do not. They are less likely to get STDs. Because they are less likely to get an STD, they are also less likely to become infertile or develop cervical cancer.

What are the disadvantages of abstinence?

There are few disadvantages to abstinence. People may find it difficult to abstain for long periods of time and may end their period of abstinence without being prepared to protect themselves against pregnancy or infection.

How do I talk with my partner about being abstinent?

Talking with your partner about your decision to abstain from sex play is important—whether or not you've had sex play before. Partners need to be honest with each other and make sexual decisions together. These are some of the best ways to keep a relationship happy. Even so, it may not be easy to do. You may feel awkward or embarrassed.

- It's best to talk about your feelings before things get sexual. For many people it's hard to be clear about what they want if they get aroused. It is helpful to think—ahead of time—about how you can say "no" to sex play. What behavior will be clear? What words will be best? You can practice saying the words out loud. Then think about how someone might respond to you.

- Take the time to consider fully what being abstinent will mean for you. It is important to know what you are thinking and feeling and what you need. Then you can tell your partner about it.

- Be straightforward about the limits you want to set.

Keep in mind that having sex is not the only way two people can get to know each other. Sex play is also not the only way couples can be close. People get closer as they build trust by:

- talking;
- listening;
- sharing;
- being honest;
- respecting each other's thoughts and feelings; and

- enjoying one another's company.

Abstinence can only work when both partners agree to it. So it is also helpful to keep talking with each other about why you've agreed to abstain from sex play. Your relationship may change. And your decision to be abstinent may change, too.

How can I stay abstinent?

Staying abstinent is a choice you make every day. There are ways to help yourself with that choice.

- Remind yourself why you chose to be abstinent.
- Think about the consequences.
- Don't reevaluate your decision to stay abstinent during sexually charged situations—stick with your decision until you can think about it with a clear head.

Abstinence can be difficult for some people. Women and men need to be clear about their reasons to stay abstinent. If you are tempted to have sex play, it helps to remember why you made the decision to be abstinent in the first place. How can you stay abstinent? Think about your answers to these questions:

- Am I clear about why I want to be abstinent?
- Am I aware of situations that could make staying abstinent difficult for me? Can I avoid them?
- Alcohol and other drugs can affect my judgment and decision-making ability. How do I feel about not using them?
- Are there people in my life I can talk to about my decision to be abstinent? Will they be supportive?

Most people stop being abstinent at some point in their lives. When you decide not to be abstinent, ask yourself:

- Do I have information about other methods of birth control and do I have access to them?
- Do I know how to protect myself from STDs?

Chapter 27

Birth Control Methods (Contraception)

Choosing Birth Control (Contraception)

There is no best method of birth control. Each method has its pros and cons.

All women and men can have control over when, and if, they become parents. Making choices about birth control, or contraception, isn't easy. There are many things to think about. To get started, learn about birth control methods you or your partner can use to prevent pregnancy. You can also talk with your doctor about the choices.

Before choosing a birth control method, think about the following:

- Your overall health

- How often you have sex

- The number of sex partners you have

- If you want to have children someday

- How well each method works to prevent pregnancy

- Possible side effects

- Your comfort level with using the method

Excerpted from "Frequently Asked Questions about Birth Control Methods," by the Office on Women's Health (www.womenshealth.gov), part of the U.S. Department of Health and Human Services, March 6, 2009.

Keep in mind, even the most effective birth control methods can fail. But your chances of getting pregnant are lowest if the method you choose always is used correctly and every time you have sex.

Types of Birth Control

You can choose from many methods of birth control. They are grouped by how they work:

Continuous Abstinence

This means not having sex (vaginal, anal, or oral) at any time. It is the only sure way to prevent pregnancy and protect against sexually transmitted diseases (STDs), including human immunodeficiency virus (HIV).

Natural Family Planning/Rhythm Method

This method is when you do not have sex or use a barrier method on the days you are most fertile (most likely to become pregnant). You can read about barrier methods in the following text.

A woman who has a regular menstrual cycle has about 9 or more days each month when she is able to get pregnant. These fertile days are about 5 days before and 3 days after ovulation, as well as the day of ovulation.

To have success with this method, you need to learn about your menstrual cycle. Then you can learn to predict which days you are fertile or "unsafe." To learn about your cycle, keep a written record of the following:

- When you get your period

- What it is like (heavy or light blood flow)

- How you feel (sore breasts, cramps)

This method also involves checking your cervical mucus and recording your body temperature each day. Cervical mucus is the discharge from your vagina. You are most fertile when it is clear and slippery like raw egg whites. Use a basal thermometer to take your temperature and record it in a chart.

Your temperature will rise 0.4 to 0.8 degrees Fahrenheit on the first day of ovulation. You can talk with your doctor or a natural family planning instructor to learn how to record and understand this information.

Barrier Methods

These methods put up a block, or barrier, to keep sperm from reaching the egg.

Contraceptive sponge: This barrier method is a soft, disk-shaped device with a loop for taking it out. It is made out of polyurethane foam and contains the spermicide nonoxynol-9. Spermicide kills sperm.

Before having sex, you wet the sponge and place it, loop side down, inside your vagina to cover the cervix. The sponge is effective for more than one act of intercourse for up to 24 hours. It needs to be left in for at least 6 hours after having sex to prevent pregnancy. It must then be taken out within 30 hours after it is inserted.

Only one kind of contraceptive sponge is sold in the United States. It is called the Today Sponge. Women who are sensitive to the spermicide nonoxynol-9 should not use the sponge.

Diaphragm, cervical cap, and cervical shield: These barrier methods block the sperm from entering the cervix (the opening to your womb) and reaching the egg.

- The diaphragm is a shallow latex cup.

- The cervical cap is a thimble-shaped latex cup. It often is called by its brand name, FemCap.

- The cervical shield is a silicone cup that has a one-way valve that creates suction and helps it fit against the cervix. It often is called by its brand name, Lea's Shield.

The diaphragm and cervical cap come in different sizes, and you need a doctor to fit you for one. The cervical shield comes in one size, and you will not need a fitting.

Before having sex, add spermicide (to block or kill sperm) to the devices. Then place them inside your vagina to cover your cervix. You can buy spermicide gel or foam at a drug store.

All three of these barrier methods must be left in place for 6 to 8 hours after having sex to prevent pregnancy. The diaphragm should be taken out within 24 hours. The cap and shield should be taken out within 48 hours.

Female condom: This condom is worn by the woman inside her vagina. It keeps sperm from getting into her body. It is made of thin, flexible, manmade rubber and is packaged with a lubricant. It can be inserted up to 8 hours before having sex. Use a new condom each time you have intercourse. And don't use it and a male condom at the same time.

Male condom: Male condoms are a thin sheath placed over an erect penis to keep sperm from entering a woman's body. Condoms can be made of latex, polyurethane, or natural/lambskin. The natural kind do not protect against STDs. Condoms work best when used with a vaginal spermicide, which kills the sperm. And you need to use a new condom with each sex act.

Condoms come in the following types:

- Lubricated condoms can make sexual intercourse more comfortable.

- Non-lubricated condoms are a type of condom that can also be used for oral sex. It is best to add lubrication to non-lubricated condoms if you use them for vaginal or anal sex. You can use a water-based lubricant, such as K-Y jelly. You can buy them at the drug store. Oil-based lubricants like massage oils, baby oil, lotions, or petroleum jelly will weaken the condom, causing it to tear or break.

Keep condoms in a cool, dry place. If you keep them in a hot place (like a wallet or glove compartment), the latex breaks down. Then the condom can tear or break.

Hormonal Methods

These methods prevent pregnancy by interfering with ovulation, fertilization, and/or implantation of the fertilized egg.

Oral contraceptives (combined pill; also called the pill): The pill contains the hormones estrogen and progestin. It is taken daily to keep the ovaries from releasing an egg. The pill also causes changes in the lining of the uterus and the cervical mucus to keep the sperm from joining the egg.

Some women prefer the extended cycle pills. These have 12 weeks of pills that contain hormones (active) and 1 week of pills that don't contain hormones (inactive). While taking extended cycle pills, women only have their period three to four times a year.

Many types of oral contraceptives are available. Talk with your doctor about which is best for you.

Your doctor may advise you not to take the pill if the following are true:

- If you are older than 35 and smoke

- If you have a history of blood clots

- If you have a history of breast, liver, or endometrial cancer

Antibiotics may reduce how well the pill works in some women. Talk to your doctor about a backup method of birth control if you need to take antibiotics.

Oral contraceptives (progestin-only pill, also called the mini-pill): Unlike the pill, the mini-pill only has one hormone—progestin. Taken daily, the mini-pill thickens cervical mucus, which keeps the sperm from joining the egg. Less often, it stops the ovaries from releasing an egg.

Mothers who breastfeed can use the mini-pill. It won't affect their milk supply. The mini-pill is a good option for these women:

- Women who can't take estrogen
- Women who are older than 35
- Women who have a risk of blood clots

The mini-pill must be taken at the same time each day. A backup method of birth control is needed if you take the pill more than 3 hours late. Antibiotics may reduce how well the pill works in some women. Talk to your doctor about a backup method of birth control if you need to take antibiotics.

The patch: Also called by its brand name, Ortho Evra, this skin patch is worn on the lower abdomen, buttocks, outer arm, or upper body.

It releases the hormones progestin and estrogen into the bloodstream to stop the ovaries from releasing eggs in most women. It also thickens the cervical mucus, which keeps the sperm from joining with the egg. You put on a new patch once a week for 3 weeks. You don't use a patch the fourth week in order to have a period.

Shot/injection: The birth control shot often is called by its brand name Depo-Provera. With this method you get injections, or shots, of the hormone progestin in the buttocks or arm every 3 months. A new type is injected under the skin. The birth control shot stops the ovaries from releasing an egg in most women. It also causes changes in the cervix that keep the sperm from joining with the egg.

The shot should not be used more than 2 years in a row because it can cause a temporary loss of bone density. The loss increases the longer this method is used. The bone does start to grow after this method is stopped. But it may increase the risk of fracture and osteoporosis if used for a long time.

Vaginal ring: This thin, flexible ring releases the hormones progestin and estrogen. It works by stopping the ovaries from releasing eggs. It also thickens the cervical mucus, which keeps the sperm from joining the egg.

It is commonly called NuvaRing, its brand name. You squeeze the ring between your thumb and index finger and insert it into your vagina. You wear the ring for 3 weeks, take it out for the week that you have your period, and then put in a new ring.

Implantable Devices

This birth control method involves devices that are inserted into the body and left in place for a few years.

Implantable rod: This is a matchstick-size, flexible rod that is put under the skin of the upper arm. It is often called by its brand name, Implanon. The rod releases a progestin, which causes changes in the lining of the uterus and the cervical mucus to keep the sperm from joining an egg. Less often, it stops the ovaries from releasing eggs. It is effective for up to 5 years.

Intrauterine devices or IUDs: An IUD is a small device shaped like a "T" that goes in your uterus. There are two types:

- **Copper IUD:** The copper IUD goes by the brand name Para-Gard. It releases a small amount of copper into the uterus, which prevents the sperm from reaching and fertilizing the egg. It fertilization does occur, the IUD keeps the fertilized egg from implanting in the lining of the uterus. A doctor needs to put in your copper IUD. It can stay in your uterus for 5 to 10 years.

- **Hormonal IUD:** The hormonal IUD goes by the brand name Mirena. It is sometimes called an intrauterine system, or IUS. It releases progestin into the uterus, which keeps the ovaries from releasing an egg and causes the cervical mucus to thicken so sperm can't reach the egg. It also affects the ability of a fertilized egg to successfully implant in the uterus. A doctor needs to put in a hormonal IUD. It can stay in your uterus for up to 5 years.

Permanent Birth Control Methods

These methods are for people who are sure they never want to have a child or they do not want more children.

Sterilization implant (Essure): Essure is the first non-surgical method of sterilizing women. A thin tube is used to thread a tiny spring-like device through the vagina and uterus into each fallopian tube. The device works by causing scar tissue to form around the coil. This blocks the fallopian tubes and stops the egg and sperm from joining.

It can take about 3 months for the scar tissue to grow, so it's important to use another form of birth control during this time. Then you will have to return to your doctor for a test to see if scar tissue has fully blocked your tubes.

Surgical sterilization: For women, surgical sterilization closes the fallopian tubes by being cut, tied, or sealed. This stops the eggs from going down to the uterus where they can be fertilized. The surgery can be done a number of ways. Sometimes, a woman having cesarean birth has the procedure done at the same time, so as to avoid having additional surgery later.

For men, having a vasectomy keeps sperm from going to his penis, so his ejaculate never has any sperm in it. Sperm stays in the system after surgery for about 3 months. During that time, use a backup form of birth control to prevent pregnancy. A simple test can be done to check if all the sperm is gone; it is called a semen analysis.

Emergency Contraception

This method is used if a woman's primary method of birth control fails. It should not be used as a regular method of birth control.

Emergency contraception (also called the morning after pill) is used to keep a woman from getting pregnant when she has had unprotected vaginal intercourse.

Unprotected can mean that no method of birth control was used. It can also mean that a birth control method was used but did not work, like a condom breaking. Or, a woman may have forgotten to take her birth control pills, or may have been abused or forced to have sex.

Emergency contraception consists of taking two doses of hormonal pills 12 hours apart. They work by stopping the ovaries from releasing an egg or keeping the sperm from joining with the egg. For the best chances for it to work, start the pills as soon as possible after unprotected sex. It should be started within 72 hours after having unprotected sex.

Preventing Sexually Transmitted Diseases

The male latex condom is the only birth control method proven to help protect you from STDs, including HIV.

Effectiveness and Side Effects

All birth control methods work the best if used correctly and every time you have sex. Be sure you know the right way to use them.

Sometimes doctors don't explain how to use a method because they assume you already know. Talk with your doctor if you have questions. They are used to talking about birth control. So don't feel embarrassed about talking to him or her.

Some birth control methods can take time and practice to learn. For example, some people don't know you can put on a male condom inside out. Also, not everyone knows you need to leave a little space at the tip of the condom for the sperm and fluid when a man ejaculates, or has an orgasm.

Where to Get Birth Control

Where you get birth control depends on what method you choose. You can buy these forms over the counter:

- Male condoms
- Female condoms
- Sponges
- Spermicides
- Emergency contraception pills (girls younger than 18 need a prescription)

You need a prescription for these forms:
- Oral contraceptives (the pill, the mini-pill)
- Skin patch
- Vaginal ring
- Diaphragm (your doctor needs to fit one to your shape)
- Cervical cap
- Cervical shield
- Shot/injection (you get the shot at your doctor's office)
- IUD (inserted by a doctor)
- Implantable rod (inserted by a doctor)

You will need surgery or a medical procedure for male and female sterilization.

Foams and Gels

You can buy spermicides over the counter. They work by killing sperm. They come in many forms:

- Foam
- Gel
- Cream
- Film
- Suppository
- Tablet

Spermicides are put in the vagina no more than 1 hour before having sex. If you use a film, suppository, or tablet, wait at least 15 minutes before having sex so the spermicide can dissolve. Do not douche or rinse out your vagina for at least 6 to 8 hours after having sex. You will need to use more spermicide each time you have sex.

Spermicides work best if used along with a barrier method, such as a condom, diaphragm, or cervical cap. Some spermicides are made just for use with the diaphragm and cervical cap. Check the package to make sure you are buying what you need.

All spermicides contain sperm-killing chemicals. Some contain nonoxynol-9, which may raise your risk of HIV if you use it a lot. It irritates the tissue in the vagina and anus, so it can cause the HIV virus to enter the body more freely. Some women are sensitive to nonoxynol-9 and need to use spermicides without it. Medications for vaginal yeast infections may lower the effectiveness of spermicides. Also, spermicides do not protect against sexually transmitted diseases.

Withdrawal Method

Withdrawal is when a man takes his penis out of a woman's vagina (or pulls out) before he ejaculates, or has an orgasm. This stops the sperm from going to the egg. Pulling out can be hard for a man to do. It takes a lot of self-control.

Even if you use withdrawal, sperm can be released before the man pulls out. When a man's penis first becomes erect, pre-ejaculate fluid may be on the tip of the penis. This fluid has sperm in it. So you could still get pregnant.

Withdrawal does not protect you from STDs or HIV.

Chapter 28

Teen Pregnancy

Chapter Contents

Section 28.1

Statistics on Teen Pregnancy in the United States

Guttmacher Institute, "U.S. Teenage Pregnancies, Births and Abortions: National and State Trends and Trends by Race and Ethnicity." New York: Guttmacher Institute, © 2010, http://www.guttmacher.org/pubs/USTPtrends .pdf, accessed May 24, 2010.

This text contains the most current teenage pregnancy, birth, and abortion statistics available, with national estimates through 2006, and state-level estimates through 2005.

Key Findings: National Levels and Trends

* In 2006, 750,000 women younger than 20 became pregnant. The pregnancy rate was 71.5 pregnancies per 1,000 women aged 15–19, and pregnancies occurred among about 7% of women in this age group.

* In 2005, the U.S. teenage pregnancy rate reached its lowest point in more than 30 years (69.5), down 41% since its peak in 1990 (116.9). However, in 2006, the rate increased for the first time in more than a decade, rising 3%.

* The pregnancy rate among sexually experienced teenagers (those who had ever had intercourse) was 152.8 pregnancies per 1,000 women aged 15–19, reflecting the fact that the over-all teenage pregnancy rate includes a substantial proportion of young people who are not sexually active. The pregnancy rate among sexually experienced teenagers also increased for the first time in over a decade, rising 3% from 2005 to 2006.

* The teenage birthrate in 2006 was 41.9 births per 1,000 women. This was 32% lower than the peak rate of 61.8, reached in 1991, but 4% higher than in 2005.

* The 2006 teenage abortion rate was 19.3 abortions per 1,000 women. This figure was 56% lower than its peak in 1988, but 1% higher than the 2005 rate.

- From 1986 to 2006, the proportion of teenage pregnancies ending in abortion declined almost one third, from 46% to 32% of pregnancies among 15- to 19-year-olds.

National Levels by Race and Ethnicity

- Among black women aged 15–19, the nationwide pregnancy rate fell by 45% (from 223.8 per 1,000 to 122.7) between 1990 and 2005, before increasing to 126.3 in 2006.

- Among non-Hispanic white teenagers, the pregnancy rate declined 50% in the same period (from 86.6 per 1,000 to 43.3), before increasing to 44.0 in 2006.

- Among Hispanic teenagers (of any race), the pregnancy rate decreased by 26% (from 169.7 per 1,000 to 124.9) between 1992 and 2005, before rising to 126.6 in 2006.

- Among all racial and ethnic groups, the birthrate reversed its downward trend in 2006 for the first time in more than a decade.

State Levels and Trends

- Between 1988 and 2000, teenage pregnancy rates declined in every state, and between 2000 and 2005, they fell in every state except North Dakota. (State data are not yet available for 2006.)

- In general, states with the largest numbers of teenagers also had the greatest number of teenage pregnancies. California reported the highest number of teenage pregnancies (96,490), followed by Texas, New York, Florida, and Illinois (with about 30,000–70,000 each). The smallest numbers of teenage pregnancies were in Vermont, North Dakota, Wyoming, South Dakota, and New Hampshire, all of which reported fewer than 1,600 pregnancies among women aged 15–19.

- New Mexico had the highest teenage pregnancy rate (93 per 1,000), followed by Nevada, Arizona, Texas, and Mississippi. The lowest rates were in New Hampshire (33), Vermont, Maine, Minnesota, and North Dakota.

- In 2005, teenage birthrates were highest in Texas (62 per 1,000), New Mexico, Mississippi, Arkansas, and Arizona. The states with the lowest teenage birthrates were New Hampshire (18 per 1,000), Vermont, Massachusetts, Connecticut, and New Jersey.

- Teenage abortion rates were highest in New York (41 per 1,000), New Jersey, Nevada, Delaware, and Connecticut.

- By contrast, teenagers in South Dakota (6 per 1,000), Utah, Kentucky, Nebraska, and North Dakota all had abortion rates of eight or fewer per 1,000 women aged 15–19.

- More than half of teenage pregnancies ended in abortion in New Jersey, New York, and Connecticut.

- In five states, 15% or fewer teenage pregnancies ended in abortion: Kentucky, Arkansas, South Dakota, Oklahoma, and Utah.

These observations exclude the District of Columbia, which is more comparable to a city than a state.

State Levels by Race and Ethnicity

- Among states with available data, Arkansas had the highest pregnancy rate among non-Hispanic white teenagers (67 per 1,000). Pregnancy rates among this group were also high in other Southern states: Tennessee, South Carolina, Kentucky, West Virginia, and Mississippi (60–63 per 1,000). Meanwhile, Minnesota had the lowest rate among non-Hispanic white teenagers (29 per 1,000), followed by Wisconsin, North Dakota, and Pennsylvania (31–34). However, many states do not record abortions by age, race, and ethnicity, and some of these were likely to have had high or low rates.

- The states known to have the highest pregnancy rates among black teenagers aged 15–19 were New York, Pennsylvania, Wisconsin, Iowa, and Minnesota (132–149 per 1,000). The rate was lowest in Hawaii (42 per 1,000), followed by Idaho, Maine, Utah, and Alaska (52–74).

- The highest pregnancy rate among Hispanic women aged 15–19 was found in Alabama (228 per 1,000). Rates were also over 185 in Tennessee, South Carolina, Delaware, and Georgia. In contrast, pregnancy rates among Hispanic teenagers were lowest in West Virginia and Maine (43 and 47 per 1,000, respectively).

Discussion

Pregnancy rates among teenagers and young women in the United States rose steadily from the early 1970s to the early 1990s, increasing by about 21% among all women younger than 20 and 17% among women aged 20–24 during those two decades. At the same time, the birthrate among these women remained relatively unchanged until the late 1980s, when it began to rise. From 1973, when abortion was legalized, to 1990, the abortion rate rose substantially.

By 1990 or 1991, the pregnancy rate among teenagers and young women had begun a steady and consistent decline. A decrease in both birth and abortion rates among these women signaled that both intended and unintended pregnancy rates were declining among these age groups. Recent research concluded that almost all of the decline in the pregnancy rate between 1995 and 2002 among 18- to 19-year-olds was attributable to increased contraceptive use. Among women aged 15–17, about one quarter of the decline during the same period was attributable to reduced sexual activity and three quarters to increased contraceptive use.

But, for the first time since the early 1990s, overall rates of pregnancy and birth—and, to a lesser extent, rates of abortion—among teenagers and young women increased from 2005 to 2006. It is too soon to tell whether this reversal is simply a short-term fluctuation, a more lasting stabilization or the beginning of a longer-term increase. Preliminary data on births for 2007 show a further increase in the birthrate among all women, including teenagers and those aged 20–24.

Other research has noted and seeks to provide additional explanations for the longer-term trends and changes, including shifts in the racial and ethnic composition of the population, increases in poverty, the growth of abstinence-only sex education programs at the expense of comprehensive programs, and changes in public perception and attitudes toward both teenage and unintended pregnancy.

In addition to the increases in teenage pregnancy, birth, and abortion rates, the data presented here indicate that there are still large and long-standing disparities in rates by race and by state. These disparities echo those seen among unintended pregnancy rates, which are several times higher for women of color. Research underway to calculate state-level unintended pregnancy rates will soon allow us to assess whether the state disparities seen among teenagers carry over to adult women.

Section 28.2

Options for Pregnant Teens

If you are pregnant, you have three options. First, you can stay pregnant and become a parent, with or without the support of the other parent. Second, you can carry the pregnancy to term (when the baby is ready to be born), and then give the baby up for adoption. Third, you can have an abortion, ending the pregnancy.

No matter what decision you make, be responsible and find out everything you can about each of your options. Get opinions from adults that you trust and seek medical care. You have the right to confidential health care with your privacy secured. The longer you wait to make a decision, the fewer options you may have. None of the options are easy, but you should find out as much as you can from several different agencies. However, be careful when gathering information from agencies because many "Crisis Pregnancy Centers" will not present all of your options and may have their own agendas.

Do not just "let pregnancy happen." Be responsible.

Teen Parenthood

Choosing to be a parent while still a teenager is a very difficult choice that will have educational, financial, social, physical, and emotional costs. In most cases, a teen will need a very supportive partner, family, school, and community to be able to raise a child. Talk to teens who are parents and ask about their lives. Do their realities match your dreams for your future? What support do they have, and will you have? Yes, it's difficult, but if you decide to continue your pregnancy, be confident in your abilities and gather as much support and resources as you can. It's hard work, but possible.

Adoption

There are many different options available if you choose to give your baby to another family. There are "open" adoptions, in which you can visit your child and be a part of his or life. There are also adoptions that are "closed," meaning your identity is sealed and you have no relationship with your child.

People choose both options, for different reasons. You will need help making this choice—find out as much as you can from several different agencies. Be careful. Many "Crisis Pregnancy Centers" will not present all of your options—they may have their own agenda.

Abortion

Abortion means the end of pregnancy before the fetus can live independently outside the mother. If abortion happens spontaneously before 24 weeks of pregnancy it is called a miscarriage. An induced abortion is caused deliberately in order to terminate the pregnancy.

In the case of *Roe v. Wade,* 1973, the Supreme Court confirmed women's right to choose to terminate an unwanted pregnancy and since then courts have upheld this decision. However, the decision to have an abortion is extremely personal.

Stories about Choices

To read stories about girls who faced these choices, and made very different decisions, and other relevant stories, go to: Teenwire [http://www.teenwire.org], sexuality and relationship information from Planned Parenthood.

Section 28.3

Prenatal Care for Pregnant Teens

When a teen is pregnant and decides to have a child, it's likely that she'll be thinking about how things will change once the baby is born. She'll have to plan for her social life to take a serious slowdown, and any money she's got will go straight into the diaper fund.

But what a woman does during her pregnancy is just as important as what she does once the baby is born. Unfortunately, one third of pregnant teens do not receive adequate prenatal care, which means their babies are more likely to have low birth weight and childhood health problems. Low birth weight babies may face serious health problems as newborns and are at increased risk of long-term disabilities.

Having a healthy pregnancy requires some serious lifestyle changes from the minute a woman realizes she is pregnant. So, what do pregnant teens need to know? Here are a few of the most important things.

Call a Health Care Provider

First things first—if a woman is pregnant, she needs to see a health care provider as soon as possible. Contact your local Planned Parenthood health center to schedule an appointment. Don't procrastinate on this one! Prenatal care is necessary to monitor the health of the fetus and the mother.

Ditch the Smokes

The other thing a pregnant woman needs to do pronto is stop some of those bad habits like smoking. Smoking reduces the amount of oxygen the fetus receives, contributes to low birth weight, and could even cause a miscarriage. So if you're a smoker, here's another big reason to quit. Cigarettes and coffee often go together but not when a woman is pregnant. Most health care providers advise pregnant women to limit their caffeine intake. (Don't forget that chocolate contains caffeine, too.)

Pass on the Partying

Drinking alcohol during pregnancy is a serious don't. Alcohol consumption can lead to fetal alcohol syndrome (FAS) or fetal alcohol effects (FAE). FAS and FAE cause birth defects and affect a child's ability to learn, think, and move. And even a little alcohol, any kind of alcohol, can harm a fetus.

Drugs and pregnancy also don't mix. Drug use during pregnancy has been linked to low birth weight and symptoms of drug withdrawal in infants, including excessive crying and shaking. Check in with your health care provider before you take any drugs, including prescription and over-the-counter medications.

Weighing In

A woman can help prevent low birth weight by following her health care provider's recommendations and by eating right. And say goodbye to dieting—pregnant women require 300–800 additional calories a day. It's really important for a pregnant woman to get the vitamins and minerals she needs, especially folic acid, calcium, and iron. Exercise is also an important part of staying healthy, but it's important for a pregnant woman to check with her clinician about what's safe for her to do.

Having a healthy pregnancy starts from day one. Eat right, steer clear of drugs and alcohol, and make sure to get adequate prenatal care.

Chapter 29

Understanding Sexual Orientation

Sexual Orientation at a Glance

- Sexual orientation is the term used to describe whether a person feels sexual desire for people of the opposite gender (heterosexual), same gender (homosexual), or both genders (bisexual).

- We do not know for sure what causes sexual orientation.

- You cannot tell a person's sexual orientation just by looking at them.

- Homophobia—fear and hatred of lesbian, gay, and bisexual people—is very dangerous.

Many of us are curious about sexual orientation. People often wonder what makes people bisexual, heterosexual, or homosexual—and how they can determine a person's sexual orientation. If you're just curious about sexual orientation, this is also a good place to start. Here are some of the most common questions people have about sexual orientation. We hope our answers are helpful.

What Is Sexual Orientation?

Sexual orientation is the term used to describe whether a person feels sexual desire for people of the opposite gender, same gender, or both genders.

- People who feel sexual desire for members of the other gender are heterosexual—straight.
- People who feel sexual desire for people of the same gender are homosexual—gay. Gay women are also called lesbians.
- People who are attracted to both genders are bisexual.
  All these sexual orientations are perfectly normal.

What Causes Sexual Orientation?

It's not exactly known what causes a person to be straight, gay, lesbian, or bisexual, but research shows that it's based on biological factors that are in place before birth. We do know that sexual orientation is usually established before puberty. And although sexual orientation probably begins to develop before birth, it may seem to change over the course of a lifetime for some people.

One thing is clear—sexual orientation is not something that people can decide for themselves, or for others.

How Many People Are Homosexual?

There is no way to know for sure—experts can only guess how many people may be homosexual. Research by Alfred Kinsey suggested that about one in 10 people are homosexual. Other research suggests somewhat lower estimates.

What Is the Kinsey Scale?

Alfred Kinsey developed the Kinsey scale as a way of describing a person's sexual orientation. Kinsey found that many people were not exclusively straight or gay—that a person's sexual orientation can actually be somewhere in between. The Kinsey scale categories are:

- 0—exclusively heterosexual;
- 1—predominantly heterosexual, infrequently homosexual;
- 2—predominantly heterosexual, but more than infrequently homosexual;

- 3—equally heterosexual and homosexual (bisexual);
- 4—predominantly homosexual, but more than infrequently heterosexual;
- 5—predominantly homosexual, infrequently heterosexual; and
- 6—exclusively homosexual.

Today, many researchers believe the Kinsey scale is too simple. They suggest that each person's sexual orientation may be even more complex than these basic labels.

People are all different, and each person's sexual orientation is unique.

People may choose to label their sexual orientation as they wish—and many people choose not to label it at all.

How Can I Figure out Someone's Sexual Orientation?

The only way you can know is if the person tells you. Some people think they can tell people's sexual orientation by the way they walk, talk, or dress, or by the job or hobbies they have. This is not true. Those are just stereotypes—widely accepted but very simplified judgments about a group.

What If I'm Unsure about My Sexual Orientation?

You are not alone. It can take years to understand our sexual orientation. Often, people may find that they are "questioning" for quite a while, or that none of the labels used to describe sexual orientation seems to apply to them. Each of us has to answer these questions for ourselves, but it may take time before we know.

Rest assured that many other people are still figuring out their sexuality, so what you're feeling is more common than you might think. Talking with a trusted friend or family member may help you figure it out.

What Is Coming Out?

"Coming out" or "coming out of the closet" is a process of accepting and being open about one's previously hidden identity—such as being bisexual, lesbian, or gay. The first step is coming out to ourselves. This happens as we recognize our orientation and accept it. We may also decide to tell others—sometimes right away, and sometimes later on.

This decision is different for each person. Coming out isn't a one-time thing. Because many people assume that all people they meet are heterosexual, coming out can be a constant process. Every time lesbian, gay, or bisexual people meet a new person, they have to decide whether and when to come out.

The coming-out process builds self-esteem, but can be stressful. Coming out often helps us feel closer to the people we love, even though it can be risky.

If you're deciding whether or not to come out, you have much to think about. Consider all the pluses and minuses. If coming out means that you risk losing your place in the family and emotional and financial support, for example, you may want to wait until you can find a way to support yourself. You should also think about whether coming out could put you in any physical danger.

What Is Homophobia?

Homophobia is fear or hatred of people who are lesbian, gay, or bisexual. Homophobia can also be fear or hatred of people who may appear to be lesbian or gay.

When gay, lesbian, and bisexual people have fear or hatred of themselves because of their homosexuality, it's called internalized homophobia.

Homophobia comes from fear. Some people are fearful because they have the wrong information—family, friends, and religious authorities often encourage negative feelings about homosexuality. And some people are fearful because they don't have any information about homosexuality—they are not aware of gay people or issues.

What Are the Results of Homophobia?

Homophobia hurts all of us. It can prevent lesbian, gay, and bisexual people from feeling safe and from living full lives. It leads to discrimination and sometimes violence. Lesbian, gay, and bisexual people—and those who appear to be homosexual—may face verbal abuse or physical violence because of their sexual orientation. This abuse is sometimes called gay-bashing.

More subtle forms of discrimination also come from homophobia. For example, people who are, or who are perceived to be, gay, lesbian, or bisexual, may not be hired for certain jobs, be allowed to rent certain apartments, or may be treated poorly by health care providers.

The stress of homophobia can be very harmful. It can cause:

- depression;
- fear;

- isolation;

- paranoia.

Internalized homophobia can lead to suicide. Up to 30 percent of lesbian, gay, and bisexual adolescents attempt suicide.

Homophobia can also hurt straight people. It can keep straight men from forming close friendships with other men, for example.

Fighting Homophobia

No matter what your sexual orientation, there are several simple things you can do to fight homophobia:

- Challenge stereotypes about lesbians, gays, and bisexuals.

- Use inclusive language—language that acknowledges that not everyone is heterosexual. For example, if you meet a woman who wears a wedding ring, don't automatically refer to her husband.

- Treat everyone—regardless of sexual orientation—with respect and dignity.

Here are some tips that might help you challenge homophobia in your everyday life:

- First, make sure you are safe. Don't challenge someone if you fear for your safety.

- Remember it's not personal. Homophobia is a fear that makes no sense. It might feel like a personal attack, but it's not.

- Pick a good time. Some homophobic situations come up very publicly. Others happen just between a couple of friends. Sometimes you might decide to speak up right away. Other times you may say something later on. And sometimes you might choose to just walk away.

- Ask questions and stay calm. Sometimes people don't know what words are insensitive or offensive. Try to remain calm and tell them.

- Friends are important. Don't go it alone. Ask for help when you need it. Develop a support system.

- Practice different ways you could approach situations. Talk it out with a friend.

Chapter 30

Gay, Lesbian, Bisexual, Transgender, and Questioning Youth

What is sexual orientation?

Sexual orientation is the overall term that is used to describe people's physical and/or romantic attractions to other people. The most common labels are heterosexual, homosexual, or bisexual.

- Heterosexual (or straight) refers to a person who is attracted to and falls in love with someone of another gender.

- Homosexual (or gay man or lesbian woman) refers to a person who is attracted to and falls in love with someone of the same gender.

- Bisexual refers to a person who is attracted to and falls in love with someone of another or the same gender.

[Editor's Note: In this text, LGBTQ refers to lesbian, gay, bisexual, transgender, and questioning.]

What is gender identity?

Gender identity refers to the internal sense that people have that they are female, male, or some variation of these. For many people biological sex (which is based on chromosomes and sexual anatomy) and

"Questions and Answers: LGBTQ Youth Issues," published by SIECUS, the Sexuality Information and Education Council of the United States, 90 John Street, Suite 704, New York, NY 10038, www.siecus.org. © 2010. Reprinted with permission.

gender identity are the same. For others, however, they may be different. The term transgender refers to individuals whose internal feelings of being male or female differ from the sexual anatomy they were born with. Transgender people may be heterosexual, homosexual, or bisexual.

How many people identify as lesbian, gay, bisexual, or transgender?

Estimates of how many people identify as lesbian, gay, or bisexual vary widely and there is not very much research done on the subject.

The CDC [Centers for Disease Control and Prevention] periodically conducts the National Survey of Family Growth (NFSG) (http://www.cdc.gov/nchs/about/major/nsfg/abclist.htm), which asks questions about reproductive and sexual health to men and women ages 15–44. The NSFG asked respondents a number of questions about their sexual orientation and attractions. Males and females ages 18–44 were asked "Do you think of yourself as heterosexual, homosexual, bisexual, or something else?"

- 90.2% of males ages 18–44 identified as heterosexual, 2.3% identified as homosexual, 1.8% identified as bisexual, and 3.9% identified as "something else."

- 90.3% of female ages 18–44 identified as heterosexual, 1.3% identified as homosexual, 2.8% identified as bisexual, and 4 % identified as "something else."

There are some differences, however, when participants are asked who they are attracted to:

- 92.2% of males ages 18–44 reported being attracted only to females, 3.9% reported being attracted mostly to females, 1.7% reported being attracted mostly to males, 1.5% reported being attracted only to males, 1.0% reported being attracted to both males and females, and 0.7% weren't sure of who they were attracted to.

- 85.8% of female ages 18–44 reported being attracted only to males, 10.2% reported being attracted mostly to males, 1.9% reported being attracted to both males and females, 0.8% reported being attracted mostly to females, 0.7% reported being attracted only to females, and 0.8% weren't sure of who they were attracted to.

The truth is there is almost no data on how many individuals identify as transgender. Informal estimates suggest that less than 1% of the population consider themselves transgender but these are based only on those transgender individuals who have sought mental health services.

Is there good data on same-sex sexual behavior?

Unfortunately, there is a limited amount of scientific data on same-sex sexual behavior. Research designed to examine this subject is often controversial and conservatives in congress regularly oppose its funding.

The most recent National Survey of Family Growth (NSFG), conducted by the CDC in 2002 does include some questions about same-sex sexual behavior. Men and women, however, were asked dramatically different questions in this category. Women were asked about "any sexual experience of any kind" with another female, whereas men were asked only about anal or oral sex with another male.

In response, 11.2% of females ages 15–44 reported having had any sexual experience of any kind with another female. Among young women ages 15–19 the numbers were similar with 10.6% reporting same-sex sexual contact.

The numbers for males were much lower, with only 6% of males ages 15–44 reporting ever having anal or oral sex with another male and only 4.5% of males ages 15–19 reporting having done so. Again, it's possible the smaller numbers may be due to the more limited scope of the question asked to males.

Are LGBTQ youth at higher risk for contracting HIV/AIDS?

Young men who have sex with men (MSM) are at higher risk for contracting HIV/AIDS [human immunodeficiency virus/acquired immunodeficiency syndrome] than their heterosexual counterparts. Studies have shown that rates of risky sexual behavior among young MSM are higher than among older MSM and that many young MSM don't believe they are at risk.

- In the seven cities that participated in the CDC's Young Men's Survey during 1994–1998, 14% of African-American MSM and 7% of Hispanic MSM ages 15–22 were infected with HIV.

- In a recent CDC study of young MSM, 77% of those who tested HIV-positive mistakenly believed that they were not infected.

- Of the men who tested positive, most (74%) had previously tested negative for HIV infection, and 59% believed that they were at low or very low risk.

- Young black MSM were more likely to be unaware of their infection—approximately 9 of 10 young black MSM were unaware compared with 6 of 10 young white MSM.

It is important to note that the CDC counts M to F [male to female] transgender women as MSM, and that very little research exists on the specific health risks transgender individuals face. A number of studies in different U.S. cities have found HIV prevalence in transgender women ranging from 14–47% and even higher rates in transgender sex workers.

Are LGBTQ youth at higher risk of contracting other STDs?

There is very little data on STDs other than HIV that is reported by either sexual orientation or sexual behavior. Some data suggests that men who have sex with men are disproportionately affected by some STDs. For example, the CDC says that, MSM have accounted for an increasing number of estimated syphilis cases in the United States. Specifically, in 2006 64% of primary and secondary syphilis cases were among MSM.

Are LGBTQ youth disproportionately affected by mental health issues?

Discrimination and violence put LGBTQ youth in particularly vulnerable positions with respect to mental health and suicide. The most commonly cited research on LGBTQ youth and suicide is a 1989 report from the Secretary's Task Force on Youth Suicide at the United States Department of Health and Human Services which found that lesbian, gay, and bisexual youth were two to three times more likely to attempt suicide than their heterosexual peers.

Newer research shows that LGBT youth are still slightly more likely to report a suicide attempt than heterosexual youth, however, closer analysis revealed that half of the attempts by LGBT youth were suicidal ideation rather than a concrete act to end life. The researcher believes these reported attempts are a way that LGBT youth communicate the hardships of their lives.

More recent research published in the *American Psychologist* also concludes that high rates of "major depression, generalized anxiety disorder and substance use or dependence" persist in lesbian and gay youth.

Are LGBTQ youth disproportionately affected by homelessness?

A 2006 report by the National Gay and Lesbian Taskforce and the National Coalition for the Homeless estimates that between 20–40% of all homeless youth in the United States identify as LGBT. Given that only 3–5% of Americans identify as lesbian, gay, or bisexual, it's clear that homelessness disproportionately affects LGBTQ youth.

These numbers are corroborated by a 2005 study funded by the New York City Council which found that almost one third of New York's homeless youth identify as lesbian, gay, bisexual, or transgender.

The primary cause of homelessness for all youth is family conflict, and research suggests that family conflict over a young person's sexual orientation or gender identity can often lead to homelessness.

Is their an increase of public acceptance of LGBTQ individuals?

There is certainly more discussion of sexual orientation in today's popular culture and media than ever before, and surveys suggest that there is a corresponding greater acceptance of homosexuality among the public. A Gallup poll conducted in May of each year asks Americans about their attitudes related to homosexuality. In 2007, 57% of all Americans said they found homosexuality to be an acceptable lifestyle compared with 50% in 1998 and just 34% in 1982.

The survey also shows that acceptance of LGBTQ individuals is even higher among younger generations; 75% of Americans ages 18–34 found homosexuality acceptable.

Do schools teach about sexual orientation?

The content of health and sexuality education varies depending on the community and research on what topics each community teaches is quite limited.

A recent study of health education programs conducted by the CDC's Division of Adolescent and School Health, however, provides some insight into what is being taught in America's classroom. The study found that 48% of schools taught about sexual identity and sexual orientation. In comparison 86% of all high schools that taught about abstinence as the most effective way to avoid pregnancy and STDs, 69% taught about marriage and commitment, 65% taught about condom efficacy, and 39% taught students how to correctly use a condom.

Every 2 years the Gay, Lesbian, and Straight Education Network (GLSEN) surveys LGBT high school students across the country on their experiences. The 2005 National School Climate Survey asked students some questions about sexuality education curricula and found that "nearly half (44.6%) of the students surveyed reported that their school followed an abstinence-only health curriculum, and these students were more likely to have experienced verbal harassment on the basis of sexual orientation, and were more likely to have missed school in the past year because they felt unsafe." These students also reported having fewer supportive faculty/school staff at their school.

Are schools safe places for LGBTQ youth?

GLSEN's 2005 National School Climate Survey concluded that in certain schools and certain states with supportive laws, the experiences of LGBT youth in schools are improving, but overall there has been a lack of consistent progress. Most students still hear homophobic remarks and report feeling unsafe at some point, and many are still victims of physical harassment and assault. In particular the survey found [the following]:

- 75.4% of LGBT high school students reported hearing remarks such as "faggot" or "dyke" frequently or often at school.

- 89.2% of LGBT high school students reported hearing "that's so gay" or "you're so gay" (often used to indicate that someone or something is stupid or worthless) frequently or often at school.

- 18.6% of LGBT high school students reported hearing homophobic remarks from their teachers or other school staff.

- 74.2% of LGBT high school students in the survey reported feeling unsafe in school because of personal characteristics, such as their sexual orientation, gender, or religion, 64.3% reported feeling unsafe at school because of their sexual orientation specifically, and 40.7% felt unsafe because of how they expressed their gender.

- 64.1% of LGBT high school students reported that they had been verbally harassed at least some of the time in school in the past year because of their sexual orientation and 45.5% because of their gender expression.

- 37.8% of LGBT high school students had experienced physical harassment at school on the basis of sexual orientation and 26.1% on the basis of their gender expression.

- 17.6% of LGBT high school students had been physically assaulted because of their sexual orientation and 11.8% because of their gender expression.

The good news is, there are a growing number of resources and support for LGBTQ youth. The first Gay-Straight Alliance (GSA)—school clubs that promote tolerance and respect for everyone regardless of sexual orientation or gender identity—formed in 1988. GLSEN, the Gay, Lesbian, and Straight Education Network, reports that there are now over 3,000 of the student clubs registered with their organization.

Are LGBT people coming out at younger ages?

There is not a lot of research on when or why young people choose to publicly identify as gay, lesbian, or bisexual. Research by Cornell University professor Ritch Savin-Williams, however, suggests that the average LGBT youth now comes out at 16 compared to 21 in the 1970s.

Part Four

Common Health Concerns of Teens and Their Parents

Chapter 31

Dealing with a Health Problem

Living with a long-lasting health condition (also called a chronic illness) presents a person with new challenges. Learning how to meet those challenges is a process—it doesn't happen right away. But understanding more about your condition, and doing your part to manage it, can help you take health challenges in stride. Many people find that taking an active part in the care of a chronic health condition can help them feel stronger and better equipped to deal with lots of life's trials and tribulations.

What Are Chronic Illnesses?

There are two types of illnesses: acute and chronic. Acute illnesses (like a cold or the flu) are usually over relatively quickly. Chronic illnesses, though, are long-lasting health conditions (the word "chronic" comes from the Greek word chronos, meaning time).

Having a chronic condition doesn't necessarily mean an illness is critical or dangerous—although some chronic illnesses, such as cancer and AIDS [acquired immunodeficiency syndrome], can be life threatening. But chronic illnesses can also include conditions like asthma, arthritis, and diabetes. Although the symptoms of a chronic illness might go away with medical care, usually a person still has the underlying

"Dealing with a Health Condition," January 2007, reprinted with permission from www.kidshealth.org. Copyright © 2007 The Nemours Foundation. This information was provided by KidsHealth, one of the largest resources online for medically reviewed health information written for parents, kids, and teens. For more articles like this one, visit www.KidsHealth.org, or www.TeensHealth.org.

condition—even though when properly treated he or she may feel completely healthy and well much of the time.

Each health condition has its own symptoms, treatment, and course. Aside from the fact that they are all relatively long lasting, chronic illnesses aren't necessarily alike in other ways. Most people who have a chronic illness don't think of themselves as "having a chronic illness." They think of themselves as having a specific condition—such as asthma, or arthritis, or diabetes, or lupus, or sickle cell anemia, or hemophilia, or leukemia, or whatever ongoing health condition they have.

If you're living with a chronic illness, you may feel affected not just physically, but also emotionally, socially, and sometimes even financially. The way a person might be affected by a chronic illness depends on the particular illness and how it affects the body, how severe it is, and the kinds of treatments that might be involved. It takes time to adjust to and accept the realities of a long-term illness, but teens who are willing to learn, seek support from others, and participate actively in the care of their bodies usually get through the coping process.

The Coping Process

Most people go through stages in learning to cope with a chronic illness. A person who has just been diagnosed with a particular health condition may feel a lot of things. Some people feel vulnerable, confused, and worried about their health and the future. Others feel sad or disappointed in their bodies. For some, the situation seems unfair, causing them to feel angry at themselves and the people they love. These feelings are the start of the coping process. Everyone's reaction is different, but they're all completely normal.

The next stage in the coping process is learning. Most people living with a long-term illness find that knowledge is power: The more they find out about their condition, the more they feel in control and the less frightening it is.

The third stage in coping with a chronic illness is all about taking it in stride. At this stage, people feel comfortable with their treatments and with the tools (like inhalers or shots) they need to use to live a normal life.

So someone with diabetes, for example, may feel a range of emotions when the condition is first diagnosed. The person may believe he or she will never be able to go through the skin prick tests or injections that may be necessary to manage the condition. But after working with doctors and understanding more about the condition, that person will grow to be more practiced at monitoring and managing insulin levels—and it will stop feeling like such a big deal. Over time, managing diabetes will become second nature and the steps involved will seem like just another way to care for one's body, in much the same way that daily teeth brushing or showering help people stay healthy.

There's no definite time limit on the coping process. Everybody's process of coming to terms with and accepting a chronic illness is different. In fact, most people will find that emotions surface at all stages in the process. Even if treatments go well, it's natural to feel sad or worried from time to time. Recognizing and being aware of these emotions as they surface is all part of the coping process.

Tools for Taking Control

People living with chronic illnesses often find that the following actions can help them take control and work through the coping process.

Acknowledge Feelings

Emotions may not be easy to identify. For example, sleeping or crying a lot or grouchiness may be signs of sadness or depression. It's also very common for people with chronic illnesses to feel stress as they balance the realities of dealing with a health condition and coping with schoolwork, social events, and other aspects of everyday life.

Many people living with chronic illnesses find that it helps to line up sources of support to deal with the stress and emotions. Some people choose to talk to a therapist or join a support group specifically for people with their condition. It's also important to confide in those you trust, like close friends and family members.

The most important factor when seeking help isn't necessarily finding someone who knows a lot about your illness, but finding someone who is willing to listen when you're depressed, angry, frustrated—or even just plain old happy. Noticing the emotions you have, accepting them as a natural part of what you're going through, and expressing or sharing your emotions in a way that feels comfortable can help you feel better about things.

Understand Other People's Reactions

You may not be the only one who feels emotional about your illness. Parents often struggle with seeing their children sick because they want to prevent anything bad from happening to their kids. Some parents feel guilty or think they've failed their child, others may get mad about how unfair it seems. Everyone else's emotions can seem like an extra burden on people who are sick, when of course it's not their fault. Sometimes it helps to explain to a parent that, when you express anger or fear, you're simply asking for their support—not for them to cure you. Tell your parents you don't expect them to have all the answers, but that it helps if they just listen to how you feel and let you know they understand.

Because the teen years are all about fitting in, it can be hard to feel different around friends and classmates. Many people with chronic illnesses are tempted to try to keep their condition secret. Sometimes, though, trying to hide a condition can cause its own troubles as Melissa, who has Crohn's disease, discovered. Some of Melissa's medications made her look puffy, and her classmates started teasing her about gaining weight. When Melissa explained her condition, she was surprised at how accepting her classmates were. When talking to friends about your health condition, it can sometimes help to explain that everyone is made differently. For the same reason some people have blue eyes and others brown, some of us are more vulnerable to certain conditions than others.

Depending on the severity of your illness, you may find yourself constantly surrounded by well-meaning adults. Teachers, coaches, and school counselors may all try to help you—perhaps causing you to feel dependent, frustrated, or angry. Talk to these people and explain how you feel. Educating and explaining the facts of your condition can help them understand what you're capable of and allow them to see you as a student or an athlete—not a patient.

Keep Things in Perspective

It's easy for a health condition to become the main focus of someone's life—especially as that person first learns about and starts dealing with the condition. Many people find that reminding themselves that their condition is only a part of who they are can help put things back in perspective. Keeping up with friends, favorite activities, and everyday things helps a lot.

Play an Active Role in Your Health Care

The best way to learn about your condition and put yourself in control is to ask questions. There's usually a lot of information to absorb when visiting a doctor. You may need to go over specifics more than once or ask a doctor or nurse to repeat things to be sure you understand everything. This may sound basic, but lots of people hesitate to say, "Hey, can you say that again?" because they don't want to sound stupid.

But it takes doctors years of medical school and practice to learn the information they're passing on to you in one office visit!

If you've just been diagnosed with a particular condition, you may want to write down some questions to ask your doctor. For example, some of the things you might want to know are:

- How will this condition affect me?

- What kind of treatment is involved?

- Will it be painful?

- How many treatments will I get?

- Will I miss any school?

- Will I be able to play sports, play a musical instrument, try out for the school play, or participate in other activities I love?

- What can I expect—will my condition be cured? Will my symptoms go away?

- What are the side effects of the treatments and how long will they last?

- Will these treatments make me sleepy, grumpy, or weak?

- What happens if I miss a treatment or forget to take my medicine?

- What if the treatments don't work?

Even though your doctor can't exactly predict how you'll respond to treatment because it varies greatly from one person to the next, knowing how some people react may help you prepare yourself mentally, emotionally, and physically. The more you learn about your illness, the more you'll understand about your treatments, your emotions, and the best ways to create a healthy lifestyle based on your individual needs.

Living with a Health Condition

There's no doubt the teen years can be a more challenging time to deal with a health condition. In addition to the social pressures to fit in, it's a time of learning about and understanding our bodies. At a time when it's natural to be concerned with body image, it can seem hard to feel different. It's understandable that people can feel just plain sick and tired of dealing with a chronic illness once in a while.

Even teens who have lived with an illness since childhood can feel the pull of wanting to lead a "normal" life in which they don't need medicine, have any limitations, or have to care for themselves in any special way. This is a perfectly natural reaction. Sometimes teens who have learned to manage their illness feel so healthy and strong that they wonder whether they need to keep following their disease management program. A person with diabetes, for example, may consider skipping a meal when at the mall or checking his or her blood sugar after the game instead of before.

Unfortunately, easing up on taking care of yourself can have disastrous results. The best approach is to tell your doctor how you feel. Talk about what you'd like to be doing and can't. See if there's anything you can work out. This is all part of taking more control and becoming a player in your own medical care.

When you're living with a chronic health condition, it can feel hard at times to love your body. But you don't have to have a perfect body to have a great body image. Body image can improve when you care for your body, appreciate its capabilities, and accept its limitations—a fact that's true for everyone, whether they're living with a chronic condition or not.

Voicing any frustration or sadness to an understanding ear can help when a person feels sick of being sick. At times like this it's important to think of ways others could help and ask for what you'd like. Some people find they can ease their own sense of loss by reaching out and offering to help someone in need. Lending a hand to someone else can help one's own troubles seem easier to manage.

Adjusting to living with a chronic illness takes a little time, patience, support—and willingness to learn and participate. People who deal with unexpected challenges often find an inner resilience they might not have known was there before. Many say that they learn more about themselves through dealing with these challenges and feel they grow to be stronger and more self-aware than they would if they'd never faced their particular challenge. People living with chronic illnesses find that when they take an active role in taking care of their body, they grow to understand and appreciate their strengths—and adapt to their weaknesses—as never before.

Chapter 32

Acne

What is acne?

Acne is a disorder resulting from the action of hormones and other substances on the skin's oil glands (sebaceous glands) and hair follicles. These factors lead to plugged pores and outbreaks of lesions commonly called pimples or zits. Acne lesions usually occur on the face, neck, back, chest, and shoulders. Although acne is usually not a serious health threat, it can be a source of significant emotional distress. Severe acne can lead to permanent scarring.

How does acne develop?

Doctors describe acne as a disease of the pilosebaceous units (PSUs). Found over most of the body, PSUs consist of a sebaceous gland connected to a canal, called a follicle, that contains a fine hair. These units are most numerous on the face, upper back, and chest. The sebaceous glands make an oily substance called sebum that normally empties onto the skin surface through the opening of the follicle, commonly called a pore. Cells called keratinocytes line the follicle.

The hair, sebum, and keratinocytes that fill the narrow follicle may produce a plug, which is an early sign of acne. The plug prevents sebum from reaching the surface of the skin through a pore. The mixture of

Excerpted from text by the National Institute of Arthritis and Musculoskeletal and Skin Diseases (NIAMS, www.niams.nih.gov), part of the National Institutes of Health, January 2006.

oil and cells allows bacteria *Propionibacterium acnes* (*P. acnes*) that normally live on the skin to grow in the plugged follicles. These bacteria produce chemicals and enzymes and attract white blood cells that cause inflammation. (Inflammation is a characteristic reaction of tissues to disease or injury and is marked by four signs: swelling, redness, heat, and pain.) When the wall of the plugged follicle breaks down, it spills everything into the nearby skin—sebum, shed skin cells, and bacteria—leading to lesions or pimples.

People with acne frequently have a variety of lesions. The basic acne lesion, called the comedo, is simply an enlarged and plugged hair follicle. If the plugged follicle, or comedo, stays beneath the skin, it is called a closed comedo and produces a white bump called a whitehead. A comedo that reaches the surface of the skin and opens up is called an open comedo or blackhead because it looks black on the skin's surface. This black discoloration is due to changes in sebum as it is exposed to air. It is not due to dirt. Both whiteheads and blackheads may stay in the skin for a long time.

What causes acne?

The exact cause of acne is unknown, but doctors believe it results from several related factors. One important factor is an increase in hormones called androgens (male sex hormones). These increase in both boys and girls during puberty and cause the sebaceous glands to enlarge and make more sebum. Hormonal changes related to pregnancy or starting or stopping birth control pills can also cause acne.

Another factor is heredity or genetics. Researchers believe that the tendency to develop acne can be inherited from parents. For example, studies have shown that many school-age boys with acne have a family history of the disorder. Certain drugs, including androgens and lithium, are known to cause acne. Greasy cosmetics may alter the cells of the follicles and make them stick together, producing a plug.

Factors that can cause an acne flare include the following:

- Changing hormone levels in adolescent girls and adult women 2 to 7 days before their menstrual period starts

- Oil from skin products (moisturizers or cosmetics) or grease encountered in the work environment (for example, a kitchen with fry vats)

- Pressure from sports helmets or equipment, backpacks, tight collars, or tight sports uniforms

- Environmental irritants, such as pollution and high humidity

- Squeezing or picking at blemishes
- Hard scrubbing of the skin
- Stress

What are some myths about the causes of acne?

There are many myths about what causes acne. Chocolate and greasy foods are often blamed, but there is little evidence that foods have much effect on the development and course of acne in most people. Another common myth is that dirty skin causes acne; however, blackheads and other acne lesions are not caused by dirt. Stress doesn't cause acne, but research suggests that for people who have acne, stress can make it worse.

Who gets acne?

People of all races and ages get acne. It is most common in adolescents and young adults. An estimated 80 percent of all people between the ages of 11 and 30 have acne outbreaks at some point. For most people, acne tends to go away by the time they reach their thirties; however, some people in their forties and fifties continue to have this skin problem.

How is acne treated?

Acne is often treated by dermatologists (doctors who specialize in skin problems). These doctors treat all kinds of acne, particularly severe cases. Doctors who are general or family practitioners, pediatricians, or internists may treat patients with milder cases of acne.

The goals of treatment are to heal existing lesions, stop new lesions from forming, prevent scarring, and minimize the psychological stress and embarrassment caused by this disease. Drug treatment is aimed at reducing several problems that play a part in causing acne:

- Abnormal clumping of cells in the follicles
- Increased oil production
- Bacteria
- Inflammation

Depending on the extent of the problem, the doctor may recommend one of several over-the-counter (OTC) medicines and/or prescription medicines. Some of these medicines may be topical (applied to the skin), and others may be oral (taken by mouth). The doctor may suggest using more than one topical medicine or combining oral and topical medicines.

How should people with acne care for their skin?

Clean skin gently. If you have acne, you should gently wash your face with a mild cleanser, once in the morning and once in the evening, as well as after heavy exercise. Wash your face from under the jaw to the hairline and be sure to thoroughly rinse your skin. Ask your doctor or another health professional for advice on the best type of cleanser to use. Using strong soaps or rough scrub pads is not helpful and can actually make the problem worse. Astringents are not recommended unless the skin is very oily, and then they should be used only on oily spots. It is also important to shampoo your hair regularly. If you have oily hair, you may want to wash it every day.

Avoid frequent handling of the skin. Avoid rubbing and touching skin lesions. Squeezing, pinching, or picking blemishes can lead to the development of scars or dark blotches.

Shave carefully. Men who shave and who have acne should test both electric and safety razors to see which is more comfortable. When using a safety razor, make sure the blade is sharp and soften your beard thoroughly with soap and water before applying shaving cream. Shave gently and only when necessary to reduce the risk of nicking blemishes.

Avoid a sunburn or suntan. Many of the medicines used to treat acne can make you more prone to sunburn. A sunburn that reddens the skin or suntan that darkens the skin may make blemishes less visible and make the skin feel drier. However, these benefits are only temporary, and there are known risks of excessive sun exposure, such as more rapid skin aging and a risk of developing skin cancer.

Choose cosmetics carefully. While undergoing acne treatment, you may need to change some of the cosmetics you use. All cosmetics, such as foundation, blush, eye shadow, moisturizers, and hair-care products should be oil free. Choose products labeled noncomedogenic (meaning they don't promote the formation of closed pores). In some people, however, even these products may make acne worse. For the first few weeks of treatment, applying foundation evenly may be difficult because the skin may be red or scaly, particularly with the use of topical tretinoin or benzoyl peroxide.

Chapter 33

Allergies in Adolescents

Your eyes itch, your nose is running, you're sneezing, and you're covered in hives. It's allergy season again, and all you want to do is curl up into a ball of misery.

There has to be something you can do to feel better. After all, doctors seem to have a cure for everything, right? Not for allergies. But there are ways to relieve allergy symptoms or avoid getting the symptoms, even though you can't actually get rid of the allergies themselves.

What Are Allergies?

Allergies are abnormal immune system reactions to things that are typically harmless to most people. When you're allergic to something, your immune system mistakenly believes that this substance is harmful to your body. (Substances that cause allergic reactions, such as certain foods, dust, plant pollen, or medicines, are known as allergens.)

In an attempt to protect the body, the immune system produces IgE [immunoglobulin E] antibodies to that allergen. Those antibodies then cause certain cells in the body to release chemicals into the bloodstream, one of which is histamine (pronounced: his-tuh-meen).

The histamine then acts on the eyes, nose, throat, lungs, skin, or gastrointestinal tract and causes the symptoms of the allergic reaction. Future exposure to that same allergen will trigger this antibody response again. This means that every time you come into contact with that allergen, you'll have an allergic reaction.

Allergic reactions can be mild, like a runny nose, or they can be severe, like difficulty breathing. An asthma attack, for example, is often an allergic reaction to something that is breathed into the lungs by a person who is susceptible.

Some types of allergies produce multiple symptoms, and in rare cases, an allergic reaction can become very severe—this severe reaction is called anaphylaxis (pronounced: an-uh-fuh-lak-sis). Signs of anaphylaxis include difficulty breathing, difficulty swallowing, swelling of the lips, tongue, and throat or other parts of the body, and dizziness or loss of consciousness.

Anaphylaxis usually occurs minutes after exposure to a triggering substance, such as a peanut, but some reactions might be delayed by as long as 4 hours. Luckily, anaphylactic reactions don't occur often and can be treated successfully if proper medical procedures are followed.

Why Do People Get Allergies?

The tendency to develop allergies is often hereditary, which means it can be passed down through your genes. (Thanks a lot, Mom and Dad!) However, just because a parent or sibling has allergies doesn't mean you will definitely get them, too. A person usually doesn't inherit a particular allergy, just the likelihood of having allergies.

What Things Are People Are Allergic to?

Some of the most common allergens are:

Foods: Food allergies are most common in infants and often go away as people get older. Although some food allergies can be serious, many simply cause annoying symptoms like an itchy rash, a stuffy nose, and diarrhea. The foods that people are most commonly allergic to are milk and other dairy products, eggs, wheat, soy, peanuts and tree nuts, and seafood.

Insect bites and stings: The venom (poison) in insect bites and stings can cause allergic reactions, and can be severe and even cause an anaphylactic reaction in some people.

Airborne particles: Often called environmental allergens, these are the most common allergens. Examples of airborne particles that can cause allergies are dust mites (tiny bugs that live in house dust); mold spores; animal dander (flakes of scaly, dried skin, and dried saliva from your pets); and pollen from grass, ragweed, and trees.

Medicines: Antibiotics—medications used to treat infections—are the most common type of medicines that cause allergic reactions. Many other medicines, including over-the-counter medications (those you can buy without a prescription), also can cause allergic-type reactions.

Chemicals: Some cosmetics or laundry detergents can make people break out in an itchy rash (hives). Usually, this is because someone has a reaction to the chemicals in these products. Dyes, household cleaners, and pesticides used on lawns or plants also can cause allergic reactions in some people.

How Do Doctors Diagnose and Treat Allergies?

If your family doctor suspects you might have an allergy, he or she might refer you to an allergist (a doctor who specializes in allergy treatment) for further testing. The allergist will ask you about your own allergy symptoms (such as how often they occur and when) and about whether any family members have allergies. The allergist also will perform tests to confirm an allergy—these will depend on the type of allergy someone has and may include a skin test or blood test.

The most complete way to avoid allergic reactions is to stay away from the substances that cause them (called avoidance). Doctors can also treat some allergies using medications and allergy shots.

Avoidance

In some cases, like food allergies, avoiding the allergen is a life-saving necessity. That's because, unlike allergies to airborne particles that can be treated with shots or medications, the only way to treat food allergies is to avoid the allergen entirely. For example, people who are allergic to peanuts should avoid not only peanuts, but also any food that might contain even tiny traces of them.

Avoidance can help protect people against non-food or chemical allergens, too. In fact, for some people, eliminating exposure to an allergen is enough to prevent allergy symptoms and they don't need to take medicines or go through other allergy treatments.

Here are some things that can help you avoid airborne allergens:

- Keep family pets out of certain rooms, like your bedroom, and bathe them if necessary.

- Remove carpets or rugs from your room (hard floor surfaces don't collect dust as much as carpets do).

- Don't hang heavy drapes and get rid of other items that allow dust to accumulate.

- Clean frequently (if your allergy is severe, you may be able to get someone else to do your dirty work!)

- Use special covers to seal pillows and mattresses if you're allergic to dust mites.

- If you're allergic to pollen, keep windows closed when pollen season's at its peak, change your clothing after being outdoors—and don't mow lawns.

- If you're allergic to mold, avoid damp areas, such as basements, and keep bathrooms and other mold-prone areas clean and dry.

Medications

Medications such as pills or nasal sprays are often used to treat allergies. Although medications can control the allergy symptoms (such as sneezing, headaches, or a stuffy nose), they are not a cure and can't make the tendency to have allergic reactions go away. Many effective medications are available to treat common allergies, and your doctor can help you to identify those that work for you.

Another type of medication that some severely allergic people will need to have on hand is a shot of epinephrine (pronounced: eh-puh-neh-frin), a fast-acting medicine that can help offset an anaphylactic reaction. This medicine comes in an easy-to-carry container that looks like a pen. Epinephrine is available by prescription only. If you have a severe allergy and your doctor thinks you should carry it, he or she will give you instructions on how to use it.

Shots

Allergy shots are also referred to as allergen immunotherapy. By receiving injections of small amounts of an allergen, your body can gradually develop antibodies and undergo other immune system changes that help reduce the reaction to that allergen.

Immunotherapy is only recommended for specific allergies, such as allergies to things you might breathe in (like pollen, pet dander, or dust mites) or insect allergies. Immunotherapy doesn't help with some allergies, like food allergies.

Although many people find the thought of allergy shots unsettling, shots can be highly effective—and it doesn't take long to get used to them. Often, the longer someone receives allergy shots, the more they help the body build up antibodies that fight the allergies. Although the shots don't cure allergies, they do tend to raise a person's tolerance when exposed to the allergen, which means fewer or less severe symptoms.

If you're severely allergic to bites and stings, talk to a doctor about getting venom immunotherapy (shots) from an allergist.

Is It a Cold or Allergies?

If the spring and summer seasons leave you sneezing and wheezing, you might have allergies. Colds, on the other hand, are more likely to occur at any time (though they're more common in the colder months).

Colds and allergies produce similar symptoms, but colds usually last only a week or so. And although both may cause your nose and eyes to itch, colds and other viral infections can also cause a fever, aches and pains, and colored mucus. Cold symptoms often worsen as the days go on and then gradually improve, but allergies begin immediately after exposure to the offending allergen and last as long as that exposure continues.

If you're not sure whether your symptoms are caused by allergies or a cold, talk with your doctor.

Dealing with Allergies

So once you know you have allergies, how do you deal with them? First and foremost, try to avoid things you're allergic to!

If you have a food allergy, that means avoiding foods that trigger symptoms and learning how to read food labels to make sure you're not consuming even tiny amounts of allergens. People with environmental allergies should keep their house clean of dust and pet dander and watch the weather for days when pollen is high. Switching to perfume-free and dye-free detergents, cosmetics, and beauty products (you may see non-allergenic ingredients listed as hypoallergenic on product labels) also can help.

If you're taking medication, follow the directions carefully and make sure your regular doctor is aware of anything an allergist gives you (like shots or prescriptions). If you have a severe allergy, consider wearing a medical emergency ID (such as a MedicAlert bracelet), which will explain your allergy and who to contact in case of an emergency.

If you've been diagnosed with allergies, you have a lot of company. The National Institutes of Health (NIH) report that more than 50 million Americans are affected by allergic diseases. The good news is that doctors and scientists are working to better understand allergies, to improve treatment methods, and to possibly prevent allergies altogether.

Chapter 34

Asthma and Teens

Learning about Asthma

Learn about asthma and the early warning signs before asthma gets out of control. Work with your teen's doctor. Come up with an asthma action plan that works for your child.

What is asthma?

Asthma is a disease that causes the airways of the lungs to tighten and swell. It is common among children and teens.

What is an asthma attack?

An asthma attack happens when your child has asthma and their lungs aren't getting enough air to breathe. Your child may cough or wheeze during an attack.

What causes an asthma attack?

Things that cause asthma attacks are called triggers. Triggers are everywhere. Your child's home or school can be full of triggers such as pests and mold.

Excerpted from "Help Your Child Gain Control Over Asthma," by the U.S. Environmental Protection Agency (EPA, www.epa.gov), November 2004. Reviewed by David A. Cooke, MD, FACP, April 4, 2010.

Be Aware of Your Teen's Warning Signs

Often your child may show warning signs. Warning signs are clues that your child's asthma may be getting worse.

How will I know if asthma is getting worse?

Learn your child's warning signs and catch an attack before it gets worse. While warning signs differ from child to child, parents report some common signs.

Asthma Warning Signs Checklist

Warning signs you noticed may include the following:

- Coughed at night
- Had a cold or the flu
- Had a fever
- Had a stuffy or runny nose
- Had a tickle in the throat
- Sneezed and had watery eyes

Your teen may have looked or seemed to be the following:

- Acted very restless
- Face was pale
- Had dark circles under the eyes
- Had tightness in the chest
- Seemed to feel weak or tired
- Seemed to have a headache

Emergency Warning Signs

There are times when you need to take your child to the hospital or urgent care right away. Ask your child's doctor what emergency signs to look for to help you know when your child is having a medical emergency with asthma.

Some parents know their child is having a medical emergency with asthma if he or she is experiencing the following:

- Is breathing in a different way: faster, or slower, or more shallow than usual

- Is coughing or wheezing and can't stop
- Has bluish fingernails or lips

Make an Asthma Action Plan

The action plan looks at what triggers or brings on your child's asthma. The plan also includes your child's daily medicine needs. And the plan lists rescue medicines for quick relief during an attack or when asthma signs start.

Work with your child's doctor and come up with a written action plan for managing your child's asthma. Share the asthma action plan with your child's school, teachers, and family members. Talk it over with people in your child's life. In case of an asthma attack they will know what to do.

While asthma action plans may differ from doctor to doctor, most plans will address two areas: a daily program and a rescue program.

Follow the action plan. It can help lower the number of asthma attacks. Talk to your child's doctor if you need to make changes in the plan.

The action plan's daily program may list the following:

- Your child's asthma triggers
- Daily medicines and how to use them
- Peak flow meter chart

The action plan's rescue program may list:

- Your child's warning signs
- Your child's peak flow meter readings
- Names of the rescue medicines used to treat asthma as an asthma attack gets worse
- Steps to take if your child has an asthma attack and when to call the doctor
- Emergency numbers and when to take your child to the emergency room

Remember parents—make sure you know the right amount of medicine your child needs to take each day. Talk to your child's doctor if you have questions.

Does your child use an inhaler, a spacer, or a peak flow meter? Ask the doctor to show you how to use these at home. Have your child practice a few times in front of the doctor.

Learn What May Trigger Your Child's Asthma

Triggers are the things that can start your child's asthma attack or make it worse. Your child may have just one trigger or you may find that several things act as triggers.

- For some teens, being around pets or dust can trigger asthma.

- Some teens find their asthma gets worse from cigarette smoke.

- For other teens, running or spending time outdoors may bring on an asthma attack.

Be sure to work with the doctor to identify your child's asthma triggers. Once you know what triggers your child's asthma, it is important to take steps to control these triggers.

Remembering to smoke outside or keeping pests out of your home means taking action every day. The more these habits are part of your daily life, the less chance there is your child will have an asthma attack.

Chapter 35

Cancer in Childhood and Adolescence

Cancer in Children

Although cancer is a leading cause of death among children in the United States, childhood cancer deaths are declining.

In the United States, cancer is the second most common cause of death among children between the ages of 1 and 14 years, surpassed only by accidents. More than 16 out of every 100,000 children and teens in the United States were diagnosed with cancer, and nearly three of every 100,000 died from the disease. The most common cancers in children were leukemia (cancer of the bone marrow and blood) and brain and central nervous system cancers.

How many children and teens develop leukemia?

In 2005, 4.1 of every 100,000 young people under 20 years of age in the United States were diagnosed with leukemia, and 0.8 per 100,000 died from it. The number of new cases was highest among the 1–4 age group, but the number of deaths was highest among the 10–14 age group.

This chapter includes text excerpted from "Cancer in Children," by the Centers for Disease Control and Prevention (CDC, www.cdc.gov), July 30, 2009; from "Care for Children and Adolescents with Cancer," by the National Cancer Institute (NCI, www.cancer.gov), part of the National Institutes of Health, May 29, 2008; and from "Childhood Cancers: Questions and Answers," also by the NCI, January 10, 2008.

How many children and teens develop brain and central nervous system cancers?

In 2005, 2.9 of every 100,000 people 0–19 years of age were found to have cancer of the brain or central nervous system, and 0.7 per 100,000 died from it.

These cancers were found most often in children between 1 and 4 years of age, but the most deaths occurred among those aged 5–9.

Are childhood cancer deaths declining?

During the past 25 years, there have been significant improvements in the 5-year relative survival rate for all of the major childhood cancers. The 5-year relative survival rate among children for all cancer sites combined improved from 58% for patients diagnosed in 1975–1977 to 80% for those diagnosed in 1996–2004.

A CDC study found that from 1990 to 2004, childhood leukemia death rates fell by 3.0% per year, childhood brain and other nervous system cancers by 1.0% per year, and all other childhood cancers combined by 1.3% per year, likely reflecting better treatment of childhood cancers.

Care for Children and Adolescents with Cancer

Survival rates for childhood cancer have risen sharply over the past 25 years. In the United States, more than 80 percent of children with cancer are alive 5 years after diagnosis, compared with about 62 percent in the mid-1970s. Much of this dramatic improvement is due to the development of improved therapies at children's cancer centers, where the majority of children with cancer have their treatment.

Why might a family look for a specialized children's cancer center when a child or adolescent is diagnosed with cancer?

Because childhood cancer is relatively rare, it is important to seek treatment in centers that specialize in the treatment of children with cancer. Specialized cancer programs at comprehensive, multidisciplinary cancer centers follow established protocols (step-by-step guidelines for treatment). These protocols are carried out using a team approach. The team of health professionals is involved in designing the appropriate treatment and support program for the child and the child's family. In addition, these centers participate in specially designed and monitored research studies that help develop more effective treatments and address issues of long-term childhood cancer survival.

When children go to a specialized cancer center, does it mean their treatment will be part of a research study?

Not necessarily. Participation in research studies is always voluntary. Parents and patients may choose to receive treatment as part of a clinical trial (research study); only patients and parents who wish to do so take part. However, a large number of children who go to pediatric cancer centers take part in clinical trials. About 55 to 65 percent of children diagnosed with cancer by or before age 14 enter an NCI-sponsored clinical trial. However, this percentage decreases to about 10 percent for children diagnosed between ages 15 and 19.

How does a family find a children's cancer center?

A child's pediatrician or family doctor often can provide a referral to a children's cancer center. Families and health professionals can also call the NCI's Cancer Information Service (CIS) at 800-4-CANCER to learn about children's cancer centers that belong to the Children's Oncology Group (COG). All of the cancer centers that participate in these groups have met strict standards of excellence for childhood cancer care. A directory of COG institutions by state is also available at http://www.curesearch.org/resources/cog.aspx on the internet.

Childhood Cancers: Questions and Answers

What are the most common types of childhood cancer?

Among the 12 major types of childhood cancers, leukemias (blood cell cancers) and cancers of the brain and central nervous system account for more than half of the new cases. About one third of childhood cancers are leukemias. The most common type of leukemia in children is acute lymphoblastic leukemia. The most common solid tumors are brain tumors (e.g., gliomas and medulloblastomas), with other solid tumors (e.g., neuroblastomas, Wilms tumors, and sarcomas such as rhabdomyosarcoma and osteosarcoma) being less common.

How many children are diagnosed with cancer in the United States annually?

In the United States in 2007, approximately 10,400 children under age 15 were diagnosed with cancer and about 1,545 children will die from the disease. Although this makes cancer the leading cause of death by disease among U.S. children 1 to 14 years of age, cancer is still relatively rare in this age group. On average, one to two children develop the disease each year for every 10,000 children in the United States.

What are the known or suspected causes of childhood cancer?

The causes of childhood cancers are largely unknown. A few conditions, such as Down syndrome, other specific chromosomal and genetic abnormalities, and ionizing radiation exposures, explain a small percentage of cases.

Environmental causes of childhood cancer have long been suspected by many scientists but have been difficult to pin down, partly because cancer in children is rare and because it is difficult to identify past exposure levels in children, particularly during potentially important periods such as pregnancy or even prior to conception. In addition, each of the distinctive types of childhood cancers develops differently—with a potentially wide variety of causes and a unique clinical course in terms of age, race, gender, and many other factors.

A number of studies are examining suspected or possible risk factors for childhood cancers, including early-life exposures to infectious agents; parental, fetal, or childhood exposures to environmental toxins such as pesticides, solvents, or other household chemicals; parental occupational exposures to radiation or chemicals; parental medical conditions during pregnancy or before conception; maternal diet during pregnancy; early postnatal feeding patterns and diet; and maternal reproductive history.

Researchers are also studying the risks associated with maternal exposures to oral contraceptives, fertility drugs, and other medications; familial and genetic susceptibility; and risk associated with exposure to the human immunodeficiency virus (HIV).

What have studies shown about the possible causes of childhood cancer?

For several decades, the NCI, a part of the National Institutes of Health (NIH), has supported national and international collaborations devoted to studying the causes of cancer in children. Key findings from this research include the following:

- High levels of ionizing radiation from accidents or from radiotherapy have been linked with increased risk of some childhood cancers.

- Children with cancer treated with chemotherapy and/or radiation therapy may be at increased risk for developing a second primary cancer. For example, certain types of chemotherapy, including alkylating agents or topoisomerase II inhibitors (e.g., epipodophyllotoxins), can cause an increased risk of leukemia.

- Recent research has shown that children with AIDS (acquired immunodeficiency syndrome), like adults with AIDS, have an increased risk of developing certain cancers, predominantly non-Hodgkin lymphoma and Kaposi sarcoma. These children also have an additional risk of developing leiomyosarcoma (a type of muscle cancer).

- Certain genetic syndromes (e.g., Li-Fraumeni syndrome, neuro-fibromatosis, and Gorlin syndrome) have been linked to an increased risk of specific childhood cancers.

- Children with Down syndrome have an increased risk of developing leukemia.

- Low levels of radiation exposure from indoor radon have not been significantly associated with childhood leukemias.

- Ultrasound use during pregnancy has not been linked with childhood cancer in numerous large studies.

- Residential magnetic field exposure from power lines has not been significantly associated with childhood leukemias.

- Pesticides have been suspected to be involved in the development of certain forms of childhood cancer based on interview data. However, interview results have been inconsistent and have not yet been validated by physical evidence of pesticides in the child's body or environment.

- No consistent findings have been observed linking specific occupational exposures of parents to the development of childhood cancers.

- Several studies have found no link between maternal cigarette smoking before pregnancy and childhood cancers, but increased risks have been related to the father's smoking habits in studies in the United Kingdom and China.

- Little evidence has been found to link specific viruses or other infectious agents to the development of most types of childhood cancers, though investigators worldwide are exploring the role of exposures of very young children to some common infectious agents that may protect children from, or put them at risk for, developing certain leukemias.

Chapter 36

Diabetes in Children and Teens

Type 1 diabetes in U.S. children and adolescents may be increasing and many more new cases of type 2 diabetes are being reported in young people.

Diabetes mellitus is a group of diseases characterized by high levels of glucose in the blood resulting from defects in insulin production, insulin action, or both. Diabetes can be associated with serious complications and premature death, but people with diabetes can take steps to control the disease and lower the risk of complications.

Type 1 Diabetes

Type 1 diabetes is an autoimmune disease in which the immune system destroys the insulin-producing beta cells of the pancreas that help regulate blood glucose levels. Type 1 diabetes mostly has an acute onset, with children and adolescents usually able to pinpoint when symptoms began. Onset can occur at any age, but it most often occurs in children and young adults.

Since the pancreas can no longer produce insulin, people with type 1 diabetes are required to take insulin daily, either by injection or via an insulin pump. Other methods to deliver insulin are being investigated. Children with type 1 diabetes are at risk for long-term complications (damage to the cardiovascular system, kidneys, eyes, nerves, blood vessels, skin, gums, and teeth).

Excerpted from "Overview of Diabetes in Children and Adolescents," by the National Diabetes Education Program (NDEP, www.ndep.nih.gov), part of the National Institutes of Health, August 2008.

Type 1 diabetes accounts for 5 to 10 percent of all diagnosed cases of diabetes, but is the leading cause of diabetes in children of all ages, and in those less than 10 years of age, type 1 accounts for almost all diabetes. A diabetes management plan for young people includes insulin therapy, self-monitoring of blood glucose, healthy eating, and physical activity. The plan is designed to ensure proper growth and prevention of hypoglycemia. New management strategies are helping children with type 1 diabetes live long and healthy lives.

Symptoms: The immunologic process that leads to type 1 diabetes can begin years before the symptoms of type 1 diabetes develop. Symptoms become apparent when most of the beta-cell population is destroyed and develop over a short period of time. Early symptoms, which are mainly due to hyperglycemia, include increased thirst and urination, constant hunger, weight loss, and blurred vision. Children also may feel very tired.

As insulin deficiency worsens, ketoacids (formed from the breakdown of fat) build up in the blood and are excreted in the urine and breath. They cause the feeling of shortness of breath and abdominal pain, vomiting, and worsening dehydration. Elevation of blood glucose, acidosis, and dehydration comprise the condition known as diabetic ketoacidosis or DKA. If diabetes is not diagnosed and treated with insulin at this point, the individual can lapse into a life-threatening diabetic coma. Often, children with vomiting are mistakenly diagnosed as having gastroenteritis. New-onset diabetes can be differentiated from a GI infection by the frequent urination that accompanies continued vomiting, as opposed to decreased urination due to dehydration if the vomiting is caused by a GI bug.

Risk Factors: A combination of genetic and environmental factors put people at increased risk for type 1 diabetes. Researchers are working to identify these factors so that targeted treatments can be designed to stop the autoimmune process that destroys the pancreatic beta cells.

Comorbidities: Autoimmune diseases such as celiac disease and autoimmune thyroiditis are associated with type 1 diabetes.

Type 2 Diabetes

The first stage in the development of type 2 diabetes is often insulin resistance, requiring increasing amounts of insulin to be produced by the pancreas to control blood glucose levels. Initially, the pancreas responds by producing more insulin, but after several years, insulin production may decrease and diabetes develops. Type 2 diabetes used to occur mainly in adults who were overweight and older than 40 years. Now, as more children and adolescents in the United States become overweight, obese, and inactive, type 2 diabetes is occurring more often in young people. Type 2 diabetes is more common in certain racial and ethnic groups such as African Americans, American Indians, Hispanic/ Latino Americans, and some Asian and Pacific Islander Americans. The increased incidence of type 2 diabetes in youth is a "first consequence" of the obesity epidemic among young people, and is a significant and growing public health problem. Overweight and obese children are at increased risk for developing type 2 diabetes during childhood, adolescence, and later in life.

Symptoms: Type 2 diabetes usually develops slowly and insidiously in children. Symptoms may be similar to those of type 1 diabetes. A child or teen can feel very tired, thirsty, or nauseated and have to urinate often. Other symptoms may include weight loss, blurred vision, frequent infections, and slow healing of wounds or sores. Some children or adolescents with type 2 diabetes may show no symptoms at all when they are diagnosed, and others may present with vaginal yeast infection or burning on urination due to yeast infection. Some children may have extreme elevation of the blood glucose level associated with severe dehydration and coma. Therefore, it is important for health care providers to identify and test children or teens who are at high risk for the disease.

Signs of Diabetes: Physical signs of insulin resistance include acanthosis nigricans, where the skin around the neck or in the armpits appears dark and thick, and feels velvety. High blood pressure and dyslipidemia also are associated with insulin resistance. Girls can have polycystic ovary syndrome with infrequent or absent periods and excess hair and acne.

Risk Factors: Being overweight, having a family member who has type 2 diabetes, being a member of a high risk racial or ethnic group, having signs of insulin resistance, being older than 10 years of age, and experiencing puberty are risk factors for the disease.

Comorbidities: Children with type 2 diabetes also are at risk for the long-term complications of diabetes and the comorbidities associated with insulin resistance (lipid abnormalities and hypertension).

Timely diagnosis and treatment of type 2 diabetes can prevent or delay the onset of diabetes complications. The cornerstone of diabetes management for children with type 2 diabetes is healthy eating, with portion control, and increased physical activity. To control their diabetes, children with type 2 diabetes also may need to take glucose-lowering medications. However, few of the available medications have been approved for use in children and youth.

Hybrid or Mixed Diabetes

While for the most part it is easy to determine if a child or teenager has type 1 or type 2 diabetes, some teens have elements of both kinds of diabetes. This phenomenon may be called hybrid or mixed diabetes. It is not surprising that some youth have elements of both type 1 and type 2 diabetes, given the fact that more children are becoming overweight and obese. Youth with hybrid diabetes are likely to have both insulin resistance that is associated with obesity and type 2 diabetes, and antibodies against the pancreatic islet cells that are associated with autoimmunity and type 1 diabetes.

Signs and symptoms: The signs and symptoms are the same as those for type 1 and type 2 diabetes.

Management: At the time of diagnosis, the clinician should attempt to determine which type of diabetes is present. Measuring antibodies against islet cells and assessing insulin production by measuring C-peptide levels help make the distinction. C-peptide levels are best determined about a year after diagnosis. The presence of hybrid diabetes may affect how the child or teen is treated. Insulin injections are likely to be needed (as for type 1), and oral diabetes medications may be used to improve insulin resistance (as for type 2). It is important to counsel the child or teen about healthy eating habits and the need for daily physical activity so he or she can reach a healthy weight. Weight loss and physical activity independently increase the body's sensitivity to insulin.

Statistics

Diabetes is one of the most common diseases in school-aged children. According to the National Diabetes Fact Sheet, about 186,300 young people in the United States under age 20 had diabetes in 2007. This represents 0.2% of all people in this age group.

Based on data from 2002–2003, the SEARCH for Diabetes in Youth study reported that approximately 15,000 United States youth under 20 years of age are diagnosed annually with type 1 diabetes, while 3,700 are newly diagnosed with type 2 diabetes. Type 2 diabetes is rare in children younger than 10 years of age, regardless of race or ethnicity. After 10 years of age, type 2 diabetes becomes increasingly common, especially in minority populations, representing 14.9% of newly diagnosed cases of diabetes in non-Hispanic whites, 46.1% in Hispanic youth, 57.8% in African Americans, 69.7 % in Asian/Pacific Islanders, and 86.2% in American Indian youth.

Results from the 2005–2006 National Health and Nutrition Examination Survey (NHANES), using measured heights and weights, indicate that an estimated 16–17 percent of children and adolescents ages 2–19 years had a BMI [body mass index] greater than or equal to 95th percentile of the age- and sex-specific BMI—about double the number of two decades ago. Overweight in youth contributes to the increasing numbers of young people who have type 2 diabetes.

Treatment Strategies

The basic elements of type 1 diabetes management are insulin administration, nutrition management, physical activity, blood glucose testing, and the avoidance of hypoglycemia. Algorithms are used for insulin dosing based on blood glucose level and food intake.

Children receiving fixed insulin doses of intermediate- and rapid-acting insulins must have food given at the time of peak action of the insulin. Children receiving a long-acting insulin analogue or using an insulin pump receive a rapid-acting insulin analogue just before meals, with the amount of pre-meal insulin based on carbohydrate content of the meal using an insulin:carbohydrate ratio and a correction scale for hyperglycemia. Further adjustment of insulin or food intake may be made based on anticipation of special circumstances such as increased exercise and intercurrent illness. Children on these regimens are expected to check their blood glucose levels routinely before meals and at bedtime.

Management of type 2 diabetes involves nutrition management, increased physical activity, and blood glucose testing. If this is not sufficient to normalize blood glucose levels, glucose-lowering medication and/or insulin therapy are used as well. There are a variety of different diabetes medications, some that are taken orally, and some taken by injection (or via a subcutaneous pump), such as insulin. Youth with type 2 diabetes may take one or more different glucose-lowering medications. Glucose lowering medications differ by their mechanism of actions. Overall, they can enhance endogenous insulin secretion, inhibit excessive hepatic glucose production, enhance insulin sensitivity in muscle and adipose tissue, inhibit gastrointestinal carbohydrate absorption, delay gastric emptying, inhibit glucagon secretion, and enhance satiety. The most frequently used oral glucose-lowering medication in children and adolescents is metformin. Glimepiride is also approved for children 8 years of age and older. All aspects of the regimen are individualized.

There is no single recipe to manage diabetes that fits all children. Blood glucose targets, frequency of blood glucose testing, type, dose and frequency of insulin, use of insulin injections with a syringe or a pen or pump, use of oral glucose-lowering medication and details of nutrition management all may vary among individuals. The family and diabetes care team determine the regimen that best suits each child's individual characteristics and circumstances.

Chapter 37

Growing Pains and Growth Disorders

Chapter Contents

Section 37.1

Growing Pains

Growing pains is a harmless condition of unknown cause that affects 10 to 20 percent of growing children. It is somewhat more common in girls. Despite the name, growing pains do not occur during the time of most rapid growth, such as the adolescent growth spurt, do not occur at specific sites of growth, and do not affect the growth of children who have them. Approximately one third of children with growing pains also experience other forms of recurrent pain, such as headaches or abdominal pain.

Growing pains are characterized by the symptoms listed below.

- Occurs in children 3 to 12 years of age

- Pain usually occurs in the both legs, especially thighs and calves, but may affect one leg at a time and vary which leg or part of the leg is affected (Pain in the arms is less common, but may occur in conjunction with leg pain. If the pain is localized to a single specific joint, it probably is not growing pains.)

- Pain occurs almost exclusively in the evenings and nighttime, often causing awakening during the night (To ease the discomfort, try a massage, heating pad, or a mild nonprescription pain medication.)

- Pain does not occur consistently during daytime activities or interfere with usual playground, recreational, or sports activities (However, children may complain more frequently in the nights following days during which they are very active. Growing pains do not cause limping.)

- Pain may occur for months or years, as frequently as almost every night, often with symptom-free intervals of weeks or months (Symptoms may wax and wane but usually remain stable with time. Most children outgrow growing pains within several years.)

- Children with growing pains have normal physical exam results. The results of X-rays and lab tests, although usually not needed, are also normal.

- Stretching the large muscle groups of the legs, such as the calves and thighs, can lessen symptoms, but is often impractical for young children.

If any of the following are present, the diagnosis of growing pains is unlikely and you and your doctor should look for other causes.

- Symptoms of general illness, such as fever or weight loss

- Pain specific to a single joint

- Pain worsening with time

- Pain interfering with usual daytime activities

- Limping

- Abnormal joint symptoms, such as restricted motion, redness, swelling, warmth, or tenderness in the related area

Section 37.2

Growth Disorders

Growth disorders affect thousands of people each year. A person may be diagnosed as a child or as an adult. Different types of growth disorders may be caused by imbalances in different types of hormones.

Overview

One of the remarkable roles of the endocrine system—a network of glands and organs that produce, store, and secrete hormones—is the regulation of growth and development. This work is directed by the pituitary gland, sometimes called the "master gland" of the endocrine system.

A small pea-sized organ at the base of the brain, the pituitary gland releases many types of hormones into the bloodstream. One of these is growth hormone (GH), also called somatotropin. The hypothalamus, part of the brain located just above the pituitary, produces growth hormone-releasing hormone (GHRH), which in turn stimulates the pituitary to produce GH. Once in the blood, GH travels to bone, muscle, and other tissues where it has many effects.

In children, for example, GH stimulates linear growth, or height. It is also important for the development of muscle and bone and the distribution of body fat throughout the body. In adults, GH affects energy, muscle strength, bone health, and psychological well-being. Having either too much or too little GH can cause health problems.

In some cases, individuals may have too much GH, a condition called acromegaly in adults. Acromegaly is usually caused by a non-cancerous tumor of the pituitary gland. In the rare instances when it occurs, too much GH in children is called gigantism.

A more common growth disorder is growth hormone deficiency (GHD). This is the condition of having too little GH. A child can be born with GHD (congenital GHD) or it may develop later during childhood, adolescence, or adulthood (acquired GHD). GHD may occur for several reasons:

- Structural abnormalities within the brain (organic GHD)

- Damage to the hypothalamus or pituitary gland because of a tumor, an infection, head trauma, or radiation—usually for the treatment of a tumor (also called organic GHD)

- An undefined cause (idiopathic GHD)

Pituitary disorders, such as GH excess or GHD, are evaluated and treated by endocrinologists—medical specialists in hormone-related conditions. Because the diagnosis and treatment of such disorders require special expertise, primary care physicians who suspect patients have GH abnormalities should refer them to an endocrinologist.

How Common Are Growth Hormone Disorders?

Growth Hormone Excess

Gigantism is extremely rare, occurring in fewer than 100 children in the United States.

Acromegaly most commonly occurs in middle-aged men and women. About 60 out of every million Americans have acromegaly.

Growth Hormone Deficiency

Estimates for the number of children with GHD vary. Some countries have reported one in 10,000 children with GHD while others have reported one in 3,500 children.

For adult-onset GHD, an estimated 35,000 adults have GHD, with about 6,000 newly diagnosed cases each year.

Growth Hormone Excess

Signs and Symptoms

In children with gigantism, the main sign is increased linear growth causing extremely tall stature. Other signs include obesity, increased head size (macrocephaly), and a prominent forehead.

Adults with acromegaly usually have large hands and feet, thick lips, coarse facial features, a protruding forehead and jaw, and widely spaced teeth. Often patients perspire excessively. Many of the signs and symptoms evolve slowly, so the diagnosis is often made years after the symptoms begin.

Numerous symptoms may be associated with acromegaly:

- Headaches

- Numbness or burning of the hands or feet, carpal tunnel syndrome
- Glucose intolerance, which puts one at risk for type 2 diabetes
- Cardiac dysfunction (heart attack, heart failure, or enlarged heart)
- High blood pressure
- Goiter (enlarged thyroid gland)
- Sleep apnea
- Tiredness
- Menstrual disorders (irregular bleeding, absence of periods)
- Decreased libido (low sex drive)
- Vision problems (tunnel vision, vision loss)
- Psychological problems (depression, anxiety)

Diagnostic Tests

GH stimulates the production of another molecule called insulin-like growth factor-1 (IGF-1) by the liver and many body tissues. Because of the link between excess GH and excess IGF-1, measuring the level of IGF-1 in the blood is an effective screening test for GH excess. Another diagnostic test measures GH during an oral glucose tolerance test. Still another test is a magnetic resonance imaging (MRI) scan of the pituitary and hypothalamus. An MRI can determine whether a tumor is the cause of the excess hormone secretion.

Sometimes tests confirm that a patient has GH excess, but the MRI shows no obvious hypothalamus or pituitary gland tumor. In this case, studies are undertaken to find a tumor elsewhere in the body that produces growth hormone-releasing hormone. This "ectopic" or abnormal hormone production stimulates excessive release of growth hormone by the pituitary gland. Ectopic tumors usually can be diagnosed by measuring GHRH [growth hormone releasing hormone] in the blood and by a computed tomography (CT) scan of possible tumor sites.

Treatment Options

Because excess GH—acting alone or together with excess IGF-1—produces adverse health effects, reducing the hormone levels to normal is desirable. Surgery, medication, and/or irradiation of the pituitary gland may be appropriate to achieve these goals.

Surgery: The most common cause of excess GH secretion is a non-cancerous tumor of the pituitary gland that produces GH. For these patients, surgery to remove the tumor is the treatment of choice. Rarely, excess GH is caused by a generalized enlargement of the pituitary gland called pituitary hyperplasia. This makes surgery impossible since there is not a discrete area to be removed.

If surgery does not normalize the GH level, or if a patient is not a candidate for surgery, other therapies are used. Medication and irradiation of the pituitary gland are options as primary or supplemental therapy.

Medications: Three types of drugs are now available for the treatment of GH excess—somatostatin analogues, GH receptor antagonists, and dopamine agonists. These medications do not "cure" the disorder but act, instead, to reduce levels of GH and IGF-1. These medications must be taken for life if surgery or irradiation fails to eliminate the cause of GH excess.

Pituitary irradiation: Radiation therapy is another therapeutic approach for people with acromegaly who have undergone pituitary surgery and still have excess GH. This remaining overproduction of GH may occur if the tumor removed during surgery had spread beyond the pituitary gland. Because complete removal of invasive tumors is often challenging, additional therapy may be needed to achieve normal GH and IGF-1 levels.

Although pituitary irradiation can lead to complete remission (absence of symptoms), it takes time to reach that goal. Conventional radiation therapy may take 10 years or longer to be fully effective. Newer methods of delivery—such as gamma knife, proton beam, or linear accelerator—allow precise targeting of the tumor with a high dose of radiation and often lead to an earlier remission than the conventional method. Still, there may be a significant delay.

Although it takes longer to attain remission with irradiation than with medications, once remission is reached, the effects of irradiation are permanent. Patients may need to take medication until the radiation therapy achieves its effect.

Unlike in adults, radiation is considered a last resort in children with GH excess, because of concerns about its effects on the developing brain.

Long-Term Follow-Up and Prognosis

People treated for acromegaly need to be monitored to make sure that GH excess does not return. They also need to be watched for signs of hypopituitarism—multiple pituitary hormone deficiencies. Patients should also be monitored for medical problems associated with acromegaly, including heart disease, high blood pressure, colon polyps, and high blood sugar.

Hypopituitarism can result from the pituitary gland tumor mass, or can be a complication of surgery or radiation therapy. Pituitary dysfunction is treated by giving back to the body the hormones that are not being produced (hormone replacement therapy).

Treating acromegaly to reduce excess GH helps patients live longer. People with untreated acromegaly have a death rate that is two to three times higher than the general population, mostly due to cardiovascular and respiratory complications. Premature death is more likely when the GH level is higher and when diabetes is present. Reducing the hormone imbalance so the levels of GH and IGF-1 are normal may offer a return to normal life expectancy.

Growth Hormone Deficiency

Signs and Symptoms

Children: Most children with GHD grow less than 2 inches per year, whereas children with normal GH usually grow at least 2 inches annually. Some children with congenital GHD may grow normally until age 2 or 3, but then their growth rate slows. Others may have slow growth starting soon after birth. If GHD goes undiagnosed, their growth rate will continue to worsen.

Some children with GHD have extra fat in the abdomen and face. During infancy, their blood sugar levels may be low. Without treatment, puberty may be delayed. All children with a persistently below-average growth rate should be referred to a pediatric endocrinologist for evaluation.

Adults: Adults with GHD fall into two general categories. Some individuals may have had GHD as a child and continue to have the deficiency. Others may have acquired the deficiency after reaching maturity. The consequences of GHD in adults result from a lack of both GH and IGF-1.

The disorder has several possible symptoms in adults:

- Increased body fat (particularly at the waist and in the face)

- Decreased muscle and bone mass

- Thinning skin with fine wrinkles

- Poor sweating or impaired temperature regulation

- Reduced strength and endurance
- Low energy level
- Decreased well-being (moodiness, mild depression)
- Loss of interest in sex
- Poor sleep
- Higher cholesterol levels, especially LDL ([low-density lipoprotein] "bad") cholesterol
- Overproduction of insulin (a hormone produced by the pancreas that regulates the levels of sugar in the blood), resulting from overweight

Diagnostic Tests

Although there is no gold standard for the diagnosis of GHD, GH stimulation tests are commonly used in patients who have symptoms, low IGF-1, and normal levels of other pituitary hormones. Because the pituitary gland secretes GH in bursts throughout the day and night, random measurements of levels in the blood are useless.

If a patient's GH levels in blood remain below the normal range in response to a growth hormone stimulation test, it is likely he or she has GHD. GH stimulation tests are not perfect, however, and some endocrinologists question their utility. For example, some children with all the clinical signs of GHD have stimulated GH concentrations in the blood that are normal.

Although no stimulation test is perfect, the insulin tolerance test tends to be an excellent predictor of GHD. The test involves giving the patient insulin after an overnight fast to lower their blood sugar. Failure to produce GH in response to insulin-induced hypoglycemia is a strong indication of GHD. This test is not appropriate for patients who have seizures or coronary artery disease.

A good alternative to the insulin tolerance test is a stimulation test that uses GH-releasing hormone together with arginine—an amino acid necessary for the release of GH. This test is inappropriate for patients with liver or kidney disease. Other stimulation tests use the medications carbidopa/levodopa or clonidine, or the hormone glucagon, all of which normally stimulate the pituitary to release GH.

Treatment

Synthetic GH is usually administered as a daily injection under the skin. Because adults tend to have more side effects than children, their treatment often begins at a low dose and then is raised gradually.

The doses of GH used to treat children—especially adolescents—are often much higher than those in adults. Younger adult patients require higher doses than older ones, and women require more than men. Women taking estrogen by mouth may need a higher dose of GH.

Long-Term Follow-Up and Prognosis

Children: Children should be evaluated every 3 to 6 months to monitor their GH treatment. The best indicators are gains in height and rate of growth. Follow-up is important to assure compliance with the daily injections, to detect and manage possible side effects, monitor growth progress, and to adjust dosage periodically.

If patients have been compliant with their injections and their growth remains lower than desirable, the GH dose may be increased within the guidelines approved by the U.S. Food and Drug Administration (FDA). If the patient's IGF-1 levels are well above the normal range at any time, then a decreased dose should be considered.

The children with the best chance of reaching their height potential are those who start GH therapy as soon as the diagnosis is made, and continue it through adolescence. With the current GH products, most children with GHD reach normal adult stature. When children with GHD reach late adolescence, tests should be done to see if they still need GH therapy into adulthood.

Undesirable effects of growth hormone therapy in childhood are exceedingly rare. The most troubling side effect in children is increased intracranial pressure (a rise in normal brain pressure) causing severe headaches and vomiting. Because of changes in the blood vessels of the eyes, this condition is typically diagnosed by an ophthalmologist. In all reported cases, the problem was temporary and went away when GH therapy was stopped. Restarting GH at a lower dose and gradually increasing the dose has resulted in no further problems.

Curvature of the spine (scoliosis) and a hip disorder called slipped capital femoral epiphysis (a condition in which the growing end of the thigh bone—the ball that fits into the hip socket—slips off the neck of the thigh bone) have been reported in children receiving GH therapy. Any child suspected of having one of these conditions is referred to an orthopedic specialist.

Adults: Monthly follow-up visits are usual for adults starting growth hormone replacement therapy. Patients require continued monitoring for side effects, optimal replacement dosage, and long-term treatment results. Some adults taking GH report joint pain and edema, an abnormal build-up of fluid in joints and tissues. Decreasing the dosage temporarily can relieve these problems.

Blood sugar levels may need to be monitored as well because GH therapy can decrease a patient's sensitivity to insulin. Patients with type 2 diabetes need special attention because GH therapy hinders control of that disease until the patient loses excess abdominal fat. Follow-up visits, even for those on lifetime replacement therapy, should be scheduled at least twice a year. While GH therapy may "unmask" underlying type 2 diabetes, there is no evidence that GH causes diabetes.

Lifestyle and Prevention

For children: Because growth hormone is taken for years, parents of children with GHD should be aware of some safety precautions:

- Carefully follow the directions for taking GH.

- Tell all doctors who care for your child that he or she is undergoing growth hormone therapy.

- Make sure your child takes any other prescription drugs exactly as prescribed.

- Contact your child's doctor immediately if you have any questions about treatment or signs or symptoms which suggest a complication of GH treatment.

In addition, encourage your child to have a healthy lifestyle. Eating a variety of healthy foods will help your child to grow and respond to growth hormone therapy. Be sure that your child gets regular exercise and plenty of sleep, too.

For adults: Adults receiving GH treatment should also eat a balanced diet, get regular exercise, and get plenty of sleep.

Some adults find their lives are much better after taking GH alone. Others may find they still need some help, particularly with the psychological symptoms of GHD. You may need medication to control anxiety or lift your mood.

Counseling may be helpful, too. Some forms of therapy, such as cognitive-behavior therapy, can allow you to correct negative thoughts you may be having. You also may want to join a support group with other adults who have GHD. Talking to others who have been through the same thing can be healing.

Chapter 38

Juvenile Arthritis

What is juvenile arthritis?

Arthritis means joint inflammation. This term refers to a group of diseases that cause pain, swelling, stiffness, and loss of motion in the joints.

Arthritis is also used more generally to describe the more than 100 rheumatic diseases that may affect the joints but can also cause pain, swelling, and stiffness in other supporting structures of the body such as muscles, tendons, ligaments, and bones. Some rheumatic diseases can affect other parts of the body, including various internal organs.

Juvenile arthritis (JA) is a term often used to describe arthritis in children and teens. Children and teens can develop almost all types of arthritis that affect adults, but the most common type that affects children is juvenile idiopathic arthritis.

Prevalence statistics for JA vary, but according to a 2008 report from the National Arthritis Data Workgroup, about 294,000 children age 0 to 17 are affected with arthritis or other rheumatic conditions.

What is juvenile idiopathic arthritis?

JIA is currently the most widely accepted term to describe various types of chronic arthritis in children. In general, the symptoms of

Excerpted from "Juvenile Arthritis," by the National Institute of Arthritis and Musculoskeletal and Skin Diseases (NIAMS, www.niams.nih.gov), part of the National Institutes of Health, September 2008.

JIA include joint pain, swelling, tenderness, warmth, and stiffness that last for more than 6 continuous weeks. It is divided into seven separate subtypes, each with characteristic symptoms. The subtypes include systemic arthritis (sometimes referred to as systemic juvenile rheumatoid arthritis, or JRA), oligoarthritis, polyarthritis rheumatoid factor negative, polyarthritis rheumatoid factor positive, psoriatic arthritis, enthesitis-related arthritis, and undifferentiated arthritis.

What causes juvenile arthritis?

Most forms of juvenile arthritis are autoimmune disorders, which means that the body's immune system—which normally helps to fight off bacteria or viruses—mistakenly attacks some of its own healthy cells and tissues. The result is inflammation, marked by redness, heat, pain, and swelling. Inflammation can cause joint damage. Doctors do not know why the immune system attacks healthy tissues in children who develop JA. Scientists suspect that it is a two-step process. First, something in a child's genetic makeup gives him or her a tendency to develop JA; then an environmental factor, such as a virus, triggers the development of the disease.

Not all cases of JA are autoimmune, however. Recent research has demonstrated that some people, such as many with systemic arthritis, have what is more accurately called an autoinflammatory condition. Although the two terms sound somewhat similar, the disease processes behind autoimmune and autoinflammatory disorders are different.

When the immune system is working properly, foreign invaders such as bacteria and viruses provoke the body to produce proteins called antibodies. Antibodies attach to these invaders so that they can be recognized and destroyed. In an autoimmune reaction, the antibodies attach to the body's own healthy tissues by mistake, signaling the body to attack them. Because they target the self, these proteins are called autoantibodies.

Like autoimmune disorders, autoinflammatory conditions also cause inflammation. And like autoimmune disorders, they also involve an overactive immune system. However, autoinflammation is not caused by autoantibodies. Instead, autoinflammation involves a more primitive part of the immune system that in healthy people causes white blood cells to destroy harmful substances. When this system goes awry, it causes inflammation for unknown reasons. In addition to inflammation, autoinflammatory diseases often cause fever and rashes.

What are its symptoms and signs?

The most common symptom of all types of juvenile arthritis is persistent joint swelling, pain, and stiffness that is typically worse in the morning or after a nap. The pain may limit movement of the affected joint, although many children, especially younger ones, will not complain of pain. JA commonly affects the knees and the joints in the hands and feet. One of the earliest signs of JA may be limping in the morning because of an affected knee. Besides joint symptoms, children with systemic JA have a high fever and a skin rash. The rash and fever may appear and disappear very quickly. Systemic arthritis also may cause the lymph nodes located in the neck and other parts of the body to swell. In some cases (fewer than half), internal organs including the heart and (very rarely) the lungs, may be involved.

Eye inflammation is a potentially severe complication that commonly occurs in children with oligoarthritis but can also be seen in other types of JA. All children with JA need to have regular eye exams, including a special exam called a slit lamp exam. Eye diseases such as iritis or uveitis can be present at the beginning of arthritis but often develop some time after a child first develops JA. Very commonly, JA-associated eye inflammation does not cause any symptoms and is found only by performing eye exams.

Typically, there are periods when the symptoms of JA are better or disappear (remissions) and times when symptoms "flare," or get worse. JA is different in each child; some may have just one or two flares and never have symptoms again, while others experience many flares or even have symptoms that never go away.

Some children with JA have growth problems. Depending on the severity of the disease and the joints involved, bone growth at the affected joints may be too fast or too slow, causing one leg or arm to be longer than the other. Overall growth also may be slowed. Doctors are exploring the use of growth hormone to treat this problem. JA may also cause joints to grow unevenly.

How is it treated?

The main goals of treatment are to preserve a high level of physical and social functioning and maintain a good quality of life. To achieve these goals, doctors recommend treatments to reduce swelling, maintain full movement in the affected joints, relieve pain, and prevent, identify, and treat complications. Most children with JA need a combination of medication and nonmedication treatments to reach these goals.

Chapter 39

Infections Often Spread in Schools

Chapter Contents

Section 39.1

Preventing Influenza in Schools

This section contains text excerpted from "Key Facts About Seasonal Influenza (Flu)," by the Centers for Disease Control and Prevention (CDC, www.cdc.gov), October 16, 2009; excerpted from "2009 H1N1," by the CDC, February 10, 2010; and excerpted from "Questions and Answers about CDC Guidance for State and Local Public Health Officials and School Administrators for School (K-12) Responses to Flu during the 2009-2010 School Year," by the CDC (www.flu.gov), February 2010.

Key Facts about Seasonal Influenza

What Is Influenza (Also Called Flu)?

The flu is a contagious respiratory illness caused by influenza viruses. It can cause mild to severe illness, and at times can lead to death. The best way to prevent seasonal flu is by getting a seasonal flu vaccination each year.

Every year in the United States, on average, the following are true:

- Five percent to 20 percent of the population gets the flu.
- More than 200,000 people are hospitalized from flu-related complications.
- About 36,000 people die from flu-related causes.

Some people, such as older people, young children, pregnant women, and people with certain health conditions (such as asthma, diabetes, or heart disease), are at increased risk for serious complications from seasonal flu illness.

Symptoms of Flu

Symptoms of seasonal flu include the following:

- Fever (often high)
- Headache

- Extreme tiredness

- Dry cough

- Sore throat

- Runny or stuffy nose

- Muscle aches

Stomach symptoms, such as nausea, vomiting, and diarrhea, also can occur but are more common in children than adults. Some people who have been infected with the new H1N1 flu virus have reported diarrhea and vomiting.

How Flu Spreads

Flu viruses are thought to spread mainly from person to person through coughing or sneezing of people with influenza. Sometimes people may become infected by touching something with flu viruses on it and then touching their mouth or nose. Most healthy adults may be able to infect others beginning 1 day before symptoms develop and up to 5–7 days after becoming sick. That means that you may be able to pass on the flu to someone else before you know you are sick, as well as while you are sick.

Preventing Seasonal Flu: Get Vaccinated

The single best way to prevent seasonal flu is to get a seasonal flu vaccination each year. There are two types of flu vaccines:

- The flu shot is an inactivated vaccine (containing killed virus) that is given with a needle. The seasonal flu shot is approved for use in people 6 months of age and older, including healthy people and people with chronic medical conditions.

- The nasal-spray flu vaccine is a vaccine made with live, weakened flu viruses that do not cause the flu (sometimes called LAIV for "Live Attenuated Influenza Vaccine"). LAIV is approved for use in healthy people 2–49 years of age who are not pregnant.

About 2 weeks after vaccination, antibodies develop that protect against influenza virus infection. Flu vaccines will not protect against flu-like illnesses caused by non-influenza viruses.

H1N1 Flu

What is H1N1 (swine flu)?

H1N1 (sometimes called "swine flu") is a new influenza virus causing illness in people. This new virus was first detected in people in the United States in April 2009. This virus is spreading from person-to-person worldwide, probably in much the same way that regular seasonal influenza viruses spread. On June 11, 2009, the World Health Organization (WHO) declared that a pandemic of H1N1 flu was underway.

Is the H1N1 virus contagious?

The H1N1 virus is contagious and is spreading from human to human.

How does the H1N1 virus spread?

Spread of the H1N1 virus is thought to occur in the same way that seasonal flu spreads. Flu viruses are spread mainly from person to person through coughing, sneezing, or talking by people with influenza. Sometimes people may become infected by touching something—such as a surface or object—with flu viruses on it and then touching their mouth or nose.

What are the signs and symptoms of this virus in people?

The symptoms of H1N1 flu virus in people include fever, cough, sore throat, runny or stuffy nose, body aches, headache, chills, and fatigue. Some people may have vomiting and diarrhea. People may be infected with the flu, including H1N1 and have respiratory symptoms without a fever. Severe illnesses and deaths have occurred as a result of illness associated with this virus.

What can I do to protect myself from getting sick?

There is a seasonal flu vaccine to protect against seasonal flu viruses and a H1N1 vaccine to protect against the H1N1 influenza virus (sometimes called "swine flu"). A flu vaccine is by far the most important step in protecting against flu infection.

There are also everyday actions that can help prevent the spread of germs that cause respiratory illnesses like the flu. Take these everyday steps to protect your health:

- Cover your nose and mouth with a tissue when you cough or sneeze. Throw the tissue in the trash after you use it.

- Wash your hands often with soap and water. If soap and water are not available, use an alcohol-based hand rub.

- Avoid touching your eyes, nose, or mouth. Germs spread this way.

- Try to avoid close contact with sick people.

- If you are sick with flu-like illness, CDC recommends that you stay home for at least 24 hours after your fever is gone except to get medical care or for other necessities. (Your fever should be gone without the use of a fever-reducing medicine.) Keep away from others as much as possible to keep from making others sick.

Other important actions that you can take are the following:

- Follow public health advice regarding school closures, avoiding crowds, and other social distancing measures.

- Be prepared in case you get sick and need to stay home for a week or so; a supply of over-the-counter medicines, alcohol-based hand rubs (for when soap and water are not available), tissues, and other related items could help you to avoid the need to make trips out in public while you are sick and contagious.

Influenza at School

Why should we be concerned about the spread of flu in schools?

Students can get sick with flu and schools may act as a point of spread, where students can easily spread flu to other students and their families. So far, with 2009 H1N1 flu, the largest number of cases has been in people between the ages of 5 and 24 years old.

Which students and staff are at higher risk for complications from flu?

Anyone can get the flu (even healthy people), and serious problems from the flu can happen at any age. However, children younger than 5 years old, but especially children younger than 2 years old; people aged 65 years or older; pregnant women; adults and children who have asthma, neurological and neurodevelopmental conditions; chronic lung disease; heart disease; blood disorders; endocrine disorders, such as diabetes; kidney, liver, and metabolic disorders; weakened immune system due to disease or medication; and people younger than 19 years of age who are receiving long-term aspirin therapy are more likely to get complications from the flu.

What can families, students, and school personnel do to keep from getting sick and spreading flu?

Families, students, and school staff can keep from getting sick with flu in three ways:

- **Practicing good hand hygiene:** Students and staff members should wash their hands often with soap and water, especially after coughing or sneezing. Alcohol-based hand rubs are also useful.

- **Cover your mouth and nose when you cough or sneeze:** The main way that the flu spreads is from person to person in the droplets produced by coughs and sneezes, so it's important to cover your mouth and nose with a tissue when you cough or sneeze. If you don't have a tissue, cough or sneeze into your elbow or shoulder, not into your hands.

- **Staying home if you're sick:** Keeping sick students at home means that they keep their viruses to themselves rather than sharing them with others.

Students, staff, and their families must take personal responsibility for helping to slow the spread of the virus by practicing these steps to keep from getting sick with flu and protecting others from getting the flu.

What is the best way to practice good hand hygiene?

Washing your hands with soap and water for at least 20 seconds (the time it takes to sing "Happy Birthday" twice) is the best way to keep your hands from spreading the virus.

Alcohol-based hand rubs containing at least 60% alcohol are also useful.

If soap and water are not available and alcohol-based products are not allowed in the school, other hand rubs that do not contain alcohol may be useful for cleaning hands. However, they may not be as useful as alcohol-based rubs.

Section 39.2

Meningococcal Infection on Campus

Meningococcal disease is a rare but sometimes deadly disease, often called meningitis, that strikes adolescents and young adults.

The disease spreads quickly and within hours of the first symptoms and can cause organ failure, brain damage, amputations of limbs, or death.

Parents and their adolescent children should learn more about meningococcal disease and prevention. Vaccination can prevent most cases of the disease.

Facts about Meningococcal Disease

- Adolescents and young adults have an increased incidence of meningococcal disease, accounting for nearly 30 percent of all U.S. cases. One out of four cases among adolescents will result in death.

- The majority of meningococcal disease cases among adolescents and young adults are potentially vaccine-preventable.

- The number of cases changes from year to year. About 1,500 Americans were infected annually from 1998–2007. Each year, meningococcal disease strikes between 900 to nearly 3,000 Americans, and about 11% percent of those infected will die.

- Nearly 20 percent of survivors have long-term disabilities, such as brain damage, limb amputations, hearing loss, or organ damage/failure.

- The disease can take one of two forms: swelling of membranes that surround the brain and spinal cord (meningococcal meningitis), or the more deadly meningococcemia, an infection of the blood.

- Meningococcal disease is caused by bacteria called *Neisseria meningitidis.*

Adolescents, Young Adults at Increased Risk

Lifestyle factors common among adolescents and young adults seem to be linked to the disease. These include crowded living situations such as dormitories, boarding schools and sleep-away camps, going to bars, smoking, and irregular sleep habits.

Immunization Information

The Centers for Disease Control and Prevention recommends meningococcal immunization (one shot) for all adolescents 11 through 18 years of age.

Others who wish to be immunized against the disease should speak to their health care provider.

Vaccination offers the best protection against the disease.

Consider Vaccination

Immunization can prevent the majority of meningococcal disease cases in adolescents and young adults:

- The meningococcal conjugate vaccine is expected to provide long-term immunity and decrease carriage of meningococcal bacteria among adolescents, preventing the spread of the disease.

- Vaccination protects against four of the five major strains of the bacteria responsible for meningococcal disease in the United States. The majority of cases in adolescents and young adults are vaccine-preventable.

- As with all vaccines, there may be minor reactions (pain and redness at the injection site or a mild fever).

Be Alert: Early Flu-Like Symptoms

Meningococcal disease often is misdiagnosed because its early signs are much like those of the flu or migraines. Symptoms may include high fever, headache, stiff neck, confusion, nausea, vomiting, and exhaustion.

Later, after the disease has taken hold, a rash may appear. If any of these symptoms are present and are unusually sudden and severe, call a physician.

Don't wait.

How Meningitis Is Spread

The disease is spread through air droplets and direct contact with someone who is infected. That includes coughing, kissing, and through close personal contact.

Adolescents and young adults can reduce their risk by being vaccinated.

Most cases occur in late winter to early spring.

Find out More

For more information about meningococcal disease and immunization, visit the following websites:

- National Meningitis Association, www.nmaus.org

- American Academy of Family Physicians, www.aafp.org

- American Academy of Pediatrics, www.aap.org

- Centers for Disease Control and Prevention, www.cdc.gov

- National Foundation for Infectious Diseases, www.nfid.org

For medical advice about meningococcal immunization, consult your physician, college health service, or local public health department.

Section 39.3

Methicillin-Resistant Staphylococcus Aureus *in Schools*

Excerpted from "Questions and Answers about Methicillin-Resistant
Staphylococcus aureus in Schools," by the Centers for Disease Control
and Prevention (CDC, www.cdc.gov), October 9, 2007.

What type of infections does MRSA cause?

In the community most MRSA infections are skin infections that may
appear as pustules or boils which often are red, swollen, painful, or have
pus or other drainage. These skin infections commonly occur at sites of visible skin trauma, such as cuts and abrasions, and areas of the body covered
by hair (e.g., back of neck, groin, buttock, armpit, beard area of men).

Almost all MRSA skin infections can be effectively treated by drainage of pus with or without antibiotics. More serious infections, such as
pneumonia, bloodstream infections, or bone infections, are very rare
in healthy people who get MRSA skin infections.

How is MRSA transmitted?

MRSA is usually transmitted by direct skin-to-skin contact or contact with shared items or surfaces that have come into contact with
someone else's infection (e.g., towels, used bandages).

How do I protect myself from getting MRSA?

You can protect yourself by doing the following:

- Practicing good hygiene (e.g., keeping your hands clean by washing with soap and water or using an alcohol-based hand sanitizer, and showering immediately after participating in exercise)

- Covering skin trauma such as abrasions or cuts with a clean dry
  bandage until healed

- Avoiding sharing personal items (e.g., towels, razors) that come
  into contact with your bare skin, and using a barrier (e.g., clothing

or a towel) between your skin and shared equipment such as weight-training benches

- Maintaining a clean environment by establishing cleaning procedures for frequently touched surfaces and surfaces that come into direct contact with people's skin

I have a MRSA skin infection. How do I prevent spreading it to others?

Cover your wound. Keep wounds that are draining or have pus covered with clean, dry bandages until healed. Follow your healthcare provider's instructions on proper care of the wound. Pus from infected wounds can contain staph, including MRSA, so keeping the infection covered will help prevent the spread to others. Bandages and tape can be discarded with the regular trash.

Clean your hands frequently. You, your family, and others in close contact should wash their hands frequently with soap and water or use an alcohol-based hand sanitizer, especially after changing the bandage or touching the infected wound.

Do not share personal items. Avoid sharing personal items, such as towels, washcloths, razors, clothing, or uniforms, that may have had contact with the infected wound or bandage. Wash sheets, towels, and clothes that become soiled with water and laundry detergent. Use a dryer to dry clothes completely.

Section 39.4

Mononucleosis

"Mononucleosis," © 2010 A.D.A.M., Inc. Reprinted with permission.

Mononucleosis is a viral infection causing fever, sore throat, and swollen lymph glands, especially in the neck.

Causes

Mononucleosis, or mono, is often spread by saliva and close contact. It is known as "the kissing disease," and occurs most often in those age 15 to 17. However, the infection may develop at any age.

Mono is usually linked to the Epstein-Barr virus (EBV), but can also be caused by other organisms such as cytomegalovirus (CMV).

Symptoms

Mono may begin slowly with fatigue, a general ill feeling, headache, and sore throat. The sore throat slowly gets worse. Your tonsils become swollen and develop a whitish-yellow covering. The lymph nodes in the neck are frequently swollen and painful.

A pink, measles-like rash can occur and is more likely if you take the medicines ampicillin or amoxicillin for a throat infection. (Antibiotics should **not** be given without a positive Strep test.)

Symptoms of mononucleosis include:

- drowsiness;
- fever;
- general discomfort, uneasiness, or ill feeling;
- loss of appetite;
- muscle aches or stiffness;
- rash;
- sore throat;
- swollen lymph nodes, especially in the neck and armpit;
- swollen spleen.

Less frequently occurring symptoms include:

- chest pain;
- cough;
- fatigue;
- headache;
- hives;
- jaundice (yellow color to the skin);
- neck stiffness;
- nosebleed;
- rapid heart rate;
- sensitivity to light;
- shortness of breath.

Exams and Tests

During a physical examination, the doctor may find swollen lymph nodes in the front and back of your neck, as well as swollen tonsils with a whitish-yellow covering.

The doctor might also feel a swollen liver or swollen spleen when pushing on your belly. There may be a skin rash.

Blood work often reveals a higher-than-normal white blood cell (WBC) count and unusual-looking white blood cells called atypical lymphocytes, which are seen when blood is examined under a microscope. Atypical lymphocytes and abnormal liver function tests are a hallmark sign of the disease.

- A monospot test will be positive for infectious mononucleosis.
- A special test called an antibody titer can help your doctor distinguish a current (acute) EBV infection from one that occurred in the past.

Treatment

The goal of treatment is to relieve symptoms. Medicines such as steroids (prednisone) and antivirals (such as acyclovir) have little or no benefit.

To relieve typical symptoms:

- drink plenty of fluids;
- gargle with warm salt water to ease a sore throat;

- get plenty of rest;
- take acetaminophen or ibuprofen for pain and fever.

You should also avoid contact sports while the spleen is swollen (to prevent it from rupturing).

Outlook (Prognosis)

The fever usually drops in 10 days, and swollen lymph glands and spleen heal in 4 weeks. Fatigue usually goes away within a few weeks, but may linger for 2 to 3 months.

Possible Complications

- Death in persons with weakened immune systems
- Hemolytic anemia
- Hepatitis with jaundice (more common in patients older than 35)
- Inflammation of the testicles (orchitis)
- Neurological complications (rare), including:
  - Guillain-Barré syndrome
  - Meningitis
  - Seizures
  - Temporary facial paralysis (Bell palsy)
  - Uncoordinated movements (ataxia)
- Secondary bacterial throat infection
- Spleen rupture (rare; avoid pressure on the spleen)

When to Contact a Medical Professional

The initial symptoms of mono feel very much like a typical viral illness. It is not necessary to contact a health care provider unless symptoms last longer than 10 days or you develop the following:

- Abdominal pain
- Breathing difficulty
- Persistent high fevers (more than 101.5 degrees F)
- Severe headache
- Severe sore throat or swollen tonsils
- Weakness in the arm or legs
- Yellow discoloration of your eyes or skin

Call 911 or go to an emergency room if you develop:

- sharp, sudden, severe abdominal pain;
- significant difficulty swallowing or breathing;
- stiff neck or severe weakness.

Prevention

Persons with mononucleosis may be contagious while they have symptoms and for up to a few months afterward. How long someone with the disease is contagious varies. The virus can live for several hours outside the body. Avoid kissing or sharing utensils if you or someone close to you has mono.

Section 39.5

Staphylococcal Infections in Teens

"Staph Infections," January 2008, reprinted with permission from www
.kidshealth.org. Copyright © 2008 The Nemours Foundation. This information
was provided by KidsHealth, one of the largest resources online for medically
reviewed health information written for parents, kids, and teens. For more
articles like this one, visit www.KidsHealth.org, or www.TeensHealth.org.

Amy was used to the occasional outbreak of zits, but the bump on her neck was different. It started out fairly small and itchy, but now was big and red and sore. Amy's mom took her to the doctor and they were surprised to hear that the bump was a boil, an infection usually caused by staph bacteria.

What Is a Staph Infection?

Staph (pronounced: staff) is the shortened name for *Staphylococcus* (pronounced: staf-uh-low-kah-kus), a type of bacteria. These bacteria can live harmlessly on many skin surfaces, especially around the nose, mouth, genitals, and anus. But when the skin is punctured or broken for any reason, staph bacteria can enter the wound and cause an infection.

There are more than 30 species in the staph family of bacteria, and they can cause different kinds of illnesses—for example, one kind of staph can cause urinary tract infections. But most staph infections are caused by the species *Staphylococcus aureus* (*S. aureus*).

S. aureus most commonly causes skin infections like folliculitis, boils, impetigo, and cellulitis that are limited to a small area of a person's skin. *S. aureus* can also release toxins (poisons) that may lead to illnesses like food poisoning or toxic shock syndrome.

How Do People Get Staph Infections?

In teens, most staph infections are minor skin infections. People with skin problems like burns or eczema may be more likely to get staph skin infections.

People can get staph infections from contaminated objects, but staph bacteria often spread through skin-to-skin contact—the bacteria can be spread from one area of the body to another if someone touches the infected area.

Staph infections can spread from person to person among those who live close together in group situations (such as in college dorms). Usually this happens when people with skin infections share things like bed linens, towels, or clothing. Warm, humid environments can contribute to staph infections, so excessive sweating can increase someone's chances of developing an infection.

Serious Staph Infections

Although it's very rare, infections caused by *S. aureus* can occasionally become serious. This happens when the bacteria move from a break in the skin into the bloodstream. This can lead to infections in other parts of the body, such as the lungs, bones, joints, heart, blood, and central nervous system.

Staph infections in other parts of the body are less common than staph skin infections. They are more likely in people whose immune systems have been weakened by another disease—or by certain medications, like chemotherapy for cancer.

Occasionally patients having surgery may get more serious types of staph infections. The good news is that hospital staff take many precautions to avoid infection in someone having surgery. That's why they carefully clean the area being operated on, use sterile equipment, and sometimes give a person antibiotics.

You may also have heard about methicillin-resistant *Staphylococcus aureus* or MRSA for short. MRSA is a type of staph that has built up an immunity to the antibiotics doctors usually use to treat staph infections. Although MRSA can be harder to treat, in most cases the infection heals with the right treatment.

What Are the Signs of a Staph Skin Infection?

Staph skin infections show up in lots of different ways. Some of the more common conditions often caused by *S. aureus* skin infections are:

- **Folliculitis** (pronounced: fuh-lih-kyoo-lie-tus) is an infection of the hair follicles, the tiny pockets under the skin where hair shafts (strands) grow. In folliculitis, tiny white-headed pimples appear at the base of hair shafts, sometimes with a small red area around each pimple. This occurs often where people shave or have irritated skin from rubbing against clothing.

- A **furuncle** (pronounced: fyoor-un-kul), commonly known as a boil, is a swollen, red, painful lump in the skin, usually due to an infected hair follicle. The lump usually fills with pus, growing larger and more painful until it ruptures and drains. Furuncles often begin as folliculitis and then worsen. They are most frequently found on the face, neck, buttocks, armpits, and inner thighs, where small hairs can often be irritated. A cluster of several furuncles is called a carbuncle (pronounced: kar-bun-kul). A person with a carbuncle may feel ill and feverish.

- **Impetigo** (pronounced: im-puh-tie-go) is a superficial skin infection that mostly happens in young children, but it can sometimes affect teens and adults. Most impetigo infections affect the face or extremities like the hands and feet. An impetigo skin infection begins as a small blister or pimple, and then develops a honey-colored crust. Impetigo doesn't usually cause pain or fever, although the blisters may itch and can be spread to other parts of the body by scratching.

- **Cellulitis** (pronounced: sell-yuh-lie-tus) is an infection involving the skin and areas of tissue below the skin surface. It begins as a small area of redness, pain, swelling, and warmth on the skin. As this area begins to spread, a person may feel feverish and ill. Cellulitis can affect any area of the body, but it's most common on the legs.

- A **hordeolum** (pronounced: hore-dee-oh-lum), commonly known as a stye, is a staph infection in the eyelid. It develops when glands connected to the base of the eyelash become swollen and irritated.

A person with a stye will usually notice a red, warm, uncomfort-able, and sometimes painful swelling near the edge of the eyelid.

Many of these staph infections are minor and can be treated at home. If a minor infection gets worse—for example, you start feeling feverish or ill or the area spreads and gets very red or and hot—it's a good idea to see a doctor.

Wound infections generally show up two or more days after the injury or surgery. The signs of a wound infection (redness, pain, swelling, and warmth) are similar to those found in cellulitis. A wound infection may be accompanied by fever and a generally ill feeling. Pus or a cloudy fluid can drain from the wound and a yellow crust (like that in impetigo) can develop. If you think you have a wound infection after surgery, or you have a serious wound that seems to be infected, call your doctor.

Can I Prevent a Staph Skin Infection?

Staphylococcus aureus bacteria are everywhere. Many healthy peo-ple carry staph bacteria without getting sick. Cleanliness and good hygiene are the best way to protect yourself against getting staph (and other) infections—including MRSA. You can help prevent staph skin infections by washing your hands frequently and by bathing or showering daily.

Keep areas of skin that have been injured (such as cuts, scrapes, eczema, and rashes caused by allergic reactions or poison ivy) clean and covered. Use any antibiotic ointments or other treatments that your doc-tor suggests. If someone in your family has a staph infection, don't share towels, sheets, or clothing until the infection has been fully treated.

If you develop a staph infection, you can prevent spreading it to other parts of your body by being careful not to touch the infected skin, keeping it covered whenever possible, and using a towel only once when you clean the area (wash the towel in hot water afterward or use disposable towels).

What Can I Do to Feel Better?

How long it takes for a staph skin infection to heal depends on the type of infection and whether a person gets treatment for it. A boil, for example, may take 10 to 20 days to heal without treatment, but treatment may speed up this process. Most styes, on the other hand, go away on their own within several days.

To help relieve pain from a skin infection, and to help pus drain out, try soaking the affected area in warm water or applying warm, moist washcloths. Use a clean washcloth each time—wash used cloths in soap and hot water and dry them fully in a clothes dryer. You can also apply a heating pad or a hot water bottle to the skin for about 20 minutes, three or four times a day.

Pain relievers like acetaminophen or ibuprofen can help reduce pain until the infection subsides. For some skin infections, it can also help to wash the area with an antibacterial cleanser and apply an antibiotic ointment. Cover the skin with a clean dressing.

Styes can be treated using warm compresses over the eye (with the eye closed) three or four times a day. Be sure you always use a clean washcloth each time. Occasionally, a stye will require a topical antibiotic. See your doctor if a stye doesn't go away in a few days.

If you get a staph infection on skin areas that you normally shave, avoid shaving, if possible, until the infection clears up. If you do have to shave the area, use a clean disposable razor or clean your electric razor after each use.

Staph infections can be a nuisance, but the good news is that they are usually not serious.

Chapter 40

Malocclusion, Braces, and Orthodontics

Malocclusion means the teeth are not aligned properly.

Causes

Occlusion refers to the alignment of teeth and the way that the upper and lower teeth fit together (bite). Ideally, all upper teeth fit slightly over the lower teeth. The points of the molars fit the grooves of the opposite molar.

The upper teeth keep the cheeks and lips from being bitten and the lower teeth protect the tongue.

Malocclusion is most often hereditary, which means the condition is passed down through families. There may be a difference between the size of the upper and lower jaws or between jaw and tooth size, resulting in overcrowding of teeth or in abnormal bite patterns.

Variations in size or structure of either jaw may affect its shape, as can birth defects such as cleft lip and palate. Other causes of malocclusion include:

- childhood habits such as thumb sucking, tongue thrusting, pacifier use beyond age 3, and prolonged use of a bottle;

- extra teeth, lost teeth, impacted teeth, or abnormally shaped teeth;

- ill-fitting dental fillings, crowns, appliances, retainers, or braces;

- misalignment of jaw fractures after a severe injury; and

- tumors of the mouth and jaw.

There are different categories of malocclusion.

- Class 1 malocclusion is the most common. The bite is normal, but the upper teeth slightly overlap the lower teeth.

- Class 2 malocclusion, called retrognathism or overbite, occurs when the upper jaw and teeth severely overlap the bottom jaw and teeth.

- Class 3 malocclusion, called prognathism or underbite, occurs when the lower jaw protrudes or juts forward, causing the lower jaw and teeth to overlap the upper jaw and teeth.

Symptoms

- Abnormal alignment of teeth
- Abnormal appearance of the face
- Difficulty or discomfort when biting or chewing
- Speech difficulties (rare) including lisp
- Mouth breathing (breathing through the mouth without closing the lips)

Exams and Tests

Most problems with teeth alignment are discovered by a dentist during a routine exam. The dentist may pull your cheek outward and ask you to bite down to check how well your back teeth come together. If there is any problem, the dentist will usually refer you to an orthodontist for diagnosis and treatment.

Dental x-rays, head or skull x-rays, or facial x-rays may be required. Plaster or plastic molds of the teeth are often needed.

Treatment

Very few people have perfect teeth alignment. However, most problems are so minor that they do not require treatment.

Malocclusion is the most common reason for referral to an orthodontist.

By treating moderate or severe malocclusion, the teeth are easier to clean and there is less risk of tooth decay and periodontal diseases (gingivitis or periodontitis). Treatment eliminates strain on the teeth, jaws, and muscles, which lessens the risk of breaking a tooth and may reduce symptoms of temporomandibular joint disorders.

The goal is to correct the positioning of the teeth. Braces or other appliances may be used. Metal bands are placed around some teeth, or metal, ceramic, or plastic bonds are attached to the surface of the teeth. Wires or springs apply force to the teeth.

One or more teeth may need to be removed if overcrowding is part of the problem. Rough or irregular teeth may be adjusted down, reshaped, and bonded or capped. Misshapen restorations and dental appliances should be repaired. Surgery may be required on rare occasions. This may include surgical reshaping to lengthen or shorten the jaw (orthognathic surgery). Wires, plates, or screws may be used to stabilize the jawbone, in a similar manner to the surgical stabilization of jaw fracture.

It is important to brush and floss your teeth every day and have regular visits to a general dentist. Plaque accumulates on braces and may permanently mark teeth or cause tooth decay if not properly cared for.

Retainers (used to stabilize the teeth) may be required for an indefinite time to maintain the new position of the teeth.

Outlook (Prognosis)

Problems with teeth alignment are easier, quicker, and less expensive to treat when they are corrected early. Treatment is most successful in children and adolescents because their bone is still soft and teeth are moved more easily. Treatment may last 6 months to 2 or more years, depending on the severity of the case.

Treatment of orthodontic disorders in adults is often successful but may require longer use of braces or other devices.

Possible Complications

- Tooth decay
- Discomfort during treatment
- Irritation of mouth and gums (gingivitis) caused by appliances
- Chewing or speaking difficulty during treatment

When to Contact a Medical Professional

Call your orthodontist if toothache, mouth pain, or other new symptoms develop during orthodontic treatment.

Prevention

Many types of malocclusion are not preventable. Control of habits such as thumb sucking may be necessary in some cases. However, early detection and treatment may optimize the time and method of treatment needed.

Chapter 41

Scoliosis

Chapter Contents

Section 41.1

Scoliosis: A Guide for Teens

What is scoliosis?

Scoliosis means that your spine, or backbone, is curved.

What causes scoliosis?

There are different types of scoliosis and different reasons that might cause your spine to curve. The most common type of scoliosis is called idiopathic scoliosis and has no known cause, but does occur more in girls and in families. The back just doesn't grow as straight as it should, and no one knows why. There are also other less common causes of scoliosis. Sometimes, the spine appears to be curved because of a difference in leg length. And rarely, some babies are born with spinal defects that cause the spine to grow unevenly. This last type of scoliosis is called congenital scoliosis.

Who gets scoliosis?

Anyone can get scoliosis. But the most common type of scoliosis, idiopathic scoliosis, usually occurs after age 10. Girls are more likely to develop idiopathic scoliosis then boys are. Check out the list of some famous people with scoliosis.

- Sarah Michelle Gellar—Actress/model

- Janet Evans—Olympic swimmer

- Alexandra Marinescu—Olympic gymnast

- Renee Russo—Actress/model

- Melanie Blatt—All Saints star

- Liza Minelli—Singer/Broadway actress
- Isabella Rossellini—Actress/model
- Chloe Sevigny—Actress
- Daryl Hannah—Actress

Everyone between fifth and ninth grade should be checked for scoliosis by their health care provider. It is especially important to be checked regularly if you have a parent, sister, or brother with scoliosis, since scoliosis can run in families.

How is scoliosis diagnosed?

An examination to check for scoliosis usually includes a physical examination, and sometimes may include an X-ray evaluation and curve measurement.

Physical examination: Your health care provider will look at your back, chest, hips, legs, feet, and skin. He or she will check to see if your shoulders are even, whether your head is centered over your shoulders, and whether opposite sides of your body look even. He or she will also examine your back muscles, while you are bending forward, to see if one side of your rib cage is higher than the other.

If there is a significant asymmetry (a big difference between opposite sides of your body), your health care provider may suggest an x-ray or a referral to an orthopedic spine specialist (a doctor who has experience treating people with scoliosis).

X-ray evaluation: If you have a medium or large spinal curve, unusual back pain, or you still have a lot of growing to do, your health care provider will arrange for you to have an X-ray. You will be asked to stand facing the X-ray machine. An X-ray is a detailed picture of your spine. Your health care provider will be able to see any curves in your spine and can figure out if they need to be watched or treated.

Curve measurement: The doctor measures the curve on the X-ray image. He or she finds your vertebrae at the beginning and end of the curve and measures the angle of the curve. Curves that are greater than 20 degrees may need treatment.

What kinds of treatment are available?

Depending on the location, degree (severity) of the curves, and growth remaining, your health care provider will recommend observation, bracing, or surgery.

Observation: Some curves get worse with growth. Others don't change and some may even get better. Some curves require no treatment. However, your health care provider will want to watch your curve carefully to make sure that it does not get worse as you grow.

Bracing: If your curve is large enough and you are growing, your doctor may recommend a brace. The scoliosis brace is designed for you and your particular curve. It holds your spine in a straighter position, and it helps prevent your curve from getting worse while you are growing. A brace will not make your spine straight, but it can help improve the curve or prevent it from getting worse.

Your doctor will give you specific directions about how to put on your brace, when to wear it, and how long to wear it. The brace needs to be worn for the full number of hours prescribed by your doctor until you finish growing. Generally, braces can be removed for activities such as showering, swimming, and sports. The braces are made of firm plastic and fit closely over the hips. Almost all braces can be hidden beneath clothing, and you can continue to do all athletic activities.

Surgery: Bracing does not work for everyone and every curve. If you have a very large curve or one that does not stop getting worse with a brace, your doctor will probably recommend surgery. There are different types of surgery. Some may be better for your specific curve than other types. The main purpose of scoliosis surgery is to fuse (join together) the bones of your curve. The fusion keeps your spine straight. Your surgeon will talk to you about your options, the different types of surgery, and the different types of implants available. Implants are devices that are inserted during surgery. They remain in your back after surgery and help keep your spine straight.

If you are considering surgery you should be sure to ask your surgeon the following questions:

- What will happen if I don't have surgery?
- What type of surgery will work best for me?
- What implants will be used?
- How straight will my spine be after surgery?
- How long will the operation take?
- What are the risks of this surgery?
- What are the benefits to getting this type of surgery?
- What is the scar like?

- How long will I have to remain in the hospital after the surgery?
- How long will it take to recover?
- When can I start being as active as I was before surgery?
- What permanent restrictions are there on activity?
- Can I talk to another patient/family who had the surgery?

What will happen if I ignore my scoliosis?

After you have been diagnosed with scoliosis, you may not think that treatment is that important. However, it is very important to treat scoliosis since spinal curves can become worse and cause physical changes to your spine. In the worst cases, scoliosis can cause changes in your chest and lungs and difficulty breathing. It is also important to treat curves since treatment is much more successful before curves become severe.

How do I cope with scoliosis?

If you are diagnosed with scoliosis, it doesn't mean you can't live a healthy and active life. Most teens with scoliosis are able to exercise, take part in sports and athletics, drive, and be involved in friendships and relationships.

Teens with scoliosis can do pretty much everything that teens without scoliosis can do. It is also important to remember that if you are diagnosed with scoliosis, it is not your fault. Nothing you did caused the scoliosis, and there is nothing you could have done to prevent it. If you have scoliosis, the important thing is for you and your health care provider to choose and follow the best treatment plan for you.

Section 41.2

Setting Young Spines Straight

For youngsters whose spines are bent with scoliosis, the approaches coming out of Cincinnati Children's Spine Center are nothing short of life-changing.

Early Detection Is Important

Scoliosis often develops unnoticed—and worsens with teenage growth spurts. It is often painless, making detection difficult. That is why many schools provide screenings; if not, your family doctor can check for it. Once detected, a physical and X-rays can determine the extent of the problem. Whether and how to treat it depends on many factors, including a child's age, the nature of the curve, and how much a child may continue to grow. If you suspect your child has curvature in the spine, have it checked out as early as possible.

"We look for early assessment so we can identify the curves that may ultimately require intervention," says Alvin Crawford, MD, director of Cincinnati Children's Spine Center.

Improved, Less Invasive Options

When intervention is necessary, new treatments are available that are more effective and less invasive. Some children can be helped with video-assisted thoracoscopic surgery (VATS). Dr. Crawford is an international authority on this minimally invasive technique, which replaces the 15-inch incision of traditional fusion surgery with four 1-inch incisions on a patient's side.

Other patients may be better suited for growing rods, which reduce the need for braces. "When we diagnose children at 8 or 10 years old," Dr. Crawford says, "they could face 7 or 8 years of bracing. Instead, I can use growing rods with hooks or screws as anchors. These children have a surgery every 6 months or so to lengthen the rods as they grow. This avoids fusion, and children can remain fairly active, living without a brace most of that time."

For other patients, the treatment of choice remains the traditional surgical fusion of vertebrae, stabilizing the spine with a corrective metal rod and hooks or screws. This method helps prevent the progression of scoliosis.

Bracing a Thing of the Past?

Researchers here are re-examining the merits of traditional bracing to realign the spine. Cincinnati Children's is Ohio's only center in the multisite Bracing in Adolescent Idiopathic Scoliosis (AIS) Trial of the National Institutes of Health to study the value of bracing. Researchers are comparing the risk of curve progression in teens with AIS who wear a brace to the risk of those who do not.

A minimally invasive technique developed by spine surgeons here could revolutionize treatment of early onset scoliosis. It eliminates extensive spinal fusion to correct an abnormal curvature. "This new technique staples together the growth plates on the actively growing side of the deformity and allows the other side of the spine to catch up," says Dr. Crawford. The method is currently under review by the Food and Drug Administration and is not yet available to patients.

Other research involves locating the genes responsible for scoliosis and evaluating a less invasive posterior spinal fusion technique.

Morgan's Back

Tammy Cluff had never noticed the curve in her daughter Morgan's back. But after their pediatrician's nurse pointed it out, Tammy could see, especially during cheerleading workouts, that Morgan, then 12, would need help to straighten her spine. "I started noticing that she was always crooked. Nothing I did or she did would straighten her out," Tammy says.

At Cincinnati Children's, orthopedic surgeon and Spine Center director Alvin Crawford, MD, recommended surgery to correct Morgan's severe scoliosis. In February 2007, he inserted two rods next to her spine, fusing the vertebrae to prevent further curvature, and adjusted some ribs below her shoulder blade to help minimize protrusion.

The road to recovery was long: 8 days in the hospital; 6 weeks in a brace full-time and another 4 weeks of wearing a brace at night; a year without sports or jumping of any kind. But Morgan is now an active, 15-year-old high school freshman who will try out for cheerleading later this year.

Delighted with the surgery's results, Morgan and Tammy offer the following suggestions for other families facing scoliosis surgery:

- **Ask your doctor for reliable information sources.** "Dr. Crawford's office gave us all the information we needed, and I did additional research. My goal was to stay positive. I didn't want to hear negative stories," Tammy says.

- **Ask a lot of questions.** Tammy made sure she got answers from Dr. Crawford before the surgery, during the hospitalization, and even now, in Morgan's yearly followup visits.

- **Keep your child involved with friends as much as possible.** "It's hard for a teenager to have such major surgery, because sometimes friends shy away. Try to schedule time often for your child's friends to visit."

- **Find the support you need.** Family, friends and even strangers who recognized she was wearing a brace shared their experiences with scoliosis surgery to help Morgan during her recovery.

Part Five

Emotional, Social, and Mental Health Concerns in Adolescents

Chapter 42

Adolescent Stress

Stress is a common problem among teens, and as a parent, you have a role in helping the teen in your life cope with it. So what exactly is stress? According to the Centers for Disease Control and Prevention (CDC), stress is the body's physical and psychological response to anything perceived as overwhelming. This may be viewed as a result of life's demands—pleasant or unpleasant—and the body's lack of resources to meet them.

While stress is a natural part of life, it often creates imbalance in the body, especially a teen's body, which is already experiencing so many changes. Girls also report feeling "frequently stressed" more than boys.[1] A certain amount of stress can be helpful as a way of keeping your teen motivated. But too much or too little may render them ineffective and interfere with their relationships at home and socially, as well as their physical well-being. According to a recent survey, 43 percent of 13- to 14-year-olds say they feel stressed every single day; by ages 15 to 17, the number rises to 59 percent.[2] The day-to-day pressures teens experience, such as the pressure to fit in and to be successful, can lead to stress. Jobs and family economics can also prove stressful for teens, as nearly two thirds of them say they are "somewhat" or "very concerned" about their personal finances.[3]

If stress becomes unmanageable and teens are left to their own devices without guidance from a parent or caregiver, they may find

From "Teen Stress: Helping Your Teen Cope," by the National Youth Anti-Drug Media Campaign (www.theantidrug.com), 2009.

their own ways of coping. Sometimes these coping mechanisms involve unhealthy behaviors such as drinking, smoking marijuana, and engaging in other risky behaviors.[4] Here's how you can help the teen in your life with healthy, productive coping strategies.

- **Recognize when your teen is stressed out.** Is your teen getting adequate rest? Is he or she eating well-balanced meals? Does he or she ever get to take breaks to restore energy? If these needs are unmet, your teen will show it through chronic moodiness, irritability, anxiety, and/or long bouts of sadness. If you have a teen daughter, be particularly aware if she is obsessing about looks or weight.

- **Introduce positive coping strategies to your teen.** Let's face it, stress will be a part of your teen's life. Help him or her identify ways to relieve stress in a healthy way. It can be as simple as having your teen talk to you about problems or pressures. Other ideas include exercising, getting enough sleep, listening to music, writing in a journal, keeping a healthy diet, seeing a counselor, and reminding your teen of his or her accomplishments.

- **Be a good example.** Young people often pick up their coping strategies by watching their parents. If a child sees a parent drink an alcoholic beverage or smoke a cigarette every time he or she is overwhelmed, he or she is more likely to imitate the same behavior. So, be mindful of your own reactions to stress and set a good example for your children.

If signs of stress persist, ask for help. Some sources you can consult include a health care provider, mental health center, social worker, counselor, nurse, therapist, or clergy.

Warning Signs

Physical symptoms include the following:

- Allergies
- Chronic fatigue
- Racing heartbeat
- Nightmares
- Sleeping problems
- Dizziness

- Change in appetite
- Headaches
- Muscle tension
- Restlessness
- Stomachaches
- Gastrointestinal problems

Emotional symptoms include the following:

- Anger
- Denial of a problem
- Loneliness
- Feeling powerless
- Feeling trapped
- Constant worry
- Anxiety
- Depression
- Nervousness
- Feeling rejected
- Difficulty making decisions
- Being easily upset

References

1. Associated Press/MTV survey, "Academic performance top cause of teen stress." August 23, 2007. http://www.msnbc.msn .com/id/20322801.

2. SADD, Unpublished data from Teens Today survey.

3. TRU 3rd Wave, February 2009.

4. SADD, Unpublished data from Teens Today survey.

Chapter 43

School Pressures

Chapter Contents

Section 43.1

Test Anxiety

Your child went to class, completed homework, and studied. He or she arrived at the exam confident about the material. But if he or she has test anxiety, a type of performance anxiety, taking the test is the most difficult part of the equation.

Causes

- **Fear of failure:** While the pressure to perform can act as a motivator, it can also be devastating to individuals who tie their self-worth to the outcome of a test.

- **Lack of preparation:** Waiting until the last minute or not studying at all can leave individuals feeling anxious and overwhelmed.

- **Poor test history:** Previous problems or bad experiences with test taking can lead to a negative mindset and influence performance on future tests.

Symptoms

- **Physical symptoms:** Headache, nausea, diarrhea, excessive sweating, shortness of breath, rapid heartbeat, light-headedness, and feeling faint can all occur. Test anxiety can lead to a panic attack, which is the abrupt onset of intense fear or discomfort in which individuals may feel like they are unable to breathe or having a heart attack.

- **Emotional symptoms:** Feelings of anger, fear, helplessness, and disappointment are common emotional responses to test anxiety.

- **Behavioral/cognitive symptoms:** Difficulty concentrating, thinking negatively, and comparing yourself to others are common symptoms of test anxiety.

Tips for Managing Test Anxiety

Share these tips with your child if he or she is anxious about an upcoming exam:

- **Be prepared.** Develop good study habits. Study at least a week or two before the exam, in smaller increments of time and over a few days (instead of pulling an "all-nighter"). Try to simulate exam conditions by working through a practice test, following the same time constraints.

- **Develop good test-taking skills.** Read the directions carefully, answer questions you know first, and then return to the more difficult ones. Outline essays before you begin to write.

- **Maintain a positive attitude.** Remember that your self-worth should not be dependent on or defined by a test grade. Creating a system of rewards and reasonable expectations for studying can help to produce effective studying habits. There is no benefit to negative thinking.

- **Stay focused.** Concentrate on the test, not other students during your exams. Try not to talk to other students about the subject material before taking an exam.

- **Practice relaxation techniques.** If you feel stressed during the exam, take deep, slow breaths and consciously relax your muscles, one at a time. This can invigorate your body and will allow you to better focus on the exam.

- **Stay healthy.** Get enough sleep, eat healthy, exercise, and allow for personal time. If you are exhausted—physically or emotionally—it will be more difficult for you to handle stress and anxiety.

- **Visit the counseling center.** Schools are aware of the toll exams can take on students. They have offices or programs specifically dedicated to helping you and providing additional educational support so that you can be successful.

Section 43.2

Cheating

Excerpted from "Cheating: New Alarm about an Old Problem," by the Substance Abuse and Mental Health Services Administration (SAMHSA, family.samhsa.gov), part of the U.S. Department of Health and Human Services, September 6, 2006.

Stealing answers or copying someone else's work—some students probably have cheated since schools started handing out grades. While cheating may be nothing new, it has become more common and often uses new technology. Parents and school officials face the hard question of what to do about dishonesty and the shortcuts to success that many students take.

Most students cheat. In nationwide surveys on college campuses, about seven in 10 students admitted to some cheating. Three in five high school students admitted that they had cheated on an exam, and more than four in five admitted copying another student's homework in the past 12 months.

Many students see the world as a harsh place where people do whatever it takes to get ahead. If young people believe that cheating can make the difference between winning and losing in life, they may see little reason not to take the "easy route."

New Methods

The old ways of cheating—using crib notes, whispering answers, and copying homework—are alive and well. Some students don't bother cheating at their desks—instead, they make sure to be absent on test day so they can get the questions from friends before taking a makeup exam. These simple schemes still account for a large share of today's cheating.

However, cheating also has gone high-tech. Students seeking an edge in their schoolwork are taking cheating to new levels using computers, cell phones, personal digital assistants (PDAs), and powerful calculators. At home or in computer labs, students can find conclusions, well-written text, and even whole term papers to drop into their assignments without showing where the work came from. In class, students can use phones and PDAs to retrieve stored information, get it from the internet, or send it to a friend. During an exam, one student can send a friend the answers while they both take the test.

High-tech cheating creates a vicious circle. As technology advances and students get better at using the latest devices, teachers and school officials find it harder to keep up with cheaters. The more that cheating goes uncaught, the freer students feel to do it.

Many Reasons

Why do so many students cheat? Is it because they are lazy or the subject matter is hard to grasp? While these motives surely fuel much of the cheating among students, the problem is not confined to low-achieving and unmotivated students. Boys, girls, athletes, smart kids, student leaders, and those with "strong religious beliefs"—cheating is common among most types of students.

- **A need to succeed:** Pressure for grades—to win parents' approval and gain admission to colleges—leads many students to cheat. While many students are pushed to succeed by parents and a grade-based system that starts naming winners at an early age, students also feel pulled by a desire to get on a path to top colleges and high-paying jobs.

- **Hazy standards:** You may think that cheating is a clear matter of right and wrong—a student's work should be his own. Yet, for many students, cheating is a fuzzy idea. Some think it is okay to work together on an assignment. Confusion rises as schools and teachers emphasize teamwork. The ease of finding information on the internet and pasting it into one's homework also blurs the line between research and lifting someone else's words. One study found that three in 10 college students saw nothing wrong with this practice.

- **Lack of time:** Getting up early to get to school, staying late with teams and clubs, having a job, and doing homework at night means a full schedule for many teens. As a result, they may be tempted to cheat to give themselves more time for a social life or to sleep.

- **Lack of interest:** Some students may cheat because they simply don't like schoolwork, but for many, the decision to cut corners may be more subtle. A student who is interested in math may not care much about history. Another—attracted to art, literature, or languages—may not be inclined to put much effort into a science class. As a result, a student who is bored by a subject or thinks it has no bearing on her life may view cheating as a harmless way to save time and avoid a headache while getting a better grade.

Needed Answers

So what can parents do to stem the tide of cheating? Starting at preschool age, parents can teach their kids the value of honesty—explaining it, expecting it, and demonstrating it. Providing youth with the tools to make good decisions will make students less likely to cheat. Emphasizing that learning is a steppingstone—rather than a detour—on the road to success can help a student to rely on his own effort. Besides, cheating to get a good grade can backfire when a child is expected to know something that he never learned or didn't bother to memorize.

Still, messages about the meaning of honor and knowledge may mean little to young people who fear being left behind by peers who are willing to play the cheating game. Getting a student to stay on the path of honesty is more likely when parents practice what they preach about the value of learning by easing off on pressure for high grades, honors classes, and admission to top colleges. Parents also can help without doing their child's assignments—this only fosters the idea that it is okay to get a good grade when someone else does the work.

Both parents and educators can step up their efforts to uncover cheating. Parents can become savvy about what wireless devices can do and what resources are available on the internet. Checking the websites a student visits and reviewing his work to see if it looks too polished can cut down on cheating and provide opportunities to address it.

Educators are becoming more aware of the latest cheating methods and are responding with technology such as software that matches the text in student papers against material available on the internet.

However, guarding against cheating must go hand in hand with clear standards about what cheating includes. Honor codes (a pledge to be honest) also can help. Yet, while honor codes call for doing the right thing, they may not give students a clear idea of why honesty matters.

School staff and parents may get students to pay more attention to their pleas for truth by appealing to students' sense of fairness. Showing that cheating threatens an equal shot at success for everyone can give new meaning to an idea that many students may find hard to apply.

In sum, cheating in school is widespread, aided by technology, and often seen by students as normal or even necessary. As a result, parents must be alert to cheating and start early in teaching their children about fairness and showing them that honesty is worth the effort.

Section 43.3

Helping Your Child Feel Connected to School

From "Helping Your Child Feel Connected to School," by the Centers for Disease Control and Prevention (CDC, www.cdc.gov), July 2009.

As a parent, you want your child to do well in school. You also want your child to be healthy and avoid behaviors that are risky or harmful. Through your guidance and support, you can have great influence on your child's health and learning. But you also have important allies in this effort—the caring adults in your child's school.

Research shows that students who feel a genuine sense of belonging at school are more likely to do well in school, stay in school, and make healthy choices. This sense of belonging is often described as school connectedness. Connected students believe their parents, teachers, school staff, and other students in their school care about them and about how well they are learning.

Why is it important for your child to feel connected to school?

Scientists who study youth health and behavior have learned that strong connections at school can help young people:

- get better grades;
- have higher test scores;
- stay in school longer; and
- attend school more regularly.

In addition, students who feel connected to their school are less likely to:

- smoke cigarettes;
- drink alcohol;
- have sexual intercourse;
- carry a weapon or become involved in violence;

- be injured from drinking and driving or not wearing seat belts;
- have emotional distress or eating disorders; or
- consider or attempt suicide.

What can you do to increase your child's connection to school?

Here are some actions that you can take, at home and at school, to help your child become more connected to his or her school.

1. Encourage your child to talk openly with you, teachers, counselors, and other school staff about his or her ideas, needs, and worries.

2. Find out what the school expects your child to learn and how your child should behave in school by talking to teachers and staff, attending school meetings, and reading information the school sends home. Then, support these expectations at home.

3. Help your child with homework, and teach your child how to use his or her time well. Make sure your child has the tools—books, supplies, a quiet place to work—he or she needs to do homework at home, at the library, or at an afterschool program.

4. Encourage your child to help adults at home, at school, and in the community, such as helping with chores, serving as a library aide, volunteering at a hospital or clinic, or tutoring younger students after school.

5. Read school newsletters, attend parent-teacher-student conferences, and check out the school's website to learn what is going on at the school. Encourage your child to participate in school activities.

6. Meet regularly with your child's teachers to discuss his or her grades, behavior, and accomplishments.

7. Ask teachers if your child can participate in or lead parent-teacher conferences.

8. As your schedule allows, help in your child's classroom, attend afterschool events, or participate in a school committee, such as a health team or parent organization. Ask whether your school offers babysitting or transportation for parents who need them.

9. Offer to share important aspects of your culture with your child's class.

10. If your first language is not English, ask for materials that are translated into the language you speak at home, and ask for interpreters to help you at school events.

11. Learn whether community organizations provide dental services, health screenings, child care, or health promotion programs at school. If not, advocate having those services offered at your school or in your school district.

12. Get involved with your child's school to help plan school policies and school-wide activities.

13. Ask whether your school or school district provides—or could offer—programs or classes to help you become more involved in your child's academic and school life. For example, the school or school district might offer:

    • training to help you talk with your child and to help manage his or her behavior;

    • programs to help you to talk with your child's teachers and help your child learn;

    • educational programs for parents by telephone or online; or

    • general education development (GED), English as a second language, or other classes to help you work better with your child and with the adults at school.

14. Talk with teachers and school staff to suggest simple changes that can make the school a more pleasant and welcoming place. For example, the school might decorate the eating area with student-made posters, allow families to use the school gym or other facilities during out-of-school times, or create a place in the school or on school grounds for kids and families to socialize.

Chapter 44

Adolescent Social Development and Concerns

Chapter Contents

Section 44.1

Developing Friendships: Tips to Help Your Child

From "Making Friends in School," by the Substance Abuse and Mental Health Services Administration (SAMHSA, family.samhsa.gov), part of the U.S. Department of Health and Human Services, August 28, 2008.

Making good grades probably tops your list of goals for your middle or high school student, but making friends is also important. Middle or high school is a new chapter in your child's life. She's moving away from childhood and into the beginning of adolescence. Your child's friends will help shape many of her values and actions—including what your daughter thinks about alcohol and whether she drinks before her 21st birthday.

Fitting In

As children approach adolescence, friends and "fitting in" often become very important. Young teens increasingly look to friends and the media for clues on how to behave, and many begin to question adults' values and rules. Children want to be noticed and accepted by their fellow students. Peer acceptance often is one factor in your child's choice about whether to use alcohol, tobacco, and drugs. If your child wants to be part of a group that steers clear of harmful substances, odds are she'll choose to be drug free, too. But if your child wants to be part of a group that uses alcohol, tobacco, or drugs, she may try them in order to fit in with that group.

Feeling Good

Your child is more likely to make wise choices when she feels good about herself, so help your child build her self-esteem. When she succeeds or has made a great choice, tell her you're proud of her. When she does not succeed, help her feel better and urge her to keep trying. Your student is going through many changes and may feel like she isn't "good enough" or doesn't measure up. Building her self-esteem will help her feel more confident and will make it easier for her to form healthy friendships.

Clueing In

You also can help your child by being a good listener and spending time with him. Talk with your child every day and listen to his concerns. Stay clued in about what's going on in your child's world. Give him your full attention when he talks, and really listen to what he has to say. Be open to exploring different activities with your child to find something that she enjoys. She might like programs at a local museum or art gallery, or perhaps she has other interests that can be expanded.

Helping Out

You cannot choose your child's friends for him, but you can help him learn to choose friends wisely. You can give him tools to find friends who do not drink alcohol and who will have a positive impact on him. Some ways you can help your middle or high schooler to choose and make friends include the following:

- Discuss with your child the qualities in a friend that matter most, such as being trustworthy and kind, and making good choices when it comes to steering clear of risky behaviors.

- Help your child make plans with potential friends. Urge him to invite them over to study in the evening or watch a movie on the weekend. If a child needs a ride to your house or an activity, be willing to pick him up. Not only will your child begin to develop friendships, but you'll be able to keep an eye on their activities and get to know his friends.

- Introduce your child to new groups of people who share her interests. After-school clubs, faith-based activities, and sports programs are good places for meeting new people. The more teens participate in school-based, community-based, church- or faith-based activities, the less likely they are to use cigarettes, alcohol, or illicit drugs.

- Don't judge your child's choice of friends without talking with them and finding out what they like to do—and whether it's illegal, unsafe, or risky. Looks can be deceiving, so try not to judge your child's friends based on how they dress.

- Get to know the friends' parents. In this way, you can create a "network" of parents whom you trust to monitor your child when he is at his friends' houses.

- Warn your child about instant messaging (IM), text messaging, or e-mails. Whatever is sent electronically can be sent to other children, so they shouldn't participate in bullying or gossip, or send private or personal information.

Making friends in school is important to your child, so let her know it's important to you, too. Giving your child your support will boost her confidence and help her develop positive friendships.

Section 44.2

Cliques

"The Ins and Outs of Teen Cliques" is reprinted with permission from the Cincinnati Children's Hospital Medical Center website, http://www.cincinnati childrens.org. © 2005 Cincinnati Children's Hospital Medical Center. All rights reserved. Reviewed by David A. Cooke, MD, FACP, March 16, 2010.

When it comes to fierce hierarchy in social packs, teenagers could teach wolves a thing or two.

Every parent recalls the thrill of being in the in crowd or the pain of being on the outside. Many find it difficult to watch their own children go through this signature turmoil of adolescence.

"Teenagers need a sense of belonging to a peer group," says Paul Chirlin, MD, a pediatrician at Springdale Mason Pediatrics. "The job of adolescence is to break the parent-child link and create more peer links and community involvement."

"Teenagers have always tended to gather with like-minded peers, and that's not unhealthy. Every teen needs peer support. The issue is whether that group is seen as positive or negative, and if it's exclusionary."

Assessing the Group

While the word "clique" may be negative, the alternative "club" can be positive. "Think of the anti-smoking club or Key Club, dedicated to community service," says Dr. Chirlin.

"Teens may have tattoos, piercings, and different hairdos, but don't jump to quick assumptions. Determine first if the group is exerting positive peer pressure or negative," he advises.

"Look at your child's friends: When are they out, where are they going, what are they doing? Find out about their parents, if possible. Ask about the group's values, and hope that your child will answer honestly. Reinforce that it's good to have peer support."

Warning bells go off, however, when a peer group accepts some teens and rejects others because of class, religion, race, or appearance, and requires members to dislike people dissimilar to them.

"This is very destructive, because it reinforces negative stereotypes," says Dr. Chirlin. "Also, our social conscience is formed when we're young, and it's hard to change the way we feel about certain people when we're adults. It's isolating behavior, so that the friends we have when we're older will be the same friends we had in high school."

When It's Time to Step In

Most alarming is a peer group that requires behaviors with permanent negative consequences, such as those involving drugs, teen pregnancy, or crimes. "Parents should lay down the law and push for the child to find some other friends," he says.

More often, teens struggle with the age-old divisions among the nerds, geeks, jocks, and cheerleaders. If a child tries to join one of the established groups and is rejected, the pain is very real.

"It's important to let teens express disappointment and anger," Dr. Chirlin says. "Then, you can point out all the things they do well and all the good friends they've had over the years. It's important, too, that teens learn that rejection is a part of life, and learning to accept disappointment is part of growing up."

Spurred on by rejection, some teens work harder to make a sports team or academic society. Parents also can encourage a rebuffed child to find opportunities in other groups that would be more egalitarian.

"Suggest a service or religious organization that is open to all comers, such as Habitat for Humanity, environmental groups, and Key Club at school," he advises.

If, however, a daughter is only interested in being a cheerleader and didn't make the squad, "There's little you can do except say you love her, give her a big hug and tell her that tomorrow will be a better day," says Dr. Chirlin. "Parents generally do a very good job at this."

Section 44.3

Peer Pressure

Excerpted from "Peer Pressure," by the National Institute on Alcohol Abuse and Alcoholism (NIAAA, www.niaaa.nih.gov), part of the National Institutes of Health. This text is undated. Reviewed by David A. Cooke, MD, FACP, April 4, 2010.

Your classmates keep asking you to have them over because you have a pool, everyone at school is wearing silly hats so you do, too, and your best friend begs you to go running with her because you both need more exercise, so you go, too. These are all examples of peer pressure. Don't get it yet?

- Pressure is the feeling that you are being pushed toward making a certain choice—good or bad.

- A peer is someone in your own age group.

- Peer pressure is—you guessed it—the feeling that someone your own age is pushing you toward making a certain choice, good or bad.

Why Peer Pressure Can Work

Have you ever given in to pressure? Like when a friend begs to borrow something you don't want to give up or to do something your parents say is off limits? Chances are you probably have given into pressure at sometime in your life.

How did it feel to give into pressure? If you did something you wish you hadn't, then most likely you didn't feel too good about it. You might have felt the following:

- Sad

- Anxious

- Guilty

- Like a wimp or pushover

- Disappointed in yourself

Everyone gives in to pressure at one time or another, but why do people sometimes do things that they really don't want to do? Here are a few reasons:

- They are afraid of being rejected by others.
- They want to be liked and don't want to lose a friend.
- They want to appear grown-up.
- They don't want to be made fun of.
- They don't want to hurt someone's feelings.
- They aren't sure of what they really want.
- They don't know how to get out of the situation.

When you face pressure you can stand your ground.

How Peers Pressure

Almost everyone faces peer pressure once in a while. Friends have a big influence on our lives, but sometimes they push us to do things that we may not want to do. Unless you want to give in every time you face this, you're going to need to learn how to handle it.

The first step to standing up to peer pressure is to understand it.

Peer Pressure Can Be Good

Peer pressure isn't all bad. You and your friends can pressure each other into some things that will improve your health and social life and make you feel good about your decisions.

Think of a time when a friend pushed you to do something good for yourself or to avoid something that would've been bad.

Here are some good things friends can pressure each other to do:

- Be honest.
- Avoid alcohol.
- Avoid drugs.
- Not smoke.
- Be nice.
- Respect others.
- Work hard.
- Exercise (together!).

You and your friends can also use good peer pressure to help each other resist bad peer pressure.

If you see a friend taking some heat, try some of these lines:

- We don't want to drink.
- We don't need to drink to have fun.
- Let's go and do something else.
- Leave her alone. She said she didn't want any.

The Right to Resist

If someone is pressuring you to do anything that's not right or good for you, you have the right to resist. You have the right to say no, the right not to give a reason why, and the right to just walk away from a situation.

Resisting pressure can be hard for some people. Why?

- They are afraid of being rejected by others.
- They want to be liked and don't want to lose a friend.
- They don't want to be made fun of.
- They don't want to hurt someone's feelings.
- They aren't sure of what they really want.
- They don't know how to get out of the situation.

Sometimes resisting isn't easy, but you can do it with practice and a little know-how. Keep trying, even if you don't get it right at first.

Quick tips on resisting pressure:

- Say no and let them know you mean it.
- Stand up straight.
- Make eye contact.
- Say how you feel.
- Don't make excuses.
- Stick up for yourself.

Resisting Spoken Pressure

Spoken pressure—when someone pressures you with words—can be difficult to resist. Most people don't want to risk making others feel bad, but it's important to stand up for yourself. Check out these strategies for dealing with spoken pressure.

Do the following:

- Say no assertively.
- Stay alcohol free.
- Suggest something else to do.
- Stand up for others.
- Walk away from the situation.
- Find something else to do with other friends.

Don't

- Attend a party unprepared to resist alcohol
- Be afraid to say no
- Mumble
- Say no too aggressively
- Act like a know-it-all when saying no

Resisting Unspoken Pressure

Sometimes you can feel pressure just from watching how others act or dress, without them saying a word to you. This "unspoken pressure" is especially hard to resist, because instead of standing up to a friend, you're standing up to how you feel inside.

Unspoken pressure may come from role models like your parents, your older siblings, teachers, coaches, or celebrities you see in movies and on TV. Unspoken pressure may also come from peers—your friends or other people your age.

Here are some tips for resisting unspoken pressure:

- Take a reality check—most teens don't drink.
- Remember it's risky—alcohol can be dangerous.
- Walk away from the situation.
- Find something else to do with other friends.

Chapter 45

Facts about Mental Health Disorders in Youth

Mental health is an essential component of young peoples' overall health and wellbeing. It affects how young people think, feel, and act; their ability to learn and engage in relationships; their self-esteem and ability to evaluate situations, options, and make choices. A person's mental health influences their ability to handle stress, relate to other people, and make decisions.

Many people experience mental health problems at some time during their lives. At least one in five children and adolescents may express a mental health problem in any year and in the United States, it is estimated that one in 10 children and adolescents suffer from mental illness severe enough to cause some level of impairment. However, in any given year, it is estimated that fewer than one in five of such children receives needed treatment.

When young people's mental health problems go untreated, they can affect their development, school performance, and relationships. The state of their mental health affects how they view themselves and others, how they evaluate and react to situations, and what choices they make and actions they take. Because mental health problems can affect a young person's judgment, in the rare case, emotional disturbances and mental disorders can be a risk factor for violence.

From "Child and Adolescent Mental Health Fact Sheet," from the National Youth Violence Prevention Resource Center (www.safeyouth.org), February 26, 2008.

Overview

Mental health problems include all diagnosable emotional, behavioral, and mental disorders. Behavioral and mental disorders can create a chain of events contributing to violent or suicidal behavior. Particularly if not recognized and treated, these problems may affect a young person's self-esteem, ability to maintain relationships, and their success in school. It is the co-occurrence of behavioral and mental disorders that can be most risky—for example, antisocial conduct co-existing with depression—that may result in violent or suicidal behavior. Left unaddressed, early mental health issues may also develop into severe problems in the adult years.

Risk Factors

Mental health problems in children and adolescents can be caused by biological factors, environmental factors, or their combination.

Biological causes may include genetics, chemical imbalances in the body, and damage to the central nervous system. The relationship of genes to mental health is complex. Researchers have not yet isolated all of the genes that might contribute to vulnerability for specific mental disorders, or determined how environmental factors might trigger that vulnerability.

Family violence is an example of an environmental factor that can increase the possibility of developing a serious behavioral disorder. For example, a young person's exposure to childhood victimization such as child abuse and neglect places them at increased risk for delinquency, adult criminality, and violent criminal behavior.

Prevention and Intervention

Results from a government-funded study find that a nurturing social environment in childhood, good early education, and academic success in school are related to protecting the mental health of youth. The influence of peers is also critical. Having delinquent or antisocial friends may increase the likelihood of developing emotional or behavioral problems. Therefore, placing delinquent or antisocial youth together—as is done in many current youth programs—may, in fact, worsen problems. In fact, many effective intervention models are designed to separate youth with problem behaviors and/or surround troubled youth with peers who do not have behavior problems. It also suggests that increased adult or parental supervision can serve as a preventative measure. With more supervision, youth are less likely to socialize with delinquent peers who can affect their behavior.

Treatment

An estimated one in five of all young people with mental disorders are not receiving any treatment. This is a result of several factors. Most often, children's and adolescents' mental health problems are not recognized or diagnosed properly, and effective treatment is not employed.

Children and adolescents with mental health problems are most often handled by the school or juvenile justice systems, which are generally ill-equipped to recognize and address mental disorders. Recent studies have indicated that between 70 and 80 percent of children with diagnosable mental disorders who receive mental health services are served within the school system, primarily by school psychologists and guidance counselors.

A number of treatment models have been found to be effective in addressing mental health problems of children and adolescents. These prevention and intervention strategies, however, are often underutilized. While they can require significant time and investment, many prevention and intervention models are economically efficient when compared to the cost mental health problems exact from youth, their families, and communities.

Research supported by the National Institutes of Mental Health (NIMH) has found that successful programs involve long-term intense interventions and address an array of factors such as family conflict, depression, social isolation, school failure, substance abuse, delinquency, and violence.

In treating serious offending delinquents, research has found two treatment models successful. One is multi-systemic therapy (MST), in which specially trained therapists work with the youth and family in their home, with a particular focus on changing the peers with whom the young people associate. MST therapists identify strengths in the family and use these strengths to develop natural support systems and to improve parenting.

The other model is therapeutic foster care. This model offers a community-based intervention for serious and chronic offending delinquents. Therapeutic foster parents are carefully selected and supported with research-based procedures for working with serious and chronic delinquents in their homes.

Chapter 46

Treating Mental Health Disorders in Teens

Research shows that half of all lifetime cases of mental illness begin by age 14. Scientists are discovering that changes in the body leading to mental illness may start much earlier, before any symptoms appear.

Through greater understanding of when and how fast specific areas of children's brains develop, we are learning more about the early stages of a wide range of mental illnesses that appear later in life. Helping teens and their parents manage difficulties early in life may prevent the development of disorders. Once mental illness develops, it becomes a regular part of your teen's behavior and more difficult to treat. Even though we know how to treat (though not yet cure) many disorders, many teens with mental illnesses are not getting treatment.

What should I do if I am concerned about mental, behavioral, or emotional symptoms in my teen?

Talk to your child's doctor or health care provider. Ask questions and learn everything you can about the behavior or symptoms that worry you. Ask the teacher if your child has been showing worrisome changes in behavior. Share this with your child's doctor or health care provider. Keep in mind that every teen is different. Ask if your child needs further evaluation by a specialist with experience in child behavioral problems.

Excerpted from "Treatment of Children with Mental Illness," by the National Institute of Mental Health (NIMH, www.nimh.nih.gov), part of the National Institutes of Health, 2009.

Specialists may include psychiatrists, psychologists, social workers, psychiatric nurses, and behavioral therapists. Educators may also help evaluate your child.

If you take your child to a specialist, ask, "Do you have experience treating the problems I see in my child?" Don't be afraid to interview more than one specialist to find the right fit. Continue to learn everything you can about the problem or diagnosis. The more you learn, the better you can work with your child's doctor and make decisions that feel right for you, your child, and your family.

How do I know if my teen's problems are serious?

Not every problem is serious. In fact, many everyday stresses can cause changes in your child's behavior. It is important to be able to tell the difference between typical behavior changes and those associated with more serious problems. Pay special attention to behaviors that include the following:

- Problems across a variety of settings, such as at school, at home, or with peers
- Changes in appetite or sleep
- Social withdrawal, or fearful behavior toward things your child normally is not afraid of
- Signs of being upset, such as sadness or tearfulness
- Signs of self-destructive behavior
- Repeated thoughts of death

Can symptoms be caused by a death in the family, illness in a parent, family financial problems, divorce, or other events?

Yes. Every member of a family is affected by tragedy or extreme stress. It's normal for stress to cause a teen to be upset. Remember this if you see mental, emotional, or behavioral symptoms in your child. If it takes more than one month for your teen to get used to a situation, or if your teen has severe reactions, talk to your child's doctor.

Check your teen's response to stress. Take note if he or she gets better with time or if professional care is needed. Stressful events are challenging, but they give you a chance to teach your child important ways to cope.

Will my teen get better with time?

Some teens get better with time. But other teens need ongoing professional help. Talk to your child's doctor or specialist about problems that are severe, continuous, and affect daily activities. Also, don't delay seeking help. Treatment may produce better results if started early.

What are psychotropic medications?

Psychotropic medications are substances that affect brain chemicals related to mood and behavior. In recent years, research has been conducted to understand the benefits and risks of using psychotropics in children and teens. Still, more needs to be learned about the effects of psychotropics. While researchers are trying to clarify how early treatment affects a growing body, families and doctors should weigh the benefits and risks of medication. Each teen has individual needs, and each teen needs to be monitored closely while taking medications.

Are there treatments other than medications?

Yes. Psychosocial therapies can be very effective alone and in combination with medications. Psychosocial therapies are also called "talk therapies" or "behavioral therapy," and they help people with mental illness change behavior. Therapies that teach parents and children coping strategies can also be effective.

Cognitive behavioral therapy (CBT) is a type of psychotherapy that can be used with teens. It has been widely studied and is an effective treatment for a number of conditions, such as depression, obsessive-compulsive disorder, and social anxiety. A person in CBT learns to change distorted thinking patterns and unhealthy behavior. Teens can receive CBT with or without their parents, as well as in a group setting. CBT can be adapted to fit the needs of each teen. It is especially useful when treating anxiety disorders.

Additionally, therapies for ADHD are numerous and include behavioral parent training and behavioral classroom management. Some teens benefit from a combination of different psychosocial approaches. An example is behavioral parent management training in combination with CBT for the teen. In other cases, a combination of medication and psychosocial therapies may be most effective. Psychosocial therapies often take time, effort, and patience. However, sometimes teens learn new skills that may have positive long-term benefits.

How should medication be included in an overall treatment plan?

Medication should be used with other treatments. It should not be the only treatment. Consider other services, such as family therapy, family support services, educational classes, and behavior management techniques. If your child's doctor prescribes medication, he or she should evaluate your child regularly to make sure the medication is working. Teens need treatment plans tailored to their individual problems and needs.

What medications are used for which kinds of childhood mental disorders?

Psychotropic medications include stimulants, antidepressants, anti-anxiety medications, antipsychotics, and mood stabilizers. Dosages approved by the U.S. Food and Drug Administration (FDA) for use in children and teens depend on body weight and age.

What else can I do to help my teen?

Teens with mental illness need guidance and understanding from their parents and teachers. This support can help your child achieve his or her full potential and succeed in school. Before a teen is diagnosed, frustration, blame, and anger may have built up within a family. Parents and teens may need special help to undo these unhealthy interaction patterns. Mental health professionals can counsel the child and family to help everyone develop new skills, attitudes, and ways of relating to each other.

Parents can also help by taking part in parenting skills training. This helps parents learn how to handle difficult situations and behaviors. Training encourages parents to share a pleasant or relaxing activity with their teen, to notice and point out what their teen does well, and to praise their teen's strengths and abilities. Parents may also learn to arrange family situations in more positive ways. Also, parents may benefit from learning stress-management techniques to help them deal with frustration and respond calmly to their child's behavior.

Sometimes, the whole family may need counseling. Therapists can help family members find better ways to handle disruptive behaviors and encourage behavior changes. Finally, support groups help parents and families connect with others who have similar problems and concerns. Groups often meet regularly to share frustrations and successes, to exchange information about recommended specialists and strategies, and to talk with experts.

Where can I go for help?

If you are unsure where to go for help, ask your family doctor. Others who can help include the following:

- Mental health specialists, such as psychiatrists, psychologists, social workers, or mental health counselors
- Health maintenance organizations
- Community mental health centers
- Hospital psychiatry departments and outpatient clinics
- Mental health programs at universities or medical schools
- State hospital outpatient clinics
- Family services, social agencies, or clergy
- Peer support groups
- Private clinics and facilities
- Employee assistance programs
- Local medical and/or psychiatric societies

You can also check the phone book under "mental health," "health," "social services," "hotlines," or "physicians" for phone numbers and addresses. An emergency room doctor can also provide temporary help and can tell you where and how to get further help. More information on mental health is at the NIMH website at www.nimh.nih.gov. For the latest information on medications, see the U.S. Food and Drug Administration website at www.fda.gov.

Chapter 47

Depression

Chapter Contents

Section 47.1

Depression in Teens

Excerpted from "Depression," by the National Institute of Mental Health (NIMH, www.nimh.nih.gov), part of the National Institutes of Health, October 2, 2009.

Everyone occasionally feels blue or sad, but these feelings are usually fleeting and pass within a couple of days. When a person has a depressive disorder, it interferes with daily life, normal functioning, and causes pain for both the person with the disorder and those who care about him or her. Depression is a common but serious illness, and most who experience it need treatment to get better.

Many people with a depressive illness never seek treatment. But the vast majority, even those with the most severe depression, can get better with treatment. Intensive research into the illness has resulted in the development of medications, psychotherapies, and other methods to treat people with this disabling disorder.

What are the different forms of depression?

There are several forms of depressive disorders. The most common are major depressive disorder and dysthymic disorder.

Major depressive disorder, also called major depression, is characterized by a combination of symptoms that interfere with a person's ability to work, sleep, study, eat, and enjoy once-pleasurable activities. Major depression is disabling and prevents a person from functioning normally. An episode of major depression may occur only once in a person's lifetime, but more often, it recurs throughout a person's life.

Dysthymic disorder, also called dysthymia, is characterized by long-term (two years or longer) but less severe symptoms that may not disable a person but can prevent one from functioning normally or feeling well. People with dysthymia may also experience one or more episodes of major depression during their lifetimes.

Some forms of depressive disorder exhibit slightly different characteristics than those described above, or they may develop under unique circumstances. However, not all scientists agree on how to characterize and define these forms of depression. They include the following:

- **Psychotic depression** occurs when a severe depressive illness is accompanied by some form of psychosis, such as a break with reality, hallucinations, and delusions.

- **Postpartum depression** is diagnosed if a new mother develops a major depressive episode within 1 month after delivery. It is estimated that 10% to 15% of women experience postpartum depression after giving birth.

- **Seasonal affective disorder (SAD)** is characterized by the onset of a depressive illness during the winter months, when there is less natural sunlight. The depression generally lifts during spring and summer. SAD may be effectively treated with light therapy, but nearly half of those with SAD do not respond to light therapy alone. Antidepressant medication and psychotherapy can reduce SAD symptoms, either alone or in combination with light therapy.

What are the symptoms of depression?

People with depressive illnesses do not all experience the same symptoms. The severity, frequency, and duration of symptoms will vary depending on the individual and his or her particular illness.

- Persistent sad, anxious, or "empty feelings

- Feelings of hopelessness and/or pessimism

- Feelings of guilt, worthlessness, and/or helplessness

- Irritability and restlessness

- Loss of interest in activities or hobbies once pleasurable, including sex

- Fatigue and decreased energy

- Difficulty concentrating, remembering details, and making decisions

- Insomnia, early morning wakefulness, or excessive sleeping

- Overeating or appetite loss

- Thoughts of suicide or suicide attempts

- Persistent aches or pains, headaches, and cramps or digestive problems that do not ease even with treatment

How do children and adolescents experience depression?

Scientists and doctors have begun to take seriously the risk of depression in children. Research has shown that childhood depression often persists, recurs, and continues into adulthood, especially if it goes untreated. The presence of childhood depression also tends to be a predictor of more severe illnesses in adulthood.

A child with depression may pretend to be sick, refuse to go to school, cling to a parent, or worry that a parent may die. Older children may sulk, get into trouble at school, be negative and irritable, and feel misunderstood. Because these signs may be viewed as normal mood swings typical of children as they move through developmental stages, it may be difficult to accurately diagnose a young person with depression.

Before puberty, boys and girls are equally likely to develop depressive disorders. By age 15, however, girls are twice as likely as boys to have experienced a major depressive episode.

Depression in adolescence comes at a time of great personal change—when boys and girls are forming an identity distinct from their parents, grappling with gender issues and emerging sexuality, and making decisions for the first time in their lives. Depression in adolescence frequently co-occurs with other disorders such as anxiety, disruptive behavior, eating disorders, or substance abuse. It can also lead to increased risk for suicide.

An NIMH-funded clinical trial of 439 adolescents with major depression found that a combination of medication and psychotherapy was the most effective treatment option. Other NIMH-funded researchers are developing and testing ways to prevent suicide in children and adolescents, including early diagnosis and treatment, and a better understanding of suicidal thinking.

How is depression detected and treated?

Depression, even the most severe cases, is a highly treatable disorder. As with many illnesses, the earlier that treatment can begin, the more effective it is and the greater the likelihood that recurrence can be prevented.

The first step to getting appropriate treatment is to visit a doctor. Certain medications, and some medical conditions such as viruses or a thyroid disorder, can cause the same symptoms as depression. A doctor can rule out these possibilities by conducting a physical examination, interview, and lab tests. If the doctor can eliminate a medical condition as a cause, he or she should conduct a psychological evaluation or refer the patient to a mental health professional.

The doctor or mental health professional will conduct a complete diagnostic evaluation. He or she should discuss any family history of depression, and get a complete history of symptoms, e.g., when they started, how long they have lasted, their severity, and whether they have occurred before and if so, how they were treated. He or she should also ask if the patient is using alcohol or drugs, and whether the patient is thinking about death or suicide.

Once diagnosed, a person with depression can be treated with a number of methods. The most common treatments are medication and psychotherapy.

Despite the relative safety and popularity of selective serotonin reuptake inhibitors (SSRIs) and other antidepressants, some studies have suggested that they may have unintentional effects on some people, especially adolescents and young adults. In 2004, the Food and Drug Administration (FDA) conducted a thorough review of published and unpublished controlled clinical trials of antidepressants that involved nearly 4,400 children and adolescents. The review revealed that 4% of those taking antidepressants thought about or attempted suicide (although no suicides occurred), compared to 2% of those receiving placebos.

This information prompted the FDA, in 2005, to adopt a "black box" warning label on all antidepressant medications to alert the public about the potential increased risk of suicidal thinking or attempts in children and adolescents taking antidepressants. In 2007, the FDA proposed that makers of all antidepressant medications extend the warning to include young adults up through age 24. A "black box" warning is the most serious type of warning on prescription drug labeling.

The warning emphasizes that patients of all ages taking antidepressants should be closely monitored, especially during the initial weeks of treatment. Possible side effects to look for are worsening depression, suicidal thinking or behavior, or any unusual changes in behavior such as sleeplessness, agitation, or withdrawal from normal social situations. The warning adds that families and caregivers should also be told of the need for close monitoring and report any changes to the physician. The latest information from the FDA can be found on their website at www.fda.gov.

Results of a comprehensive review of pediatric trials conducted between 1988 and 2006 suggested that the benefits of antidepressant medications likely outweigh their risks to children and adolescents with major depression and anxiety disorders. The study was funded in part by the National Institute of Mental Health.

Also, the FDA issued a warning that combining an SSRI or serotonin–norepinephrine reuptake inhibitor (SNRI) antidepressant with one of the commonly used triptan medications for migraine headache could cause a life-threatening "serotonin syndrome," marked by agitation, hallucinations, elevated body temperature, and rapid changes in blood pressure. Although most dramatic in the case of the monoamine oxidase inhibitors (MAOIs), newer antidepressants may also be associated with potentially dangerous interactions with other medications.

Section 47.2

Antidepressants and Teens

From "Antidepressant Medications for Children and Adolescents: Information for Parents and Caregivers," by the National Institute of Mental Health (NIMH, www.nimh.nih.gov), part of the National Institutes of Health, October 2, 2009.

Depression is a serious disorder that can cause significant problems in mood, thinking, and behavior at home, in school, and with peers. It is estimated that major depressive disorder (MDD) affects about 5 percent of adolescents.

Research has shown that, as in adults, depression in children and adolescents is treatable. Certain antidepressant medications, called selective serotonin reuptake inhibitors (SSRIs), can be beneficial to children and adolescents with MDD. Certain types of psychological therapies also have been shown to be effective. However, our knowledge of antidepressant treatments in youth, though growing substantially, is limited compared to what we know about treating depression in adults.

Recently, there has been some concern that the use of antidepressant medications themselves may induce suicidal behavior in youths. Following a thorough and comprehensive review of all the available published and unpublished controlled clinical trials of antidepressants in children and adolescents, the U.S. Food and Drug Administration (FDA) issued a public warning in October 2004 about an increased risk of suicidal thoughts or behavior (suicidality) in children and adolescents treated with SSRI antidepressant medications. In 2006, an advisory committee to the FDA recommended that the agency extend the warning to include young adults up to age 25.

More recently, results of a comprehensive review of pediatric trials conducted between 1988 and 2006 suggested that the benefits of antidepressant medications likely outweigh their risks to children and adolescents with major depression and anxiety disorders. The study, partially funded by NIMH, was published in the April 18, 2007, issue of the *Journal of the American Medical Association.*

What did the FDA review find?

In the FDA review, no completed suicides occurred among nearly 2,200 children treated with SSRI medications. However, about 4 percent of those taking SSRI medications experienced suicidal thinking or behavior, including actual suicide attempts—twice the rate of those taking placebo, or sugar pills.

In response, the FDA adopted a "black box" label warning indicating that antidepressants may increase the risk of suicidal thinking and behavior in some children and adolescents with MDD. A black-box warning is the most serious type of warning in prescription drug labeling.

The warning also notes that children and adolescents taking SSRI medications should be closely monitored for any worsening in depression, emergence of suicidal thinking or behavior, or unusual changes in behavior, such as sleeplessness, agitation, or withdrawal from normal social situations. Close monitoring is especially important during the first four weeks of treatment. SSRI medications usually have few side effects in children and adolescents, but for unknown reasons, they may trigger agitation and abnormal behavior in certain individuals.

What do we know about antidepressant medications?

The SSRIs include the following:

- Fluoxetine (Prozac)
- Sertraline (Zoloft)
- Paroxetine (Paxil)
- Citalopram (Celexa)
- Escitalopram (Lexapro)
- Fluvoxamine (Luvox)

Another antidepressant medication, venlafaxine (Effexor), is not an SSRI but is closely related.

SSRI medications are considered an improvement over older antidepressant medications because they have fewer side effects and are less likely to be harmful if taken in an overdose, which is an issue for patients with depression already at risk for suicide. They have been shown to be safe and effective for adults.

However, use of SSRI medications among children and adolescents ages 10 to 19 has risen dramatically in the past several years. Fluoxetine (Prozac) is the only medication approved by the FDA for use in treating depression in children ages 8 and older. The other SSRI medications and the SSRI-related antidepressant venlafaxine have not been approved for treatment of depression in children or adolescents, but doctors still sometimes prescribe them to children on an "off-label" basis. In June 2003, however, the FDA recommended that paroxetine not be used in children and adolescents for treating MDD.

Fluoxetine can be helpful in treating childhood depression, and can lead to significant improvement of depression overall. However, it may increase the risk for suicidal behaviors in a small subset of adolescents. As with all medical decisions, doctors and families should weigh the risks and benefits of treatment for each individual patient.

What should you do for a child with depression?

A child or adolescent with MDD should be carefully and thoroughly evaluated by a doctor to determine if medication is appropriate. Psychotherapy often is tried as an initial treatment for mild depression. Psychotherapy may help to determine the severity and persistence of the depression and whether antidepressant medications may be warranted. Types of psychotherapies include "cognitive behavioral therapy," which helps people learn new ways of thinking and behaving, and "interpersonal therapy," which helps people understand and work through troubled personal relationships.

Those who are prescribed an SSRI medication should receive ongoing medical monitoring. Children already taking an SSRI medication should remain on the medication if it has been helpful, but should be carefully monitored by a doctor for side effects. Parents should promptly seek medical advice and evaluation if their child or adolescent experiences suicidal thinking or behavior, nervousness, agitation, irritability, mood instability, or sleeplessness that either emerges or worsens during treatment with SSRI medications.

Once started, treatment with these medications should not be abruptly stopped. Although they are not habit-forming or addictive, abruptly ending an antidepressant can cause withdrawal symptoms or lead to a relapse. Families should not discontinue treatment without consulting their doctor.

All treatments can be associated with side effects. Families and doctors should carefully weigh the risks and benefits, and maintain appropriate follow-up and monitoring to help control for the risks.

Chapter 48

Other Common Mental Health Disorders Affecting Adolescents

Chapter Contents

Section 48.1

Anxiety Disorders

Excerpted from "Anxiety Disorders," by the National Institute of Mental
Health (NIMH, www.nimh.nih.gov), part of the National Institutes of
Health, September 29, 2009.

Anxiety disorders affect about 40 million American adults age 18
years and older (about 18%) in a given year, causing them to be filled
with fearfulness and uncertainty. Unlike the relatively mild, brief
anxiety caused by a stressful event (such as speaking in public or
a first date), anxiety disorders last at least 6 months and can get
worse if they are not treated. Anxiety disorders commonly occur along
with other mental or physical illnesses, including alcohol or substance
abuse, which may mask anxiety symptoms or make them worse. In
some cases, these other illnesses need to be treated before a person
will respond to treatment for the anxiety disorder.

Effective therapies for anxiety disorders are available, and research
is uncovering new treatments that can help most people with anxiety
disorders lead productive, fulfilling lives. If you think you have an anxiety disorder, you should seek information and treatment right away.

What is panic disorder?

Panic disorder is a real illness that can be successfully treated.
It is characterized by sudden attacks of terror, usually accompanied
by a pounding heart, sweatiness, weakness, faintness, or dizziness.
During these attacks, people with panic disorder may flush or feel
chilled; their hands may tingle or feel numb; and they may experience
nausea, chest pain, or smothering sensations. Panic attacks usually
produce a sense of unreality, a fear of impending doom, or a fear of
losing control.

A fear of one's own unexplained physical symptoms is also a symptom of panic disorder. People having panic attacks sometimes believe
they are having heart attacks, losing their minds, or on the verge of
death. They can't predict when or where an attack will occur, and between episodes many worry intensely and dread the next attack.

Panic attacks can occur at any time, even during sleep. An attack usually peaks within 10 minutes, but some symptoms may last much longer.

Panic disorder affects about 6 million American adults and is twice as common in women as men. Panic attacks often begin in late adolescence or early adulthood, but not everyone who experiences panic attacks will develop panic disorder. Many people have just one attack and never have another. The tendency to develop panic attacks appears to be inherited.

People who have full-blown, repeated panic attacks can become very disabled by their condition and should seek treatment before they start to avoid places or situations where panic attacks have occurred. For example, if a panic attack happened in an elevator, someone with panic disorder may develop a fear of elevators that could affect the choice of a job or an apartment, and restrict where that person can seek medical attention or enjoy entertainment.

Some people's lives become so restricted that they avoid normal activities, such as grocery shopping or driving. About one third become housebound or are able to confront a feared situation only when accompanied by a spouse or other trusted person. When the condition progresses this far, it is called agoraphobia, or fear of open spaces.

Early treatment can often prevent agoraphobia, but people with panic disorder may sometimes go from doctor to doctor for years and visit the emergency room repeatedly before someone correctly diagnoses their condition. This is unfortunate, because panic disorder is one of the most treatable of all the anxiety disorders, responding in most cases to certain kinds of medication or certain kinds of cognitive psychotherapy, which help change thinking patterns that lead to fear and anxiety.

Panic disorder is often accompanied by other serious problems, such as depression, drug abuse, or alcoholism. These conditions need to be treated separately. Symptoms of depression include feelings of sadness or hopelessness, changes in appetite or sleep patterns, low energy, and difficulty concentrating. Most people with depression can be effectively treated with antidepressant medications, certain types of psychotherapy, or a combination of the two.

What is posttraumatic stress disorder (PTSD)?

Posttraumatic stress disorder (PTSD) develops after a terrifying ordeal that involved physical harm or the threat of physical harm. The person who develops PTSD may have been the one who was harmed, the harm may have happened to a loved one, or the person may have witnessed a harmful event that happened to loved ones or strangers.

PTSD was first brought to public attention in relation to war veterans, but it can result from a variety of traumatic incidents, such as mugging, rape, torture, being kidnapped or held captive, child abuse, car accidents, train wrecks, plane crashes, bombings, or natural disasters such as floods or earthquakes.

People with PTSD may startle easily, become emotionally numb (especially in relation to people with whom they used to be close), lose interest in things they used to enjoy, have trouble feeling affectionate, be irritable, become more aggressive, or even become violent. They avoid situations that remind them of the original incident, and anniversaries of the incident are often very difficult. PTSD symptoms seem to be worse if the event that triggered them was deliberately initiated by another person, as in a mugging or a kidnapping.

Most people with PTSD repeatedly relive the trauma in their thoughts during the day and in nightmares when they sleep. These are called flashbacks. Flashbacks may consist of images, sounds, smells, or feelings, and are often triggered by ordinary occurrences, such as a door slamming or a car backfiring on the street. A person having a flashback may lose touch with reality and believe that the traumatic incident is happening all over again.

Not every traumatized person develops full-blown or even minor PTSD. Symptoms usually begin within 3 months of the incident but occasionally emerge years afterward. They must last more than a month to be considered PTSD. The course of the illness varies. Some people recover within 6 months, while others have symptoms that last much longer. In some people, the condition becomes chronic.

PTSD affects about 7.7 million American adults, but it can occur at any age, including childhood. Women are more likely to develop PTSD than men, and there is some evidence that susceptibility to the disorder may run in families. PTSD is often accompanied by depression, substance abuse, or one or more of the other anxiety disorders.

Certain kinds of medication and certain kinds of psychotherapy usually treat the symptoms of PTSD very effectively.

What is social phobia (social anxiety disorder)?

Social phobia, also called social anxiety disorder, is diagnosed when people become overwhelmingly anxious and excessively self-conscious in everyday social situations. People with social phobia have an intense, persistent, and chronic fear of being watched and judged by others and of doing things that will embarrass them. They can worry for days or weeks before a dreaded situation. This fear may become so severe that it interferes with work, school, and other ordinary activities, and can make it hard to make and keep friends.

While many people with social phobia realize that their fears about being with people are excessive or unreasonable, they are unable to overcome them. Even if they manage to confront their fears and be around others, they are usually very anxious beforehand, are intensely uncomfortable throughout the encounter, and worry about how they were judged for hours afterward.

Social phobia can be limited to one situation (such as talking to people, eating or drinking, or writing on a blackboard in front of others) or may be so broad (such as in generalized social phobia) that the person experiences anxiety around almost anyone other than the family.

Physical symptoms that often accompany social phobia include blushing, profuse sweating, trembling, nausea, and difficulty talking. When these symptoms occur, people with social phobia feel as though all eyes are focused on them.

Social phobia affects about 15 million American adults. Women and men are equally likely to develop the disorder, which usually begins in childhood or early adolescence. There is some evidence that genetic factors are involved. Social phobia is often accompanied by other anxiety disorders or depression, and substance abuse may develop if people try to self-medicate their anxiety.

Social phobia can be successfully treated with certain kinds of psychotherapy or medications.

What are specific phobias?

A specific phobia is an intense, irrational fear of something that actually poses little or no threat. Some of the more common specific phobias are heights, escalators, tunnels, highway driving, closed-in places, water, flying, dogs, spiders, and injuries involving blood. People with specific phobias may be able to ski the world's tallest mountains with ease but be unable to go above the fifth floor of an office building. While adults with phobias realize that these fears are irrational, they often find that facing, or even thinking about facing, the feared object or situation brings on a panic attack or severe anxiety.

Specific phobias affect around 19.2 million American adults and are twice as common in women as men. They usually appear in childhood or adolescence and tend to persist into adulthood. The causes of specific phobias are not well understood, but there is some evidence that the tendency to develop them may run in families.

If the feared situation or feared object is easy to avoid, people with specific phobias may not seek help; but if avoidance interferes with their careers or their personal lives, it can become disabling and treatment is usually pursued.

Specific phobias respond very well to carefully targeted psychotherapy.

What is generalized anxiety disorder (GAD)?

People with generalized anxiety disorder (GAD) go through the day filled with exaggerated worry and tension, even though there is little or nothing to provoke it. They anticipate disaster and are overly concerned about health issues, money, family problems, or difficulties at work. Sometimes just the thought of getting through the day produces anxiety.

GAD is diagnosed when a person worries excessively about a variety of everyday problems for at least 6 months. People with GAD can't seem to get rid of their concerns, even though they usually realize that their anxiety is more intense than the situation warrants. They can't relax, startle easily, and have difficulty concentrating. Often they have trouble falling asleep or staying asleep. Physical symptoms that often accompany the anxiety include fatigue, headaches, muscle tension, muscle aches, difficulty swallowing, trembling, twitching, irritability, sweating, nausea, lightheadedness, having to go to the bathroom frequently, feeling out of breath, and hot flashes.

When their anxiety level is mild, people with GAD can function socially and hold down a job. Although they don't avoid certain situations as a result of their disorder, people with GAD can have difficulty carrying out the simplest daily activities if their anxiety is severe.

GAD affects about 6.8 million American adults, including twice as many women as men. The disorder develops gradually and can begin at any point in the life cycle, although the years of highest risk are between childhood and middle age. There is evidence that genes play a modest role in the disorder.

Other anxiety disorders, depression, or substance abuse often accompany GAD, which rarely occurs alone. GAD is commonly treated with medication or cognitive behavioral therapy, but cooccurring conditions must also be treated using the appropriate therapies.

Section 48.2

Attention Deficit Hyperactivity Disorder (ADHD)

Excerpted from text by the National Institute of Mental Health (NIMH, www.nimh.nih.gov), part of the National Institutes of Health, June 15, 2009.

What is attention deficit hyperactivity disorder?

Attention deficit hyperactivity disorder (ADHD) is one of the most common childhood disorders and can continue through adolescence and adulthood. Symptoms include difficulty staying focused and paying attention, difficulty controlling behavior, and hyperactivity (over-activity).

ADHD has three subtypes:

- Predominantly hyperactive-impulsive

  - Most symptoms (six or more) are in the hyperactivity-impulsivity categories.

  - Fewer than six symptoms of inattention are present, although inattention may still be present to some degree.

- Predominantly inattentive

  - The majority of symptoms (six or more) are in the inattention category and fewer than six symptoms of hyperactivity-impulsivity are present, although hyperactivity-impulsivity may still be present to some degree.

  - Children with this subtype are less likely to act out or have difficulties getting along with other children. They may sit quietly, but they are not paying attention to what they are doing. Therefore, the child may be overlooked, and parents and teachers may not notice that he or she has ADHD.

- Combined hyperactive-impulsive and inattentive

  - Six or more symptoms of inattention and six or more symptoms of hyperactivity-impulsivity are present.

  - Most children have the combined type of ADHD.

375

Treatments can relieve many of the disorder's symptoms, but there is no cure. With treatment, most people with ADHD can be successful in school and lead productive lives. Researchers are developing more effective treatments and interventions, and using new tools such as brain imaging, to better understand ADHD and to find more effective ways to treat and prevent it.

What are the symptoms of ADHD in children?

Inattention, hyperactivity, and impulsivity are the key behaviors of ADHD. It is normal for all children to be inattentive, hyperactive, or impulsive sometimes, but for children with ADHD, these behaviors are more severe and occur more often. To be diagnosed with the disorder, a child must have symptoms for 6 or more months and to a degree that is greater than other children of the same age.

Children who have symptoms of inattention may experience the following:

- Be easily distracted, miss details, forget things, and frequently switch from one activity to another

- Have difficulty focusing on one thing

- Become bored with a task after only a few minutes, unless they are doing something enjoyable

- Have difficulty focusing attention on organizing and completing a task or learning something new

- Have trouble completing or turning in homework assignments, often losing things (e.g., pencils, toys, assignments) needed to complete tasks or activities

- Not seem to listen when spoken to

- Daydream, become easily confused, and move slowly

- Have difficulty processing information as quickly and accurately as others

- Struggle to follow instructions

Children who have symptoms of hyperactivity may experience these symptoms:

- Fidget and squirm in their seats

- Talk nonstop

- Dash around, touching or playing with anything and everything in sight

- Have trouble sitting still during dinner, school, and story time

- Be constantly in motion

- Have difficulty doing quiet tasks or activities

Children who have symptoms of impulsivity may experience the following:

- Be very impatient

- Blurt out inappropriate comments, show their emotions without restraint, and act without regard for consequences

- Have difficulty waiting for things they want or waiting their turns in games

- Often interrupt conversations or others' activities

How is ADHD treated?

Currently available treatments focus on reducing the symptoms of ADHD and improving functioning. Treatments include medication, various types of psychotherapy, education or training, or a combination of treatments.

Medications: The most common type of medication used for treating ADHD is called a "stimulant." Although it may seem unusual to treat ADHD with a medication considered a stimulant, it actually has a calming effect on children with ADHD. Many types of stimulant medications are available. A few other ADHD medications are non-stimulants and work differently than stimulants. For many children, ADHD medications reduce hyperactivity and impulsivity and improve their ability to focus, work, and learn. Medication also may improve physical coordination.

Psychotherapy: Different types of psychotherapy are used for ADHD. Behavioral therapy aims to help a child change his or her behavior. It might involve practical assistance, such as help organizing tasks or completing schoolwork, or working through emotionally difficult events. Behavioral therapy also teaches a child how to monitor his or her own behavior. Learning to give oneself praise or rewards for acting in a desired way, such as controlling anger or thinking before acting, is another goal of behavioral therapy. Parents and teachers also can give positive or negative feedback for certain behaviors. In addition, clear rules, chore lists, and other structured routines can help a child control his or her behavior.

Do teens with ADHD have special needs?

Most children with ADHD continue to have symptoms as they enter adolescence. Some children, however, are not diagnosed with ADHD until they reach adolescence. This is more common among children with predominantly inattentive symptoms because they are not necessarily disruptive at home or in school. In these children, the disorder becomes more apparent as academic demands increase and responsibilities mount. For all teens, these years are challenging. But for teens with ADHD, these years may be especially difficult.

Although hyperactivity tends to decrease as a child ages, teens who continue to be hyperactive may feel restless and try to do too many things at once. They may choose tasks or activities that have a quick payoff, rather than those that take more effort, but provide bigger, delayed rewards. Teens with primarily attention deficits struggle with school and other activities in which they are expected to be more self-reliant.

Teens also become more responsible for their own health decisions. When a child with ADHD is young, parents are more likely to be responsible for ensuring that their child maintains treatment. But when the child reaches adolescence, parents have less control, and those with ADHD may have difficulty sticking with treatment.

To help them stay healthy and provide needed structure, teens with ADHD should be given rules that are clear and easy to understand. Helping them stay focused and organized—such as posting a chart listing household chores and responsibilities with spaces to check off completed items—also may help.

Teens with or without ADHD want to be independent and try new things, and sometimes they will break rules. If your teen breaks rules, your response should be as calm and matter-of-fact as possible. Punishment should be used only rarely. Teens with ADHD often have trouble controlling their impulsivity and tempers can flare. Sometimes, a short time-out can be calming.

If your teen asks for later curfews and use of the car, listen to the request, give reasons for your opinions, and listen to your child's opinion. Rules should be clear once they are set, but communication, negotiation, and compromise are helpful along the way. Maintaining treatments, such as medication and behavioral or family therapy, also can help with managing your teenager's ADHD.

What about teens and driving?

Although many teens engage in risky behaviors, those with ADHD, especially untreated ADHD, are more likely to take more risks. In fact, in their first few years of driving, teens with ADHD are involved in nearly four times as many car accidents as those who do not have ADHD. They are also more likely to cause injury in accidents, and they get three times as many speeding tickets as their peers.

Most states now use a graduated licensing system, in which young drivers, both with and without ADHD, learn about progressively more challenging driving situations. The licensing system consists of three stages—learner's permit, during which a licensed adult must always be in the car with the driving teen; intermediate (provisional) license; and full licensure. Parents should make sure that their teens, especially those with ADHD, understand and follow the rules of the road. Repeated driving practice under adult supervision is especially important for teens with ADHD.

Section 48.3

Bipolar Disorder in Children and Teens

Excerpted from text by the National Institute of Mental Health (NIMH, www.nimh.nih.gov), part of the National Institutes of Health, 2008.

Does your child go through intense mood changes? Does your child have extreme behavior changes, too? Does your child get too excited or silly sometimes? Do you notice he or she is very sad at other times? Do these changes affect how your child acts at school or at home?

Some children and teens with these symptoms may have bipolar disorder, a serious mental illness.

What is bipolar disorder?

Bipolar disorder is a serious brain illness. It is also called manic-depressive illness. Children with bipolar disorder go through unusual mood changes. Sometimes they feel very happy or "up," and are much more active than usual. This is called mania. And sometimes children with bipolar disorder feel very sad and "down," and are much less active than usual. This is called depression.

Bipolar disorder is not the same as the normal ups and downs every kid goes through. Bipolar symptoms are more powerful than that. The illness can make it hard for a child to do well in school or get along with friends and family members. The illness can also be dangerous. Some young people with bipolar disorder try to hurt themselves or attempt suicide.

Children and teens with bipolar disorder should get treatment. With help, they can manage their symptoms and lead successful lives.

Who develops bipolar disorder?

Anyone can develop bipolar disorder, including children and teens. However, most people with bipolar disorder develop it in their late teen or early adult years. The illness usually lasts a lifetime.

How is bipolar disorder different in children and teens than it is in adults?

When children develop the illness, it is called early-onset bipolar disorder. This type can be more severe than bipolar disorder in older teens and adults. Also, young people with bipolar disorder may have symptoms more often and switch moods more frequently than adults with the illness.

What are the symptoms of bipolar disorder?

Bipolar mood changes are called mood episodes. Your child may have manic episodes, depressive episodes, or mixed episodes. A mixed episode has both manic and depressive symptoms. Children and teens with bipolar disorder may have more mixed episodes than adults with the illness.

Mood episodes last a week or two—sometimes longer. During an episode, the symptoms last every day for most of the day.

Mood episodes are intense. The feelings are strong and happen along with extreme changes in behavior and energy levels.

Children and teens having a manic episode may experience or do the following:

- Feel very happy or act silly in a way that's unusual

- Have a very short temper

- Talk really fast about a lot of different things

- Have trouble sleeping but not feel tired
- Have trouble staying focused
- Talk and think about sex more often
- Do risky things

Children and teens having a depressive episode may experience or do the following:

- Feel very sad
- Complain about pain a lot, like stomachaches and headaches
- Sleep too little or too much
- Feel guilty and worthless
- Eat too little or too much
- Have little energy and no interest in fun activities
- Think about death or suicide

How is bipolar disorder treated?

Right now, there is no cure for bipolar disorder. Doctors often treat children who have the illness in a similar way they treat adults. Treatment can help control symptoms. Treatment works best when it is ongoing, instead of on and off.

Medication: Different types of medication can help. Children respond to medications in different ways, so the type of medication depends on the child. Some children may need more than one type of medication because their symptoms are so complex. Sometimes they need to try different types of medicine to see which are best for them.

Children should take the fewest number and smallest amounts of medications as possible to help their symptoms. A good way to remember this is "start low, go slow." Always tell your child's doctor about any problems with side effects. Do not stop giving your child medication without a doctor's help. Stopping medication suddenly can be dangerous, and it can make bipolar symptoms worse.

Therapy: Different kinds of psychotherapy, or talk therapy, can help children with bipolar disorder. Therapy can help children change their behavior and manage their routines. It can also help young people get along better with family and friends. Sometimes therapy includes family members.

What can children and teens expect from treatment?

With treatment, children and teens with bipolar disorder can get better over time. It helps when doctors, parents, and young people work together.

Sometimes a child's bipolar disorder changes. When this happens, treatment needs to change too. For example, your child may need to try a different medication. The doctor may also recommend other treatment changes. Symptoms may come back after a while, and more adjustments may be needed. Treatment can take time, but sticking with it helps many children and teens have fewer bipolar symptoms.

You can help treatment be more effective. Try keeping a chart of your child's moods, behaviors, and sleep patterns. This is called a daily life chart or mood chart. It can help you and your child understand and track the illness. A chart can also help the doctor see whether treatment is working.

How can I help my child or teen?

Help your child or teen get the right diagnosis and treatment. If you think he or she may have bipolar disorder, make an appointment with your family doctor to talk about the symptoms you notice.

If your child has bipolar disorder, here are some basic things you can do:

- Be patient.
- Encourage your child to talk, and listen to him or her carefully.
- Be understanding about mood episodes.
- Help your child have fun.
- Help your child understand that treatment can help him or her get better.

Section 48.4

Borderline Personality Disorder

Excerpted from text by the National Institute of Mental Health (NIMH, www.nimh.nih.gov), part of the National Institutes of Health, May 13, 2009.

Borderline personality disorder (BPD) is a serious mental illness characterized by pervasive instability in moods, interpersonal relationships, self-image, and behavior. This instability often disrupts family and work life, long-term planning, and the individual's sense of self-identity. Originally thought to be at the "borderline" of psychosis, people with BPD suffer from a disorder of emotion regulation. While less well known than schizophrenia or bipolar disorder (manic-depressive illness), BPD is more common, affecting 2 percent of adults, mostly young women. There is a high rate of self-injury without suicide intent, as well as a significant rate of suicide attempts and completed suicide in severe cases. Patients often need extensive mental health services, and account for 20 percent of psychiatric hospitalizations. Yet, with help, many improve over time and are eventually able to lead productive lives.

What are symptoms of BPD?

While a person with depression or bipolar disorder typically endures the same mood for weeks, a person with BPD may experience intense bouts of anger, depression, and anxiety that may last only hours, or at most a day. These may be associated with episodes of impulsive aggression, self-injury, and drug or alcohol abuse. Distortions in cognition and sense of self can lead to frequent changes in long-term goals, career plans, jobs, friendships, gender identity, and values. Sometimes people with BPD view themselves as fundamentally bad, or unworthy. They may feel unfairly misunderstood or mistreated, bored, empty, and have little idea who they are. Such symptoms are most acute when people with BPD feel isolated and lacking in social support, and may result in frantic efforts to avoid being alone.

People with BPD often have highly unstable patterns of social relationships. While they can develop intense but stormy attachments, their attitudes towards family, friends, and loved ones may suddenly shift from idealization (great admiration and love) to devaluation (intense anger and dislike). Thus, they may form an immediate attachment and idealize the other person, but when a slight separation or conflict occurs, they switch unexpectedly to the other extreme and angrily accuse the other person of not caring for them at all. Even with family members, individuals with BPD are highly sensitive to rejection, reacting with anger and distress to such mild separations as a vacation, a business trip, or a sudden change in plans. These fears of abandonment seem to be related to difficulties feeling emotionally connected to important persons when they are physically absent, leaving the individual with BPD feeling lost and perhaps worthless. Suicide threats and attempts may occur along with anger at perceived abandonment and disappointments.

People with BPD exhibit other impulsive behaviors, such as excessive spending, binge eating, and risky sex. BPD often occurs together with other psychiatric problems, particularly bipolar disorder, depression, anxiety disorders, substance abuse, and other personality disorders.

How is BPD treated?

Treatments for BPD have improved in recent years. Group and individual psychotherapy are at least partially effective for many patients. Within the past 15 years, a new psychosocial treatment termed dialectical behavior therapy (DBT) was developed specifically to treat BPD, and this technique has looked promising in treatment studies. Pharmacological treatments are often prescribed based on specific target symptoms shown by the individual patient.

Antidepressant drugs and mood stabilizers may be helpful for depressed and/or labile mood. Antipsychotic drugs may also be used when there are distortions in thinking.

Section 48.5

Conduct Disorder

Excerpted from "Children and Adolescents with Conduct Disorder," by the Substance Abuse and Mental Health Services Administration (SAMHSA, mentalhealth.samhsa.gov), part of the U.S. Department of Health and Human Services, April 2003. Reviewed by David A. Cooke, MD, FACP, April 4, 2010.

What is conduct disorder?

Children with conduct disorder repeatedly violate the personal or property rights of others and the basic expectations of society. A diagnosis of conduct disorder is likely when symptoms continue for 6 months or longer. Conduct disorder is known as a "disruptive behavior disorder" because of its impact on children and their families, neighbors, and schools.

Another disruptive behavior disorder, called oppositional defiant disorder, may be a precursor of conduct disorder. A child is diagnosed with oppositional defiant disorder when he or she shows signs of being hostile and defiant for at least 6 months. Oppositional defiant disorder may start as early as the preschool years, while conduct disorder generally appears when children are older. Oppositional defiant disorder and conduct disorder are not co-occurring conditions.

What are the signs of conduct disorder?

Symptoms of conduct disorder include the following:

- Aggressive behavior that harms or threatens other people or animals
- Destructive behavior that damages or destroys property
- Lying or theft
- Truancy or other serious violations of rules
- Early tobacco, alcohol, and substance use and abuse
- Precocious sexual activity

Children with conduct disorder or oppositional defiant disorder also may experience the following:

- Higher rates of depression, suicidal thoughts, suicide attempts, and suicide

- Academic difficulties

- Poor relationships with peers or adults

- Sexually transmitted diseases

- Difficulty staying in adoptive, foster, or group homes

- Higher rates of injuries, school expulsions, and problems with the law

Section 48.6

Eating Disorders

Excerpted from text by the National Institute of Mental Health (NIMH, www.nimh.nih.gov), part of the National Institutes of Health, June 12, 2009.

What are eating disorders?

An eating disorder is marked by extremes. It is present when a person experiences severe disturbances in eating behavior, such as extreme reduction of food intake or extreme overeating, or feelings of extreme distress or concern about body weight or shape.

A person with an eating disorder may have started out just eating smaller or larger amounts of food than usual, but at some point, the urge to eat less or more spirals out of control. Eating disorders are very complex, and despite scientific research to understand them, the biological, behavioral, and social underpinnings of these illnesses remain elusive.

The two main types of eating disorders are anorexia nervosa and bulimia nervosa. A third category is "eating disorders not otherwise specified (EDNOS)," which includes several variations of eating disorders. Most of these disorders are similar to anorexia or bulimia but with slightly different characteristics. Binge-eating disorder, which has received increasing research and media attention in recent years, is one type of EDNOS.

Eating disorders frequently appear during adolescence or young adulthood, but some reports indicate that they can develop during childhood or later in adulthood. Women and girls are much more likely than males to develop an eating disorder. Men and boys account for an estimated 5% to 15% of patients with anorexia or bulimia and an estimated 35% of those with binge-eating disorder. Eating disorders are real, treatable medical illnesses with complex underlying psychological and biological causes. They frequently coexist with other psychiatric disorders such as depression, substance abuse, or anxiety disorders. People with eating disorders also can suffer from numerous other physical health complications, such as heart conditions or kidney failure, which can lead to death.

What is anorexia nervosa?

Anorexia nervosa is characterized by emaciation, a relentless pursuit of thinness and unwillingness to maintain a normal or healthy weight, a distortion of body image and intense fear of gaining weight, a lack of menstruation among girls and women, and extremely disturbed eating behavior. Some people with anorexia lose weight by dieting and exercising excessively; others lose weight by self-induced vomiting, or misusing laxatives, diuretics, or enemas.

Many people with anorexia see themselves as overweight, even when they are starved or are clearly malnourished. Eating, food, and weight control become obsessions. A person with anorexia typically weighs herself or himself repeatedly, portions food carefully, and eats only very small quantities of only certain foods. Some who have anorexia recover with treatment after only one episode. Others get well but have relapses. Still others have a more chronic form of anorexia, in which their health deteriorates over many years as they battle the illness.

According to some studies, people with anorexia are up to ten times more likely to die as a result of their illness compared to those without the disorder. The most common complications that lead to death are cardiac arrest, and electrolyte and fluid imbalances. Suicide also can result.

Many people with anorexia also have coexisting psychiatric and physical illnesses, including depression, anxiety, obsessive behavior, substance abuse, cardiovascular and neurological complications, and impaired physical development.

Other symptoms may develop over time, including the following:

- Thinning of the bones (osteopenia or osteoporosis)
- Brittle hair and nails
- Dry and yellowish skin
- Growth of fine hair over body (e.g., lanugo)
- Mild anemia and muscle weakness and loss
- Severe constipation
- Low blood pressure, slowed breathing, and pulse
- Drop in internal body temperature, causing a person to feel cold all the time
- Lethargy

Treating anorexia involves three components:

- Restoring the person to a healthy weight
- Treating the psychological issues related to the eating disorder
- Reducing or eliminating behaviors or thoughts that lead to disordered eating and preventing relapse

Some research suggests that the use of medications, such as antidepressants, antipsychotics, or mood stabilizers, may be modestly effective in treating patients with anorexia by helping to resolve mood and anxiety symptoms that often coexist with anorexia. Recent studies, however, have suggested that antidepressants may not be effective in preventing some patients with anorexia from relapsing. In addition, no medication has shown to be effective during the critical first phase of restoring a patient to healthy weight. Overall, it is unclear if and how medications can help patients conquer anorexia, but research is ongoing.

Different forms of psychotherapy, including individual, group, and family-based, can help address the psychological reasons for the illness. Some studies suggest that family-based therapies in which parents assume responsibility for feeding their afflicted adolescent are the most effective in helping a person with anorexia gain weight and improve eating habits and moods.

Shown to be effective in case studies and clinical trials, this particular approach is discussed in some guidelines and studies for treating eating disorders in younger, nonchronic patients.

Others have noted that a combined approach of medical attention and supportive psychotherapy designed specifically for anorexia patients is more effective than just psychotherapy. But the effectiveness of a treatment depends on the person involved and his or her situation. Unfortunately, no specific psychotherapy appears to be consistently effective for treating adults with anorexia. However, research into novel treatment and prevention approaches is showing some promise. One study suggests that an online intervention program may prevent some at-risk women from developing an eating disorder.

What is bulimia nervosa?

Bulimia nervosa is characterized by recurrent and frequent episodes of eating unusually large amounts of food (e.g., binge-eating), and feeling a lack of control over the eating. This binge-eating is followed by a type of behavior that compensates for the binge, such as purging (e.g., vomiting, excessive use of laxatives, or diuretics), fasting, and/or excessive exercise.

Unlike anorexia, people with bulimia can fall within the normal range for their age and weight. But like people with anorexia, they often fear gaining weight, want desperately to lose weight, and are intensely unhappy with their body size and shape. Usually, bulimic behavior is done secretly, because it is often accompanied by feelings of disgust or shame. The binging and purging cycle usually repeats several times a week. Similar to anorexia, people with bulimia often have coexisting psychological illnesses, such as depression, anxiety, and/or substance abuse problems. Many physical conditions result from the purging aspect of the illness, including electrolyte imbalances, gastrointestinal problems, and oral and tooth-related problems.

Other symptoms include the following:

- Chronically inflamed and sore throat

- Swollen glands in the neck and below the jaw

- Worn tooth enamel and increasingly sensitive and decaying teeth as a result of exposure to stomach acids

- Gastroesophageal reflux disorder

- Intestinal distress and irritation from laxative abuse

- Kidney problems from diuretic abuse

- Severe dehydration from purging of fluids

As with anorexia, treatment for bulimia often involves a combination of options and depends on the needs of the individual.

To reduce or eliminate binge and purge behavior, a patient may undergo nutritional counseling and psychotherapy, especially cognitive behavioral therapy (CBT), or be prescribed medication. Some antidepressants, such as fluoxetine (Prozac), which is the only medication approved by the U.S. Food and Drug Administration for treating bulimia, may help patients who also have depression and/or anxiety. It also appears to help reduce binge-eating and purging behavior, reduces the chance of relapse, and improves eating attitudes.

CBT that has been tailored to treat bulimia also has shown to be effective in changing binging and purging behavior and eating attitudes. Therapy may be individually oriented or group-based.

What is binge-eating disorder?

Binge-eating disorder is characterized by recurrent binge-eating episodes during which a person feels a loss of control over his or her eating. Unlike bulimia, binge-eating episodes are not followed by purging, excessive exercise, or fasting. As a result, people with binge-eating disorder often are overweight or obese. They also experience guilt, shame, and/or distress about the binge-eating, which can lead to more binge-eating.

Obese people with binge-eating disorder often have coexisting psychological illnesses including anxiety, depression, and personality disorders. In addition, links between obesity and cardiovascular disease and hypertension are well documented.

Treatment options for binge-eating disorder are similar to those used to treat bulimia. Fluoxetine and other antidepressants may reduce binge-eating episodes and help alleviate depression in some patients.

Patients with binge-eating disorder also may be prescribed appetite suppressants. Psychotherapy, especially CBT, is also used to treat the underlying psychological issues associated with binge-eating, in an individual or group environment.

How are men and boys affected?

Although eating disorders primarily affect women and girls, boys and men are also vulnerable. One in four preadolescent cases of anorexia occurs in boys, and binge-eating disorder affects females and males about equally.

Like females who have eating disorders, males with the illness have a warped sense of body image and often have muscle dysmorphia, a type of disorder that is characterized by an extreme concern with becoming more muscular. Some boys with the disorder want to lose weight, while others want to gain weight or bulk up.

Boys who think they are too small are at a greater risk for using steroids or other dangerous drugs to increase muscle mass.

Boys with eating disorders exhibit the same types of emotional, physical, and behavioral signs and symptoms as girls, but for a variety of reasons, boys are less likely to be diagnosed with what is often considered a stereotypically female disorder.

Section 48.7

Obsessive-Compulsive Disorder (OCD)

Excerpted from "When Unwanted Thoughts Take Over: Obsessive-Compulsive Disorder," by the National Institute of Mental Health (NIMH, www.nimh.nih.gov), part of the National Institutes of Health, 2009.

Everyone double-checks things sometimes—for example, checking the stove before leaving the house, to make sure it's turned off. But people with OCD feel the need to check things over and over, or have certain thoughts or perform routines and rituals over and over. The thoughts and rituals of OCD cause distress and get in the way of daily life.

The repeated, upsetting thoughts of OCD are called obsessions. To try to control them, people with OCD repeat rituals or behaviors, which are called compulsions. People with OCD can't control these thoughts and rituals.

Examples of obsessions are fear of germs, of being hurt or of hurting others, and troubling religious or sexual thoughts. Examples of compulsions are repeatedly counting things, cleaning things, washing the body or parts of it, or putting things in a certain order, when these actions are not needed, and checking things over and over.

People with OCD have these thoughts and do these rituals for at least an hour on most days, often longer. The reason OCD gets in the way of their lives is that they can't stop the thoughts or rituals, so they sometimes miss school, work, or meetings with friends, for example.

What are the symptoms of OCD?

People with OCD often experience the following:

- Have repeated thoughts or images about many different things, such as fear of germs, dirt, or intruders; violence; hurting loved ones; sexual acts; conflicts with religious beliefs; or being overly neat

- Do the same rituals over and over such as washing hands, locking and unlocking doors, counting, keeping unneeded items, or repeating the same steps again and again

- Have unwanted thoughts and behaviors they can't control

- Don't get pleasure from the behaviors or rituals, but get brief relief from the anxiety the thoughts cause

- Spend at least an hour a day on the thoughts and rituals, which cause distress and get in the way of daily life

When does OCD start?

For many people, OCD starts during childhood or the teen years. Most people are diagnosed at about age 19. Symptoms of OCD may come and go and be better or worse at different times.

Is there help?

There is help for people with OCD. The first step is to go to a doctor or health clinic to talk about symptoms. The doctor will do an exam to make sure that another physical problem isn't causing the symptoms. The doctor may make a referral to a mental health specialist.

There are different kinds of treatment for OCD. Doctors may ask people with OCD to seek psychotherapy with a psychologist, psychiatrist, or licensed social worker. A type of therapy called behavior therapy is especially useful for treating OCD. It teaches a person different ways of thinking, behaving, and reacting to situations that help them feel less anxious and fearful without having obsessive thoughts or acting compulsively.

Doctors also may prescribe medication to help treat OCD. It's important to know that some of these medicines may take several weeks to start working. The kinds of medicines used to treat OCD are antidepressants and antianxiety medicines. Some of these medicines are used to treat other problems, such as depression, but also are helpful for OCD. Although these medicines often have mild side effects, they are usually not a problem for most people, especially if the dose starts off low and is increased slowly over time.

Some people do better with therapy, while others do better with medicine. Still others do best with a combination of the two. Talk with your doctor about the best treatment for you.

Section 48.8

Schizophrenia in Teens

"Schizophrenia" is reprinted with permission from the Cincinnati Children's Hospital Medical Center website, http://www.cincinnatichildrens.org. © 2007 Cincinnati Children's Hospital Medical Center. All rights reserved.

What is schizophrenia?

Schizophrenia, one of the most complex of all mental health disorders, can be a severe, chronic, and disabling disturbance of the brain that causes distorted thinking, strange feelings, and unusual behavior and use of language and words.

What causes schizophrenia?

There is no known single cause for schizophrenia. It is believed that a chemical imbalance in the brain is an inherited factor which is necessary for schizophrenia to develop. However, it is likely that many factors—genetic, behavioral, and environmental—play a role in the development of this mental health condition.

Who is affected by schizophrenia?

Schizophrenia can occur at any age, but the majority develop symptoms between the ages of 16 and 25. Younger children can also develop this illness. Schizophrenia is uncommon in children under 12 and can be very hard to identify in the early phases. A sudden onset of the psychotic symptoms of schizophrenia frequently occurs in middle to late adolescence.

Statistics indicate that schizophrenia affects 1 percent of the population in the United States. A child born into a family with one or more schizophrenic family members has a greater chance of developing schizophrenia than a child born into a family with no history of schizophrenia.

After a person has been diagnosed with schizophrenia in a family, the chance for a sibling to also be diagnosed with schizophrenia is 7 to 8 percent.

If a parent has schizophrenia, the chance for a child to have the disorder is 10 to 15 percent. Risks increase with multiple affected family members.

What are the symptoms of schizophrenia?

In children and adolescents with schizophrenia, behavior changes may occur slowly, over time, or have a sudden onset. The child may gradually become more shy and withdrawn. They may talk about bizarre ideas or fears and begin to cling more to parents.

One of the most disturbing and puzzling characteristics of schizophrenia is the sudden onset of its psychotic symptoms.

The following are the most common symptoms of schizophrenia. However, each child may experience symptoms differently. Early warning signs of schizophrenia in children may include:

- distorted perception of reality (difficulty telling dreams or television from reality);

- confused thinking;

- detailed and bizarre thoughts and ideas;

- suspiciousness and/or paranoia unfounded (fearfulness that someone, or something, is going to harm them or is "out to get them");

- hallucinations (seeing, hearing, or feeling things that are not real such as hearing voices telling them to do something);

- delusions (ideas that seem real but are not based in reality);

- extreme moodiness;

- severe anxiety and/or fearfulness;

- flat affect (lack of emotional expression when speaking);

- difficulty in performing schoolwork;

- social withdrawal (severe problems in making and keeping friends);

- disorganized or catatonic behavior (suddenly becoming agitated and confused, or sitting and staring, as if immobilized);

- odd behaviors (an older child may regress significantly and begin acting like a younger child); or

- poor personal hygiene.

The symptoms of schizophrenia are often classified as positive (symptoms including delusions, hallucinations, and bizarre behavior), negative (symptoms including flat affect, withdrawal, and emotional unresponsiveness), disorganized speech (including speech that is incomprehensible), and disorganized or catatonic behavior (including marked mood swings, sudden aggression, or confusion, followed by sudden motionlessness and staring).

The behavior of children with schizophrenia may differ from adults with schizophrenia. Children, more often (in 80 percent of diagnosed cases), experience auditory hallucinations and typically do not experience delusions or formal thought disorders until mid-adolescence or older.

The symptoms of schizophrenia may resemble other problems or psychiatric conditions. Always consult your child's physician for a diagnosis.

How is schizophrenia diagnosed?

Schizophrenia in children and adolescents is usually diagnosed by a child and adolescent psychiatrist. Other mental health professionals usually participate in the completion of a comprehensive mental health evaluation to determine individualized treatment needs.

Treatment for Schizophrenia

Specific treatment for schizophrenia will be determined by your child's physician based on:

- overall health, and medical history;

- extent of the condition;

- type of schizophrenia;

- tolerance for specific medications, procedures, or therapies; and

- expectations for the course of the condition.

Schizophrenia is a major psychiatric illness. Treatment for schizophrenia is complex. A combination of therapies is often necessary to meet the individualized needs of the child or adolescent with schizophrenia.

There is currently no cure for schizophrenia. Treatment is aimed at reducing the symptoms associated with the disorder. When symptoms are particularly bad, a child with schizophrenia may need to be hospitalized. Types of treatment that may be helpful to a child or adolescent with schizophrenia may include [the following]:

- **Medications** (also called psychopharmacological management) include the following. Antipsychotic medications can be helpful for many of the symptoms listed above. These medications require close monitoring by a child and adolescent psychiatrist. Some examples of traditional antipsychotic medications include: Haloperidol (Haldol), Chlorpromazine (Thorazine), and Fluphenazine (Prolixin). Newer antipsychotic medications, called atypical antipsychotics include: Risperidone (Risperdal), Olanzapine (Zyprexa), Ziprasidone (Geodon), Aripiprazole (Abilify), and Quetiapine (Seroquel). The most common side effect that children report with the newer antipsychotic is weight gain. As a result, children should also be monitored for insulin resistance which could lead to the development of diabetes.

- **Individual and family psychotherapy** (Individual therapy may focus on developing social skills. Family therapy may help family members cope with the child's illness.)

- **Specialized educational and/or structured activity programs** (social skills training, vocational training, speech and language therapy, smaller classroom size, modification of academic work)

Prevention of Schizophrenia

Preventive measures to reduce the incidence of schizophrenia are not known at this time. However, identification and early intervention can improve the quality of life experienced by children and adolescents with schizophrenia.

Further, treatment is most successful when symptoms of the first psychotic episode are addressed properly and promptly. Studies suggest that early treatment may reduce the decline in functioning and other long-term problems that are usually associated with schizophrenia.

It is crucial to the success of the treated child or teen who is prescribed medications for the treatment of schizophrenia to remain compliant.

Dosages and types of medications may need to be adjusted periodically to maintain effectiveness. Always consult your child's physician for more information.

Section 48.9

Tics and Tourette Syndrome in Youth

Is It Tourette's?

Tourette syndrome is a neurological condition that begins in childhood, where individuals have a series of different repetitive movements or sounds that persist uninterrupted for greater than 1 year and usually last many years.

Tourette syndrome can run in families. It is very important for individuals with Tourette syndrome to inform themselves about this diagnosis by reading good books or websites.

Transient tic disorder is diagnosed when children have one or more tics for a short period of time, or short periods of time. Some such children will eventually have symptoms continue so that the Tourette syndrome diagnosis applies; many others will not. Brief periods of tics in childhood currently cannot be explained in most cases and often require no diagnostic testing or treatment. Particularly in children under age 8 years, these have few or no social consequences and do not interfere with the child's quality of life.

Tics in young children are common. They should usually be ignored if there are no other medical, physical, or emotional problems.

Tics are common in older children with psychiatric problems like anxiety. Sometimes medications may contribute to tics.

When Should Tics Be Treated?

Tics, even when frequent, are rarely harmful. Just because a person has tics, doesn't mean medication is needed. Often in younger children, the parents are much more upset about the tics than the child is. We do not put a child on medication to make the parents feel better. Tics should be treated if they are painful or disruptive to the person's life, such that the possible benefit is worth the risk.

Can Tics Be Treated without Medication?

Sometimes, yes, tics can improve without medication. Older children and teens are often self-conscious about their tics. Commenting on them or teasing can make this worse. A supportive environment for the child or teen may make tics better.

Non-Medical Interventions That May Help

- Helping the person realize that he/she is loved and accepted despite the tics

- Convincing siblings, grandparents, all family members that tics are OK; ignore the tics at home; no teasing about tics

- A school "in-service" by the Tourette Syndrome Association or presentation to the class to help everyone understand the symptoms

- Time outs from class, for example extra bathroom passes or errands to the office, to allow time to "let tics out" outside the classroom

- Stress reduction, physical activity, good sleep, and generally healthy diet

Medications to Suppress Tics

Tics should not be treated just because they are noticed. Tics are not harmful, and for many children, no treatment is needed. The decision to treat tics is based on the impact of the tics on the quality of life of the person with the tics. Some kids function fine at home and school despite very frequent tics. It is usually not necessary to treat tics in these cases.

Treatment with Medication May Be Helpful When Tics Are Associated

- **Pain:** Sometimes frequent tics cause muscle pains or headaches. The sensory feeling that accompanies some tics may be painful. Some children have self-injuring tics (pinching, smacking, etc.).

- **Social/psychological problems:** When tics are frequent in children in mid-to-upper elementary grades, teasing and bullying may be problems. Parents of school-aged children should discuss with the child what to say when someone asks about tics or teases. Children may say, "It's just a habit," "It's just something I do," "It's a tic," or, "I have Tourette's." Again, a presentation to the class to help everyone understand the symptoms may help. For teens, tics may cause or increase moodiness, anxiety, sadness, or depression. (Imagine how hard it is for some teens to fit in socially or ask someone on a date. Now add frequent facial tics and you can see why this is difficult for some teens.) Membership in the Tourette Syndrome Association may be helpful for meeting other kids with these symptoms and learning about successful or famous adults with Tourette's.

- **Functional interference:** When tics are very frequent, they may interfere with reading, writing, speaking, playing musical instruments, or sports. Fortunately, this is uncommon. A child may tic while waiting for a pitch; but, once the baseball is pitched, the tics usually disappear while the child focuses on hitting the ball.

- **Classroom disruption:** Occasionally, a child may develop a very loud vocal tic. If frequent, this can be disruptive to the family and classroom. Fortunately, such tics are rarely present for longer than 1 year.

Things You Should Know about Medications for Tics

- Medicines don't cure the tics. Like treatments for other common problems like asthma, medicines improve symptoms, but don't cure the condition.

- Medicines rarely reduce tics more than 50%. Even with medication, tics will likely be noticed by others.

- Adults usually tic less, whether they were treated as children or not. For most persons with tics, symptoms are more severe in childhood than in adulthood. There is no evidence that using medications for tics in childhood increases or decreases the chance of tics in adulthood.

- Choosing the right medicine is a "trial and error process." No single medicine works for everyone, and all medicines have possible side effects. The side effects are sometimes worse than the tics.

- Medications must be taken daily to work. There are no proven treatments which can be used "as needed" on a bad day. Medicines must be taken daily, and may not start to help for several weeks.

- Start low, go slow/taper off slowly. Side effects are less common when we start with a low dose and increase gradually. Once we decide to stop a medication, we taper off slowly, not all at once.

Approach to Treatment of Tics and Tourette Syndrome

Children who tic or have Tourette's commonly have other problems such as ADHD [attention deficit hyperactivity disorder], obsessive-compulsive disorder [OCD], anxiety, or learning problems. The following should all be considered when deciding on treatment(s):

1. Rank the symptoms (tics, ADHD, anxiety, obsessive-compulsive behavior, etc.). For many, the ADHD or OCD are more disruptive than the tics. Ask about the impact of symptoms (pain, social/psychological problems, functional interference, classroom disruption).

2. Consider non-medical and medical treatments, starting with the most concerning symptom.

3. If ADHD is the most concerning problem, it may still be OK to use stimulants (Ritalin/Metadate/Concerta = methylphenidate; Adderall = Dexedrine). Discuss the pros and cons with your physician.

4. Do not begin treatment with two drugs at the same time, even if there are two treatable problems. If a side effect happens, it won't be clear which drug to blame. Sometimes one medication can help two different symptoms.

5. If learning problems are significant, consider formal neuropsychological testing through the school system or a private psychologist. Although most children with tics have normal IQ, learning disabilities, and behavioral problems are still common. Neuropsychological or educational testing can help identify whether certain educational strategies are warranted. Some children who appear to have ADHD actually have other psychiatric diagnoses such as anxiety or depression.

6. If a parent has problems with anxiety, anger, depression, or substance abuse, it is unrealistic to expect the child's behavior to improve with just medications.

7. If behavior problems, impulse control, and/or rages are a bad problem, medicines alone probably won't be enough. Find a well-trained psychologist to help. This may be more important than medications for some kids, and may be needed several different times during the childhood and teenage years. Sometimes, family therapy or parent training may be needed.

Medicines to Reduce Tics

First line treatment: clonidine (Catapres) or guanfacine (Tenex).

In our clinic, we usually try clonidine or guanfacine first because they help many children and, most importantly, have mild side effects.

How Clonidine (Catapres) and Guanfacine (Tenex) Work

These medicines both act in the brain. Remember learning about the "fight or flight" response in health class in school? Our brains are "wired" to respond to danger by revving up our alertness, our heart rate, and our bodies to either "fight off" the danger or "flee (run away)" quickly. In some kids with Tourette's and/or ADHD, the brain may be overactivated. As a result there is extra movement (hyperactivity and tics), agitation or anxiety, poor attention, and/or poor sleep. Clonidine and guanfacine "turn down the volume" on this brain response.

Dosing Schedule

We start at a low dose and increase at a slow, medium, or fast rate depending on concern about side effects. The final daily dose is different for different children. Clonidine also comes in a patch, where the medicine travels continuously through the skin.

Possible Side Effects of Clonidine or Guanfacine

The number one side effect, by far, that parents call us about is excess sleepiness. For some children, this does not occur. For others, it occurs but may be temporary. For some children, it occurs, persists, and is intolerable. Mood/personality changes (depression), headaches, lightheadedness, stomach upset, and nightmares occur less commonly. The patch may cause a bad rash.

Other Possible Benefits of Clonidine or Guanfacine

In some cases, these medicines make the child calmer, improve attention, and decrease aggression or tantrums (rages).

Possible Drug-Drug Interactions

These usually do not cause problems with other medicines. If other medicines have sleepiness, lightheadedness/dizziness, or low blood pressure as a side effect, adding clonidine or guanfacine may make the problem worse. Many children take these in combination with medication for ADHD, OCD, depression, or anxiety.

Second/Third Line Treatment: Neuroleptics and Atypical Anti-Psychotics

Neuroleptics are strong medicines used for severe symptoms. Some neuroleptics (Orap, Prolixin, Haldol) and some atypical anti-psychotics (Risperdal, Geodon, Zyprexa) have been shown to decrease tics. Which to use first is controversial. All have the potential for serious side effects and should be used cautiously by physicians familiar with them.

How They Work

These medicines block dopamine in the brain. Excess dopamine appears to be involved in disorders of excess movement.

Dosing Schedule

We start at a low dose and increase at a slow, medium, or fast rate depending on concern about side effects. The final daily dose is different for different children.

Possible Side Effects of Dopamine-Blocking Medicines

These include weight gain (very common), slowing of thinking, depressed mood, feeling tired/sleepy/sluggish, muscle spasms (acute dystonic reactions), restlessness, and dangerous changes in heart rhythm. Additional risks of long-term use include tardive dyskinesia, a potentially permanent abnormal facial movement.

Other Possible Benefits of Dopamine-Blockers

For some children, these medicines decrease aggressive, impulsive behavior and tantrums.

Possible Drug-Drug Interactions

These may be dangerous. Certain antibiotics should not be taken with these medications. Always tell any doctor at each visit if you are taking these medications and use the same pharmacy for new prescriptions and refills.

Other Options

A variety of other medicines, such as muscle relaxants, antidepressants, and anti-anxiety agents appear to help some patients tic less.

Drug Studies

The Tourette Syndrome Clinic at Cincinnati Children's Hospital Medical Center is committed to finding more effective treatments for Tourette syndrome. Ask about our research registry, so you can hear about the latest research.

Tips on When You Should Call/E-mail Us

1. Call for any concerning side effect. However, you may want to hold off calling if the problem is sleepiness, because this may be temporary. If you were given a schedule to increase the dose of medication in 3 days, you may slow this down to increase every 5 to 7 days, without calling us to ask. If you can, try to put up with sleepiness for 2 weeks, and it may go away. Teachers usually understand if you warn them. If you stop the medicine before 2 weeks, you may be giving up too soon on a medicine that will eventually be helpful.

2. The tics are getting worse. You should let us know if tics are getting worse, but it may not be necessary to start, increase, or change medications. The most important factor in deciding about medication is interference. If the tics are more frequent, but aren't causing more problems, then the best approach is to wait it out. Tics increase and decrease, sometimes for no apparent reason. There is no quick fix for tics. Tics often increase when the child is stressed, when change is occurring, or even when there is an exciting event like a vacation coming up.

3. If your child develops a new movement, habit, or behavior, you may wonder whether this is a tic. Generally, tics should be brief, repetitive, partly suppressible movements or noises, which appear or sound roughly the same each time the child does it. Older children describe an urge to perform the tics. As children get older, they are more prone to other repetitive behaviors that are compulsions (not tics) or to non-repetitive, impulsive behavior. Just because the child says or feels they "can't help" something they just did doesn't mean it is a tic. Some parents make the mistake of thinking that all of their child's behaviors are tics and are out of the child's control. Sometimes, it's just bad behavior. Also, not all swearing is coprolalia (swearing tic). Most of it is just swearing. If in doubt, contact us.

What about Treating ADHD?

The most common concern people have is that stimulant medications for ADHD might worsen tics. This doesn't apply to all children. This concern was first reported in the 1970s and 1980s. Remember, however, that many children have both ADHD and tics, but the ADHD symptoms usually come first. Thus a child may have ADHD symptoms starting at age 3 years and tics starting at age 6 years. If the doctor starts a stimulant in a 6-year-old entering first grade, and the child starts to have tics, it appears that the medication caused the tics, when actually, that child was going to start having tics around that age anyway.

Stimulant medicines for ADHD may produce temporary tics in some children. Lowering the dose or stopping the medicine usually takes care of this if the problem is severe. In some children with tics and ADHD, tics improve on stimulant medication, possibly because improving ADHD symptoms reduces stress. Other non-stimulant ADHD medications can also be considered.

When Can the Medicines Be Stopped?

The decision to treat tics with medications is rarely a lifelong decision, since in most cases tics start to decrease in the teenage years. There are generally two good times to taper off of medications for tics:

1. Summertime: For many children, there is less stress in the summer. Medicines can be gradually tapered and stopped, just as they were gradually started. Consult with the doctor before tapering off of the medication.

2. After age 14 years: Studies show the peak years for tics are 7 to 14 years. We usually try to stop medications in kids over 14. Some children who have been on medicines for years are able to stop at that time.

Chapter 49

Cutting and Self-Injury

What does hurting yourself mean?

Hurting yourself, sometimes called self-injury, is when a person deliberately hurts his or her own body. Some self-injuries can leave scars that won't go away, while others leave marks or bruises that eventually will go away. These are some forms of self-injury:

- Cutting yourself (such as using a razor blade, knife, or other sharp object to cut the skin)
- Punching yourself or other objects
- Burning yourself with cigarettes, matches, or candles
- Pulling out your hair
- Poking objects through body openings
- Breaking your bones or bruising yourself
- Plucking hair for hours

Why do some teens want to hurt themselves?

Many people cut themselves because it gives them a sense of relief. Some people use cutting as a means to cope with any problem. Some

From "Cutting and Hurting Yourself," by the Office on Women's Health (www.womenshealth.gov), part of the U.S. Department of Health and Human Services, March 12, 2008.

teens say that when they hurt themselves, they are trying to stop feeling lonely, angry, or hopeless. Some teens who hurt themselves have low self-esteem, they may feel unloved by their family and friends, and they may have an eating disorder, an alcohol or drug problem, or may have been victims of abuse.

Teens who hurt themselves often keep their feelings "bottled up" inside and have a hard time letting their feelings show. Some teens who hurt themselves say that feeling the pain provides a sense of relief from intense feelings. Cutting can relieve the tension from bottled up sadness or anxiety.

Others hurt themselves in order to "feel." Often people who hold back strong emotions can begin feeling numb, and cutting can be a way to cope with this because it causes them to feel something. Some teens also may hurt themselves because they want to fit in with others who do it.

If you are hurting yourself, please get help. It is possible to overcome the urge to cut. There are other ways to find relief and cope with your emotions. Please talk to your parents, your doctor, or an adult you trust, like a teacher or religious leader.

Who are the people who hurt themselves?

People who hurt themselves come from all walks of life, no matter their age, gender, race, or ethnicity. About one in 100 people hurts himself or herself on purpose. More females hurt themselves than males. Teens usually hurt themselves by cutting with sharp objects.

What are the signs of self-injury?

These are some signs of self-injury:

- Cuts or scars on the arms or legs

- Hiding cuts or scars by wearing long-sleeved shirts or pants, even in hot weather

- Making poor excuses about how the injuries happened

Self-injury can be dangerous—cutting can lead to infections, scars, numbness, and even hospitalization and death. People who share tools to cut themselves are at risk of getting and spreading diseases like HIV [human immunodeficiency virus] and hepatitis. Teens who continue to hurt themselves are less likely to learn how to cope with negative feelings.

Are you or a friend depressed, angry, or having a hard time coping with life?

If you are thinking about hurting yourself, please ask for help. Talk with an adult you trust, like a teacher or minister or doctor. There is nothing wrong with asking for help—everyone needs help sometimes. You have a right to be strong, safe, and happy.

Do you have a friend who hurts herself or himself?

Please try to get your friend to talk to a trusted adult. Your friend may need professional counseling and treatment. Help is available—counselors can teach positive ways to cope with problems without turning to self-injury.

Have you been pressured to cut yourself by others who do it?

If so, think about how much you value that friendship or relationship. Do you really want a friend who wants you to hurt yourself, cause you pain, and put you in danger? Try to hang out with other friends who don't pressure you in this way.

Chapter 50

Teen Suicide

Chapter Contents

Section 50.1

Facts about Teen Suicide

Excerpted from "Suicide in the U.S.: Statistics and Prevention," by the
National Institute of Mental Health (NIMH, www.nimh.nih.gov), part of
the National Institutes of Health, July 2009.

Suicide is a major, preventable public health problem. In 2006, it was the eleventh leading cause of death in the United States, accounting for 33,300 deaths. The overall rate was 10.9 suicide deaths per 100,000 people. An estimated 12 to 25 attempted suicides occur per every suicide death.

Suicidal behavior is complex. Some risk factors vary with age, gender, or ethnic group and may occur in combination or change over time.

What are the risk factors for suicide?

Research shows that risk factors for suicide include the following:

- Depression and other mental disorders, or a substance-abuse disorder (often in combination with other mental disorders; more than 90 percent of people who die by suicide have these risk factors)

- Prior suicide attempt

- Family history of mental disorder or substance abuse

- Family history of suicide

- Family violence, including physical or sexual abuse

- Firearms in the home, the method used in more than half of suicides

- Incarceration

- Exposure to the suicidal behavior of others, such as family members, peers, or media figures

However, suicide and suicidal behavior are not normal responses to stress; many people have these risk factors, but are not suicidal. Research also shows that the risk for suicide is associated with changes in brain chemicals called neurotransmitters, including serotonin. Decreased levels of serotonin have been found in people with depression, impulsive disorders, and a history of suicide attempts, and in the brains of suicide victims.

Are women or men at higher risk?

Suicide was the seventh leading cause of death for males and the sixteenth leading cause of death for females in 2006.

Almost four times as many males as females die by suicide. Firearms, suffocation, and poison are by far the most common methods of suicide, overall. However, men and women differ in the method used. Men are more likely to kill themselves with firearms and suffocation, whereas females are more likely to use poisoning.

Is suicide common among children and young people?

In 2006, suicide was the third leading cause of death for young people ages 15 to 24. Of every 100,000 young people in each age group, the following number died by suicide:

- Children ages 10 to 14—1.3 per 100,000

- Adolescents ages 15 to 19—8.2 per 100,000

- Young adults ages 20 to 24—12.5 per 100,000

As in the general population, young people were much more likely to use firearms, suffocation, and poisoning than other methods of suicide, overall.

However, while adolescents and young adults were more likely to use firearms than suffocation, children were dramatically more likely to use suffocation.

There were also gender differences in suicide among young people, as follows:

- Over four times as many males as females ages 15 to 19 died by suicide.

- More than six times as many males as females ages 20 to 24 died by suicide.

What are some risk factors for nonfatal suicide attempts?

As noted, an estimated 12 to 25 nonfatal suicide attempts occur per every suicide death. Men and the elderly are more likely to have fatal attempts than are women and youth.

411

Risk factors for nonfatal suicide attempts by adults include depression and other mental disorders, alcohol and other substance abuse, and separation or divorce.

Risk factors for attempted suicide by youth include depression, alcohol or other drug use disorder, physical or sexual abuse, and disruptive behavior.

Most suicide attempts are expressions of extreme distress, not harmless bids for attention. A person who appears suicidal should not be left alone and needs immediate mental health treatment.

What should I do if I think someone is suicidal?

If you think someone is suicidal, do not leave him or her alone. Try to get the person to seek immediate help from his or her doctor or the nearest hospital emergency room, or call 911. Eliminate access to firearms or other potential tools for suicide, including unsupervised access to medications.

Section 50.2

Risk Factors and Warning Signs

From "Suicide Warning Signs," by the Substance Abuse and Mental Health Services Administration (SAMHSA, family.samhsa.gov), part of the U.S. Department of Health and Human Services, August 28, 2007.

Suicide is a serious problem among young people. You may be surprised to learn that it is the third leading cause of death for 15- to 19-year-olds in the United States. Only accidents and homicide are more common causes of death for this age group. A far greater number of youths attempt suicide each year. Suicide attempts are not easy to count because many may not be treated in a hospital or may not be recorded as self-inflicted injuries. Survey data from 2005 show that 17 percent of high school students had seriously thought about suicide, 13 percent had made plans to attempt suicide, and more than 8 percent had made a suicide attempt during the year before the survey.

Suicidal behavior is different among young women than among young men. Young women attempt suicide three times more often than young men. However, four times more young men than young women actually die from suicide. This may be because females and males tend to use different methods when attempting suicide. Young women often attempt suicide by overdosing on drugs or cutting themselves—methods that offer more opportunities for rescue. Young men often use firearms, hanging, or jumping from heights—methods which usually cause instant death and offer no chance to intervene. Suicide among young white men accounts for most suicide deaths, but the suicide rate among young black men is rising. Suicide rates for American Indians aged 15 to 19 are high (19 percent of deaths) compared to overall rates for this age group (less than 13 percent of deaths).

Risk Factors

Most youths who attempt suicide are experiencing a psychological problem such as depression or bipolar disorder, a substance abuse problem, or both. A teen's experiences and history also can increase the chance that he will attempt suicide. For instance, he has a greater risk of attempting suicide if his family has a history of suicide, if he has previously harmed himself or attempted suicide, or if he has run away. A young person also may attempt suicide in response to an extremely stressful event, loss, or conflict with another person.

Warning Signs

Most youths who attempt suicide show some warning signs beforehand. Look for signs of substance abuse or depression and get professional help for your child if she needs it.

Here are some other possible signals of suicide to watch out for:

Words

- Talks, writes, or otherwise expresses a preoccupation with suicide or death in general

- Complains of being a bad person or being "rotten inside"

- Gives verbal hints such as, "I'd be better off dead," "I won't be a problem for you much longer," "Nothing matters," "It's no use," and "I won't see you again"

Actions

- Withdraws from friends or family
- Significantly changes eating, sleeping, or appearance habits
- Experiences sudden drop in academic performance
- Puts his affairs in order; for example, gives away favorite toys, cleans his room, or throws away important belongings
- Acts in rash, hostile, or irrational ways; often expresses rage

Feelings

- Feels overwhelmingly hopeless, guilty, or ashamed
- Shows little interest in favorite activities or the future
- Becomes suddenly cheerful after a period of depression (perhaps feeling that she's found a "solution" to her problems)

A suicide of a schoolmate, friend, or even a celebrity receiving media coverage can encourage suicidal impulses in your child. Suicides sometimes occur in clusters, in which one suicide influences other people already at risk for suicide.

What to Do

If your child seems constantly depressed, angry, or withdrawn, pay attention and encourage communication. If you are worried that he's thinking about hurting or killing himself, ask, even though it may be difficult. Rather than putting dangerous thoughts into his head, asking shows him that you care and that he is not alone. If you are concerned about your child's safety, do not leave him alone. Most important, take seriously any suicide attempt. If your child or someone else you know is thinking about suicide, call 800-273-TALK (273-8255) to find a crisis center in your area.

Part Six

Substance Abuse and Adolescents

Chapter 51

Addiction and the Adolescent Brain

The brain is the command center of your body. It controls just about everything you do, even when you are sleeping.

Weighing about three pounds, the brain is made up of many parts that all work together as a team. Each of these different parts has a specific and important job to do.

When drugs enter the brain, they can interrupt the work and actually change how the brain performs its jobs. These changes are what lead to compulsive drug use, the hallmark of addiction.

Drugs of abuse affect three primary areas of the brain:

- The brain stem is in charge of all of the functions our body needs to stay alive—breathing, circulating blood, and digesting food. It also links the brain with the spinal cord, which runs down the back and is responsible for moving muscles and limbs as well as letting the brain know what's happening to the body.

- The limbic system links together a bunch of brain structures that control our emotional responses, such as feeling pleasure when we eat chocolate. The good feelings motivate us to repeat the behavior, which is good because eating is critical to our lives.

- The cerebral cortex is the mushroom-like outer part of the brain (the gray matter). In humans, it is so big that it makes up about three-fourths of the entire brain. It's divided into four areas, called lobes, which control specific functions. Some areas process

From "Brain and Addiction," by the National Institute on Drug Abuse (NIDA, teens.drugabuse.gov), part of the National Institutes of Health, 2009.

information from our senses, enabling us to see, feel, hear, and taste. The front part of the cortex, known as the frontal cortex or forebrain, is the thinking center. It powers our ability to think, plan, solve problems, and make decisions.

How does the brain communicate?

The brain is a complex communications network consisting of billions of neurons, or nerve cells. Networks of neurons pass messages back and forth within the brain, the spinal column, and the peripheral nervous system. These nerve networks control everything we feel, think, and do.

Neurons: Your brain contains about 100 billion neurons—nerve cells that work nonstop to send and receive messages. Within a neuron, messages travel from the cell body down the axon to the axon terminal in the form of electrical impulses. From there, the message is sent to other neurons with the help of neurotransmitters.

Neurotransmitters (the brain's chemical messengers): To make messages jump from one neuron to another, the neuron creates chemical messengers, called neurotransmitters. The axon terminal releases neurotransmitters that travel across the space (called the synapse) to nearby neurons. Then the transmitter binds to receptors on the nearby neuron.

Receptors (the brain's chemical receivers): As the neurotransmitter approaches the nearby neuron, it attaches to a special site on the cell called a receptor. A neurotransmitter and its receptor operate like a key and lock, in that an exquisitely specific mechanism makes sure that each receptor will forward the appropriate message only after interacting with the right kind of neurotransmitter.

Transporters (the brain's chemical recyclers): Once neurotransmitters do their job, they are pulled back into their original neuron by transporters. This recycling process shuts off the signal between the neurons.

To send a message, a brain cell releases a chemical (neurotransmitter) into the space separating two cells, called the synapse. The neurotransmitter crosses the synapse and attaches to proteins (receptors) on the receiving brain cell. This causes changes in the receiving brain cell, and the message is delivered.

What do drugs do to the brain?

Drugs are chemicals. They work in the brain by tapping into its communication system and interfering with the way nerve cells normally send, receive, and process information. Different drugs—because of their chemical structures—work differently. In fact, some drugs can change the brain in ways that last long after the person has stopped taking drugs, maybe even permanently. This is more likely when a drug is taken repeatedly.

Some drugs, such as marijuana and heroin, activate neurons because their chemical structure mimics that of a natural neurotransmitter. In fact, these drugs can "fool" receptors, can lock onto them, and can activate the nerve cells. The problem is, they don't work the same way as a natural neurotransmitter, so the neurons wind up sending abnormal messages through the brain.

Other drugs, such as amphetamine, cause nerve cells to release excessive amounts of natural neurotransmitters or prevent the normal recycling of these brain chemicals (cocaine and amphetamine). This leads to an exaggerated message in the brain, ultimately wreaking havoc on the communication channels. The difference in effect is like the difference between someone whispering in your ear versus someone shouting in a microphone.

All drugs of abuse—nicotine, cocaine, marijuana, and others—affect the brain's "reward" circuit, which is part of the limbic system. Normally, the reward circuit responds to pleasurable experiences by releasing the neurotransmitter dopamine, which creates feelings of pleasure, and tells the brain that this is something important—pay attention and remember it. Drugs hijack this system, causing unusually large amounts of dopamine to flood the system. Sometimes, this lasts for a long time compared to what happens when a natural reward stimulates dopamine. This flood of dopamine is what causes the "high" or euphoria associated with drug abuse.

How does someone become addicted to drugs?

Think about how you feel when something good happens—maybe your team wins a game or you're praised for something you've done well—that's your limbic system at work. Because natural pleasures in our lives are necessary for survival, the limbic system creates an appetite that drives you to seek out those things.

The first time someone uses a drug of abuse, he or she experiences unnaturally intense feelings of pleasure. The reward circuitry is activated—with dopamine carrying the message. Of course, drugs have other effects, too; a first-time smoker also may cough and feel nauseated from toxic chemicals in a tobacco or marijuana cigarette.

But the brain starts changing as a result of the unnatural flood of neurotransmitters. Because they sense more than enough dopamine, neurons may begin to reduce the number of dopamine receptors or simply make less dopamine. The result is less dopamine signaling in the brain, what the scientists call "down regulation." Because some drugs are toxic, some neurons also may die.

As a result, dopamine's ability to activate circuits to cause pleasure is severely weakened. The person feels flat, lifeless, and depressed. In fact, without drugs, life may seem joyless. Now the person needs drugs just to bring dopamine levels up to normal. Larger amounts of the drug are needed to create a dopamine flood, or "high"—an effect known as "tolerance."

These brain changes drive a person to seek out and use drugs compulsively, despite negative consequences such as stealing, losing friends, family problems, or other physical or mental problems brought on by drug abuse—this is addiction.

Although we know what happens to the brain when someone becomes addicted, we can't predict how many times a person must use a drug before becoming addicted. A person's genetic makeup, the genes that make each of us who we are, and the environment each play a role. What we do know is that a person who uses drugs risks becoming addicted, craving the drug despite its potentially devastating consequences.

Isn't drug addiction a voluntary behavior?

A person may start out taking drugs voluntarily, but as time passes and drug use continues, something happens that makes a person go from being a voluntary drug user to a compulsive drug user. Why? Because the continued use of drugs changes how your brain functions. It impairs your ability to think clearly, to feel OK without drugs, and to control your behaviors. These all contribute to the compulsive drug seeking and use that is addiction.

Isn't becoming addicted to a drug just a character flaw?

The first time people use drugs, it's usually a conscious decision they've made. But once people become addicted, they are dealing with a brain disease. Each drug of abuse has its own individual way of changing how the brain functions. But in most cases, it doesn't really matter which drug a person is addicted to; many of the effects it has on the brain are similar. The fact is that our brains are wired to make sure we will repeat activities, like eating, by associating those activities with pleasure or reward. Whenever this reward circuit is activated, the brain notes that something important is happening that needs to be remembered, and teaches us to do it again and again, without thinking about it. Because drugs of abuse stimulate the same circuit, we learn to abuse drugs in the same way. So while the initial decision to take drugs is a choice for some, a physical need replaces that choice. This is what's known as addiction.

Are there effective treatments for drug addiction?

Yes, although there is no cure for drug addiction yet. Addiction is a treatable, but often chronic disease. And just as with other chronic diseases, such as diabetes or heart disease, people learn to manage their condition, sometimes with the help of medications. People addicted to drugs can do the same. Drug addiction can be effectively treated with behavioral-based therapies in which people learn to change their behavior; and, for addiction to some drugs, such as tobacco, alcohol, heroin, or other opiate drugs, medications can help. Treatment will vary for each person, depending on the type of drug(s) being abused and the individual's specific circumstances. For many people with drug addictions, multiple courses of treatment may be needed to achieve success. Scientific research has revealed 13 basic principles that are the foundation for effective drug addiction treatment.

For drug treatment to work, doesn't the person have to really want it?

Most people go into drug treatment either because the court ordered them to do so, or because loved ones urged them to seek treatment. The good news is that, according to scientific studies, people who enter drug treatment programs in which they face "high" pressure" to deal with their addiction can benefit from treatment, regardless of the reason they sought treatment in the first place.

Shouldn't treatment for drug addiction be a one-shot deal?

No—it's like treating a broken bone. Like diabetes and even asthma, drug addiction typically is a chronic disorder. Some people can quit drug use "cold turkey," or they can quit after receiving treatment just one time at a rehabilitation facility. But most who have become addicted to drugs need longer term treatment and, in many instances, repeated treatments—much like a person who has developed asthma needs to constantly monitor changes in medication and exercise. The important point is that even when someone relapses, they should not give up hope. Rather they need to go back to treatment or modify their current treatment. In fact, setbacks are likely. Even people with diabetes may go off their diet or miss an insulin injection, and their symptoms will recur—that's a cue to get back on track, not to view treatment as a failure.

How do I know if someone has a drug problem?

There are questions people can ask to assess whether or not a person has a drug problem. These do not necessarily indicate that someone is addicted, but answering yes to any of these questions may suggest a developing problem, which could require follow-up with a professional drug treatment specialist. These include the following:

1. Have you ever ridden in a car driven by someone (including yourself) who had been using alcohol or drugs?

2. Do you ever use alcohol or drugs to relax, to feel better about yourself, or to fit in?

3. Do you ever use alcohol or drugs when you are alone?

4. Do you ever forget things you did while using alcohol or drugs?

5. Do family or friends ever tell you to cut down on your use of alcohol or drugs?

6. Have you ever gotten into trouble while you were using alcohol or drugs?

Chapter 52

Treating Teens for Substance Abuse

What Is Substance Abuse?

First you take a drink, then the drink takes a drink, then the drink takes you.—F. Scott Fitzgerald

In a recent study by the University of Michigan (U-M), 8th, 10th, and 12th graders across the country are continuing to show a gradual decline in the proportions reporting use of illicit drugs.

"The cumulative declines since recent peak levels of drug involvement in the mid-1990s are quite substantial, especially among the youngest students," said U-M Distinguished Research Scientist Lloyd Johnston, the principal investigator of the MTF [Monitoring the Future] study.

The proportion of 8th graders reporting use of an illicit drug at least once in the 12 months prior to the survey (called annual prevalence) was 24 percent in 1996 but has fallen to 13 percent by 2007, a drop of nearly half. The decline has been less among 10th graders, from 39 percent to 28 percent between 1997 and 2007, and least among 12th graders, a decline from the recent peak of 42 percent in 1997 to 36 percent this year.

Among the substances abused are: alcohol, tobacco, marijuana, cocaine, opiates, "club drugs" (ecstasy, etc.), stimulants, hallucinogens, inhalants, prescription drugs, and steroids.

"Teen Substance Abuse and Adolescent Substance Abuse Treatment," © National Youth Network. Reprinted with permission. This document is undated. Reviewed by David A. Cooke, MD, FACP, May 13, 2010.

Drug and substance abuse among teenagers, is substantial. Among youth age 12 to 17, about 1.1 million meet the diagnostic criteria for dependence on drugs, and about 1 million are treated for alcohol dependency.

From the National Institute of Health:

- From 2006 to 2007, the percentage of 8th graders reporting lifetime use of any illicit drug declined from 20.9% to 19.0%.

- Reported past year use among 8th graders declined from 14.8% to 13.2%.

- Past year prevalence has fallen by 44% among 8th graders since the peak year of 1996.

- Past year prevalence has fallen 27% among 10th graders and 15% among 12th graders since the peak year of 1997.

In 2007, 15.4% of 12th graders reported using a prescription drug nonmedically within the past year. Vicodin continues to be abused at unacceptably high levels. Attitudes toward substance abuse, often seen as harbingers of change in abuse rates, were mostly stable. However, among 8th graders, perceived risk of harm associated with MDMA [3,4-Methylenedioxymethamphetamine] decreased for the third year in a row. Attitudes towards using LSD [lysergic acid diethylamide] also softened among 10th graders this year.

Between 2005 and 2007, past year abuse of MDMA increased among 12th graders from 3.0% to 4.5%; and between 2004 and 2007, past year abuse of MDMA increased among 10th graders from 2.4% to 3.5%.

The remaining statistically significant increases involved teen alcohol use. The percentage of 10th graders who had been drunk in the past year rose from 38.3 in 1998 to 40.9 in 1999. Also, the percentage of 8th graders having 5+ drinks during the 2 weeks prior to being surveyed increased from 13.7 in 1998 to 15.2 in 1999.

Teenagers at risk for substance abuse include those with a family history of substance abuse, who have low self-esteem, who feel hopelessly alienated, as if they don't fit in, or who are depressed.

What Are the Symptoms of Teen Substance Abuse?

Symptoms of teen substance abuse include the following:

- Sudden personality changes that include abrupt changes in work or school attendance, quality of work, work output, grades, discipline

- Unusual flare-ups or outbreaks of temper
- Withdrawal from responsibility
- General changes in overall attitude
- Loss of interest in what were once favorite hobbies and pursuits
- Changes in friends and reluctance to have friends visit or talk about them
- Difficulty in concentration, paying attention
- Sudden jitteriness, nervousness, or aggression
- Increased secretiveness
- Deterioration of physical appearance and grooming
- Wearing of sunglasses at inappropriate times
- Continual wearing of long-sleeved garments particularly in hot weather or reluctance to wear short-sleeved attire when appropriate
- Association with known substance abusers
- Unusual borrowing of money from friends, coworkers, or parents
- Stealing small items from employer, home, or school
- Secretive behavior regarding actions and possessions; poorly concealed attempts to avoid attention and suspicion such as frequent trips to storage rooms, restroom, basement, etc.

Different substances lend themselves to different groups of symptoms. The most glaring symptom in all cases is a change, sometimes a radical one, in behavior.

Other physical signs of substance abuse are: slurred speech, memory impairment, incoordination, and impairment of attention.

How Is Substance Abuse Diagnosed?

It is sometimes difficult for mental health practitioners to arrive at a diagnosis of substance abuse alone. There are a number of practical and empirical methods to determine substance use, among them being urine or blood testing. Another method to determine use is by interviewing parents, teachers, and other caregivers regarding the history of the patient, and the current behavioral aspects that the patient has been presenting.

A major problem in the diagnosis is the consideration of dual diagnoses. A dual diagnosis is given to any person who has both a substance abuse problem and an emotional or psychiatric disorder. In order for the patient to fully recover, they must be treated for both problems. According to statistics, at least 37% of substance abusers also have a serious mental illness, and conversely, of all those diagnosed with a mental illness, 29% also abuse either drugs or alcohol.

The most common co-occurrences are depressive disorder, anxiety disorder, and psychiatric disorders such as schizophrenia and personality disorders. But any of the emotional disorders, ADHD [attention deficit hyperactivity disorder], obsessive-compulsive disorders, posttraumatic stress syndrome, can lead its sufferers down the path of self-medication and substance abuse.

There are three categories of substance abuse:

- **Use:** The occasional use of alcohol or other drugs without developing tolerance or withdrawal symptoms when not in use

- **Abuse:** The continued use of alcohol or other drugs even while knowing that the continued use is creating problems socially, physically, or psychologically

- **Dependence:** In dependence, at least three of the following factors must be present:

  - Substance is taken in larger amounts or over longer periods of time than the person intended

  - A persistent desire with unsuccessful efforts to control the use

  - Large periods of time spent obtaining, taking, or recovering from the substance

  - Frequent periods of intoxication or detoxification especially when social and major role obligations are expected (school, social situations, etc.)

  - Continued use even while knowing that the continued use is creating problems socially, physically, and/or psychologically

  - Increased tolerance

  - Withdrawal symptoms

  - Substance taken to relieve withdrawal symptoms

How Is Teen Substance Abuse Treated?

In cases of dual diagnosis, the recommended method is to primarily treat the symptomatic substance abuse and cotreat the disorder. Once stabilization is established, the full-fledged treatment for the mental disorder begins.

There are various factors that must be taken into account when considering treatment for substance abuse. Among these factors are:

- Age, developmental stage, and maturity

- Values and culture

- Gender

- Co-existing mental disorders: Without the correct treatment for the co-existing disorders, treatment for addition may not be effective because these disorders could interfere with the patient's ability to successfully participate in an addiction treatment program.

- Family factors: Family factors that could increase the patient's risks should be considered. It is considered important that parents and other family members play a large role in their family member's treatment.

Organic syndromes may be a result of substance abuse, or independent of substance abuse.

Medication

Medication varies with the manner of addiction. If a dual or co-occurring diagnosis is made, medication is administered according to the coexisting disorder. Medications are given along with other interventions. Medications that specifically treat substance abuse are:

- naltrexone (alcohol dependency and opiate dependency);

- methadone (heroin addiction); and

- Wellbutrin (smoking and marijuana abuse).

In order to begin treatment, the first thing the patient must do is detoxify. Detoxification can be done on an outpatient or inpatient basis, depending on the severity of the addiction.

Additional Methods of Substance Abuse Treatment after Detoxification

- Identify underlying co-occurring disorders and treat disorders

- Psychotherapy

- 12-step type programs like Alcoholics Anonymous

- Group therapy
- Behavior modification
- Cognitive therapy
- Residential treatment

Professionals and Programs

Professionals to Seek Out

- See your physician or pediatrician.
- Consult with your clergy to assist in spiritual and practical guidance.
- Consult with an educational consultant to help you find the right program for your child.
- Consult with a therapist or counselor.
- Consult with an educational advocate to help you with your current school situation.
- Consult with an educational consultant to find the right program for your child.

Programs

- Inpatient hospitalization
- Outpatient treatment
- Patients must be seen regularly so drug or alcohol abuse can be monitored. Some patients combine outpatient treatment with a 12-step type program. Frequent drug testing is done. In addition, outpatient treatment may include outpatient detoxification, and alcohol or drug rehabilitation.
- Day treatment
- Residential treatment center or program

Therapeutic Boarding School

These schools are usually fully accredited schools with emotional growth programs. They stress holistic education: growth of the person through holding children responsible for their actions. There is no rehabilitation or physicians on staff.

Wilderness Therapy Program

A therapeutic wilderness program does not necessarily have academics; their goal can be to introduce the children to a different role. These programs use outdoor therapy to help build low self-esteem. They make obtainable goals for them to reach. The programs vary but they are about 6 to 8 weeks long.

It is a very structured program with a goal of teaching the children coping skills and raising their self-esteem. Children go from this program to mainstream back into their public school or attend a small structured boarding school.

Residential Treatment School

A residential treatment program or school provides a full professional staff that includes therapists, psychologists, and psychiatrists. They also have a small academic program.

Many of the children in the program have been recommended there by mental health agencies that make the placements. It is a highly structured environment whose emphasis is on treatment and learning coping skills and independent living.

Chemical dependence education and rehabilitation is also provided. Outdoor therapy is sometimes used to facilitate building social skills and self-esteem. Recovery programs are also available. Residential treatment schools are secure schools.

Chapter 53

Smoking and Nicotine Use in Adolescents

Chapter Contents

431

Section 53.1

Nicotine Addiction

From "Tobacco Addiction," by the National Institute on Drug Abuse
(NIDA, teens.drugabuse.gov), part of the National Institutes of Health,
January 2010.

What is tobacco addiction?

When people are addicted, they have a compulsive need to seek
out and use a substance, even when they understand the harm it
can cause. Tobacco products—cigarettes, cigars or pipes, and smokeless tobacco—all can lead to addiction. Everyone knows that smoking is bad for you, and most people that do it want to quit. In fact,
nearly 35 million people make a serious attempt to quit each year.
Unfortunately, most who try to quit on their own relapse—often
within a week.

Is nicotine addictive?

Yes. It is actually the nicotine in tobacco that is addictive. Each
cigarette contains about 10 milligrams of nicotine. Because the smoker
inhales only some of the smoke from a cigarette, and not all of each
puff is absorbed in the lungs, a smoker gets about 1 to 2 milligrams of
the drug from each cigarette. Although that may not seem like much,
it is enough to make someone addicted.

Is nicotine the only harmful part of tobacco?

No. Nicotine is only one of more than 4,000 chemicals, many of
which are poisonous, found in the smoke from tobacco products.
Smokeless tobacco products also contain many toxins, as well as high
levels of nicotine. Many of these other ingredients are things we would
never consider putting in our bodies, like tar, carbon monoxide, acetaldehyde, and nitrosamines. Tar causes lung cancer, emphysema, and
bronchial diseases. Carbon monoxide causes heart problems, which is
one reason why smokers are at high risk for heart disease.

How is tobacco used?

Tobacco can be smoked in cigarettes, cigars, or pipes. It can be chewed or, if powdered, sniffed. "Bidis" are an alternative cigarette. They come originally from India and are hand-rolled. In the United States, bidis are popular with teens because they come in colorful packages with flavor choices. Some teens think that bidis are less harmful than regular cigarettes, but in fact they have more nicotine, which may make people smoke more, giving bidis the potential to be even more harmful than cigarettes. Hookah—or water pipe smoking—practiced for centuries in other countries, has recently become popular among teens as well. Hookah tobacco comes in many flavors, and the pipe is typically passed around in groups. Although many hookah smokers think it is less harmful than smoking cigarettes, water pipe smoking still delivers the addictive drug nicotine and is at least as toxic as cigarette smoking.

What are the common street names?

You might hear cigarettes referred to as "smokes," "cigs," or "butts." Smokeless tobacco is often called "chew," "dip," "spit tobacco," "snus," or "snuff." People may refer to hookah smoking as "narghile," "argileh," "shisha," "hubble-bubble," or "goza."

How many teens use it?

First, the good news: Smoking is at historically low levels among 8th, 10th, and 12th graders, according to NIDA's Monitoring the Future Survey. That said, in 2009, 20.1 percent of 12th graders, 13.1 percent of 10th graders, and 6.5 percent of 8th graders still reported smoking in the month prior to the survey.

Use of smokeless tobacco had been showing a decline over the past decade—until 2009, that is. According to the survey, current use of smokeless tobacco among 8th graders was 3.7 percent and 6.5 percent for 10th graders. Among 12th graders, 8.4 percent reported using smokeless tobacco in the last month, a number not seen since 1999.

How does tobacco deliver its effects?

With each puff of a cigarette, a smoker pulls nicotine and other harmful substances into the lungs, where it is absorbed into the blood. It takes just 8 seconds for nicotine to hit the brain. Nicotine happens to be shaped like the natural brain chemical acetylcholine. Acetylcholine is one of many chemicals called neurotransmitters that carry messages between brain cells. Neurons (brain cells) have specialized proteins called receptors, into which specific neurotransmitters can fit, like a key fitting into a lock. Nicotine locks into acetylcholine receptors, rapidly causing changes in the brain and body. For instance, nicotine increases blood pressure, heart rate, and respiration (breathing).

Nicotine also attaches to cholinergic receptors on neurons that release a neurotransmitter called dopamine. Dopamine is released normally when you experience something pleasurable like good food, surfing, or the company of people you love. But smoking cigarettes causes neurons to release excess dopamine, which is responsible for the feelings of pleasure experienced by the smoker. However, this effect wears off rapidly, causing smokers to get the urge to light up again for another dose of the drug.

Nicotine may be the primary addictive component in tobacco but it's not the only ingredient that is biologically important. Using advanced neuroimaging technology, scientists have found that smokers have a significant reduction in the levels of an enzyme called monoamine oxidase (MAO) in the brain and throughout the body. This enzyme is responsible for the breakdown of dopamine, other neurotransmitters involved in mood regulation, and in a variety of bodily functions. Having lower amounts of MAO in the brain may lead to higher dopamine levels and be another reason that smokers continue to smoke—to sustain the pleasurable feelings that high dopamine levels create.

Also, researchers have recently shown in animals that acetaldehyde, another chemical constituent of tobacco smoke, dramatically increases the rewarding properties of nicotine—particularly in adolescent animals—which may be one reason why teens are more vulnerable to becoming addicted to tobacco than adults.

What are adverse health effects?

Tobacco abuse harms every organ in the body. It has been conclusively linked to leukemia, cataracts, and pneumonia, and accounts for about one third of all cancer deaths. The overall rates of death from cancer are twice as high among smokers as nonsmokers, with heavy smokers having rates that are four times greater than those of nonsmokers. And, you guessed it—foremost among the cancers caused by tobacco use is lung cancer. In fact, cigarette smoking has been linked to about 90 percent of all lung cancer cases, the number-one cancer killer of both men and women. Tobacco abuse is also associated with cancers of the mouth, pharynx, larynx, esophagus, stomach, pancreas, cervix, kidney, ureter, and bladder.

Smokers also lose some of their sense of smell and taste, don't have the same stamina for exercise and sports they once did, and may smell of smoke. After smoking for a long time, smokers find that their skin ages faster and their teeth discolor or turn brown.

It's not just the smokers who are affected. Nonsmokers are exposed to "secondhand smoke," which comes from both the smoke that a smoker exhales and from the smoke floating from the end of a cigarette, cigar, or pipe. Inhaling secondhand smoke increases a person's risk of developing heart disease by 25 to 30 percent and lung cancer by 20 to 30 percent. In fact, secondhand smoke is estimated to contribute to as many as 40,000 deaths related to heart disease and about 3,000 lung cancer deaths per year among nonsmokers. Secondhand smoke also causes respiratory problems in nonsmokers, like coughing, phlegm, and reduced lung function. Children exposed to secondhand smoke are at an increased risk for sudden infant death syndrome, acute respiratory infections, ear problems, and more severe asthma. And, believe it or not, dropped cigarettes are the leading cause of residential fire fatalities, leading to more than 1,000 such deaths each year.

Each year, almost half a million Americans die from tobacco use. One of every six deaths in the United States is a result of tobacco use, making tobacco more lethal than all other addictive drugs combined.

Section 53.2

Smokeless Tobacco

From "Smokeless Tobacco and Cancer: Questions and Answers," by the National Cancer Institute (NCI, www.cancer.gov), part of the National Institutes of Health, May 30, 2003. Reviewed and revised by David A. Cooke, MD, FACP, March 16, 2010.

What is smokeless tobacco?

There are two types of smokeless tobacco—snuff and chewing tobacco. Snuff, a finely ground or shredded tobacco, is packaged as dry, moist, or in sachets (tea bag-like pouches). Typically, the user places a pinch or dip between the cheek and gum. Chewing tobacco is available in loose leaf, plug (plug-firm and plug-moist), or twist forms, with the user putting a wad of tobacco inside the cheek. Smokeless tobacco is sometimes called "spit" or "spitting" tobacco because people spit out the tobacco juices and saliva that build up in the mouth.

Recently, a third form of smokeless tobacco has become available. They are frequently described as "electronic cigarettes" or "e-cigarettes," and involve a nicotine source and a battery-operated heater. Some manufacturers claim they are a safe alternative to cigarettes, but there is no evidence to support these assertions.

What harmful chemicals are found in smokeless tobacco?

Chewing tobacco and snuff contain 28 carcinogens (cancer-causing agents). The most harmful carcinogens in smokeless tobacco are the tobacco-specific nitrosamines (TSNAs). They are formed during the growing, curing, fermenting, and aging of tobacco. TSNAs have been detected in some smokeless tobacco products at levels many times higher than levels of other types of nitrosamines that are allowed in foods, such as bacon and beer.

Other cancer-causing substances in smokeless tobacco include N-nitrosamino acids, volatile N-nitrosamines, benzo(a)pyrene, volatile aldehydes, formaldehyde, acetaldehyde, crotonaldehyde, hydrazine, arsenic, nickel, cadmium, benzopyrene, and polonium-210.

All tobacco, including smokeless tobacco, contains nicotine, which is addictive. The amount of nicotine absorbed from smokeless tobacco is three to four times the amount delivered by a cigarette. Nicotine is absorbed more slowly from smokeless tobacco than from cigarettes, but more nicotine per dose is absorbed from smokeless tobacco than from cigarettes. Also, the nicotine stays in the bloodstream for a longer time.

There has been little study of "electronic cigarettes" to far, but some research has indicated they also release toxic and carcinogenic chemicals.

What cancers are caused by or associated with smokeless tobacco use?

- Smokeless tobacco users increase their risk for cancer of the oral cavity. Oral cancer can include cancer of the lip, tongue, cheeks, gums, and the floor and roof of the mouth.

- People who use oral snuff for a long time have a much greater risk for cancer of the cheek and gum than people who do not use smokeless tobacco.

- The possible increased risk for other types of cancer from smokeless tobacco is being studied.

What are some of the other ways smokeless tobacco can harm users' health?

Some of the other effects of smokeless tobacco use include addiction to nicotine, oral leukoplakia (white mouth lesions that can become cancerous), gum disease, and gum recession (when the gum pulls away from the teeth). Possible increased risks for heart disease, diabetes, and reproductive problems are being studied.

Is smokeless tobacco a good substitute for cigarettes?

In 1986, the Surgeon General concluded that the use of smokeless tobacco "is not a safe substitute for smoking cigarettes. It can cause cancer and a number of noncancerous conditions and can lead to nicotine addiction and dependence." Since 1991, the National Cancer Institute (NCI), a part of the National Institutes of Health, has officially recommended that the public avoid and discontinue the use of all tobacco products, including smokeless tobacco. NCI also recognizes that nitrosamines, found in tobacco products, are not safe at any level. The accumulated scientific evidence does not support changing this position.

What about using smokeless tobacco to quit cigarettes?

Because all tobacco use causes disease and addiction, NCI recommends that tobacco use be avoided and discontinued. Several nontobacco methods have been shown to be effective for quitting cigarettes. These methods include pharmacotherapies such as nicotine replacement therapy and bupropion, individual and group counseling, and telephone quitlines.

Section 53.3

Hookah (Water Pipe) Smoking

"New study measures hookah use among Florida teens," © 2009 University of Florida. Reprinted with permission.

Hookah pipe smoking has gained a foothold with Florida teens, according to a new University of Florida study, which shows 11 percent of high school students and 4 percent of middle school students have tried it.

The findings were presented today (Nov. 9 [2009]) at the American Public Health Association's annual meeting in Philadelphia and appear in the November issue of the *American Journal of Public Health*. The study was conducted in collaboration with the Florida Department of Health.

Rooted in Middle Eastern culture, hookah pipes burn charcoal and tobacco, also known as shisha. Air is drawn through the tobacco and into the pipe, where it passes through water.

Hookah smokers widely but mistakenly believe that the pipe is a harmless alternative to other forms of tobacco smoking, said lead researcher Tracey Barnett, an assistant professor in the UF College of Public Health and Health Professions' department of behavioral science and community health.

"Users tend to think smoking with a hookah is safe because they believe the water in the pipe acts as a filter," Barnett said. "Many actually don't think that shisha has tobacco, while others feel it's a more pure form of tobacco that doesn't have as many chemicals, although there's really no reason to believe this."

In fact, during a typical 20- to 80-minute hookah session, users may smoke the equivalent of 100 or more cigarettes, according to the World Health Organization. Hookah smoking can deliver 11 times more carbon monoxide than a cigarette, in addition to high levels of other carcinogenic toxins and heavy metals found in cigarettes. While the water in the hookah pipes does absorb some nicotine, researchers believe smokers are exposed to enough to cause addiction.

The UF researchers' findings are based on data from the 2007 Florida Youth Tobacco Survey, an anonymous, annual survey administered by the Florida Department of Health to a random sample of public middle and high schools. The 2007 survey, completed by 9,000 students, was the first to include questions about hookah use.

There are at least 100 hookah lounges in Florida and most have opened in the past few years, Barnett said. Hookah is typically shared in groups and smoked with sweetened, flavored tobacco.

"The social nature of hookah smoking appeals to young people," Barnett said. "An 18-year-old high school senior can't get into clubs where alcohol is served, but he or she can legally smoke."

The state of Florida's minimum smoking age is 18.

While a few previous studies have estimated hookah use among college students, the UF study is only the second population-based study to examine hookah use in middle and high school students. A University of Pittsburgh study of Arizona students found that 10 percent of high school students and 2 percent of middle school students had smoked a hookah, according to data from a 2005 survey.

In addition to overall prevalence of hookah smoking, the UF researchers found that hookah usage rates were higher among boys, students who reported a history of cigarette smoking, and those who believe that cigarette smoking can relieve stress and help people feel more comfortable in social situations. Rates also increased with each advancing grade. Twelfth graders were eight times more likely to have used a hookah than 6th graders.

"Beliefs about the relative lack of harm associated with hookah use may also be held by policymakers, scientists, and the general public. This could explain the slow response to both restricting hookah use in public settings and mounting a full-scale research effort to understand its health effects," said Barbara Curbow, one of the study's co-authors and chair of the UF department of behavioral science and community health. "We hope that our work encourages policymakers and researchers to become more involved in understanding the phenomenon."

The new UF study team adds considerably to the emerging evidence of the widespread use of water pipe smoking among youth in the United States, said Dr. Wasim Maziak, an associate professor at the University of Memphis and the director of the Syrian Center for Tobacco Studies.

"Just a decade ago questions about water pipe use were not even considered in most youth tobacco surveys, and evidence suggests that water pipe smoking is no less harmful or addictive than cigarettes," Maziak said. "In fact, water pipe smoking can be the first means for introducing nicotine to tobacco-naive adolescents. All this calls for concerted efforts to continue active surveillance of this emerging tobacco-use method among U.S. youths, and to invest in research aimed at developing effective means to curb its spread."

Section 53.4

Smoking and How to Quit

Excerpted from "Smoking and How to Quit," by the Office on Women's Health (www.womenshealth.gov), part of the U.S. Department of Health and Human Services, June 17, 2009.

People smoke for different reasons. Some people smoke to deal with stress or control weight. Younger people may start smoking to rebel, show independence, or be accepted by their peers. But there is never a good reason to smoke.

When you quit, you will never again have to leave your workplace, your home, or other places to smoke. Over time, you will see some of the other benefits of quitting:

- Your teeth will be cleaner.

- You breath will smell better.

- The stain marks on your fingers will fade.

- Your skin is less wrinkled.

- You are able to smell and taste things better.

- You will also feel stronger and be able to be more active.

Make the Decision to Quit and Feel Great

If you have made the decision to quit smoking, congratulations! Not only will you improve your own health, you will also protect the health of your loved ones by no longer exposing them to secondhand smoke.

We know how hard it can be to quit smoking. Did you know that many people try to quit two or three times before they give up smoking for good? Nicotine is a very addictive drug—as addictive as heroin and cocaine. The good news is that millions of people have given up smoking for good. It's hard work to quit, but you can do it. Freeing yourself of an expensive habit that is dangerous to your health and the health of others will make you feel great!

Many people who smoke worry that they will gain weight if they quit. In fact, nearly 80 percent of people who quit smoking do gain weight, but the average weight gain is just 5 pounds. Keep in mind, however, that 56 percent of people who continue to smoke will gain weight, too. But the health benefits of quitting far exceed any risks from the weight gain that may follow quitting.

How to Quit

Research has shown that these five steps will help you to quit for good:

- **Pick a date to stop smoking.** Before that day, get rid of all cigarettes, ashtrays, and lighters everywhere you smoke. Do not allow anyone to smoke in your home. Write down why you want to quit and keep this list as a reminder.

- **Get support from your family, friends, and coworkers.** Studies have shown you will be more likely to quit if you have help. Let the people important to you know the date you will be quitting and ask them for their support. Ask them not to smoke around you or leave cigarettes out. Get more support ideas.

- **Find substitutes for smoking and vary your routine.** When you get the urge to smoke, do something to take your mind off smoking. Talk to a friend, go for a walk, or go to the movies.

- **Reduce stress with exercise, meditation, hot baths, or reading.** Try sugar-free gum or candy to help handle your cravings. Drink lots of water and juices. You might want to try changing your daily routine as well. Try drinking tea instead of coffee, eating your breakfast in a different place, or taking a different route to work.

441

- **Talk to your doctor or nurse about medicines to help you quit.** Some people have withdrawal symptoms when they quit smoking. These symptoms can include depression, trouble sleeping, feeling irritable or restless, and trouble thinking clearly. There are medicines to help relieve these symptoms. Most medicines help you quit smoking by giving you small, steady doses of nicotine, the drug in cigarettes that causes addiction. Talk to your doctor or nurse to see if one of these medicines may be right for you:

  - Nicotine patch: This is worn on the skin and supplies a steady amount of nicotine to the body through the skin.

  - Nicotine gum or lozenge: This releases nicotine into the bloodstream through the lining in your mouth.

  - Nicotine nasal spray: This is inhaled through your nose and passes into your bloodstream.

  - Nicotine inhaler: This is inhaled through the mouth and absorbed in the mouth and throat.

  - Bupropion: This is an antidepressant medicine that reduces nicotine withdrawal symptoms and the urge to smoke.

  - Varenicline (Chantix): This is a medicine that reduces nicotine withdrawal symptoms and the pleasurable effects of smoking.

- **Be prepared for relapse.** Most people relapse, or start smoking again, within the first 3 months after quitting. Don't get discouraged if you relapse. Remember, many people try to quit several times before quitting for good. Think of what helped and didn't help the last time you tried to quit. Figuring these out before you try to quit again will increase your chances for success. Certain situations can increase your chances of smoking. These include drinking alcohol, being around other smokers, gaining weight, stress, or becoming depressed. Talk to your doctor or nurse for ways to cope with these situations.

Chapter 54

Alcohol Use in Adolescents

Chapter Contents

Section 54.1

Why Do Adolescents Drink, What Are the Risks, and How Can Underage Drinking Be Prevented?

Excerpted from text by the National Institute on Alcohol Abuse and Alcoholism (NIAAA, niaaa.nih.gov), part of the National Institutes of Health, January 2006.

Alcohol is the drug of choice among youth. Many young people are experiencing the consequences of drinking too much, at too early an age. As a result, underage drinking is a leading public health problem in this country.

Each year, approximately 5,000 young people under the age of 21 die as a result of underage drinking; this includes about 1,900 deaths from motor vehicle crashes, 1,600 as a result of homicides, 300 from suicide, as well as hundreds from other injuries such as falls, burns, and drownings.

Yet drinking continues to be widespread among adolescents, as shown by nationwide surveys as well as studies in smaller populations. According to data from the 2005 Monitoring the Future (MTF) study, an annual survey of U.S. youth, three fourths of 12th graders, more than two thirds of 10th graders, and about two in every five 8th graders have consumed alcohol. And when youth drink they tend to drink intensively, often consuming four to five drinks at one time. MTF data show that 11 percent of 8th graders, 22 percent of 10th graders, and 29 percent of 12th graders had engaged in heavy episodic (or binge) drinking within the past 2 weeks. (The National Institute on Alcohol Abuse and Alcoholism [NIAAA] defines binge drinking as a pattern of drinking alcohol that brings blood alcohol concentration [BAC] to 0.08 grams percent or above. For the typical adult, this pattern corresponds to consuming five or more drinks [men], or four or more drinks [women], in about 2 hours.)

Research also shows that many adolescents start to drink at very young ages. In 2003, the average age of first use of alcohol was about 14, compared to about 17 1/2 in 1965. People who reported starting to drink before the age of 15 were four times more likely to also report meeting the criteria for alcohol dependence at some point in their lives. In fact, new research shows that the serious drinking problems (including what is called alcoholism) typically associated with middle age actually begin to appear much earlier, during young adulthood and even adolescence.

Other research shows that the younger children and adolescents are when they start to drink, the more likely they will be to engage in behaviors that harm themselves and others. For example, frequent binge drinkers (nearly 1 million high school students nationwide) are more likely to engage in risky behaviors, including using other drugs such as marijuana and cocaine, having sex with six or more partners, and earning grades that are mostly Ds and Fs in school.

Why Do Some Adolescents Drink?

As children move from adolescence to young adulthood, they encounter dramatic physical, emotional, and lifestyle changes. Developmental transitions, such as puberty and increasing independence, have been associated with alcohol use. So in a sense, just being an adolescent may be a key risk factor not only for starting to drink but also for drinking dangerously.

Risk-taking: Research shows the brain keeps developing well into the twenties, during which time it continues to establish important communication connections and further refines its function. Scientists believe that this lengthy developmental period may help explain some of the behavior which is characteristic of adolescence—such as their propensity to seek out new and potentially dangerous situations. For some teens, thrill-seeking might include experimenting with alcohol. Developmental changes also offer a possible physiological explanation for why teens act so impulsively, often not recognizing that their actions—such as drinking—have consequences.

Expectancies: How people view alcohol and its effects also influences their drinking behavior, including whether they begin to drink and how much. An adolescent who expects drinking to be a pleasurable experience is more likely to drink than one who does not. An important area of alcohol research is focusing on how expectancy influences drinking patterns from childhood through adolescence and into young adulthood. Beliefs about alcohol are established very early in life, even before the child begins elementary school. Before age 9, children generally view alcohol negatively and see drinking as bad, with adverse effects. By about age 13, however, their expectancies shift, becoming more positive. As would be expected, adolescents who drink the most also place the greatest emphasis on the positive and arousing effects of alcohol.

Sensitivity and tolerance to alcohol: Differences between the adult brain and the brain of the maturing adolescent also may help to explain why many young drinkers are able to consume much larger amounts of alcohol than adults before experiencing the negative consequences of drinking, such as drowsiness, lack of coordination, and withdrawal/hangover effects. This unusual tolerance may help to explain the high rates of binge drinking among young adults. At the same time, adolescents appear to be particularly sensitive to the positive effects of drinking, such as feeling more at ease in social situations, and young people may drink more than adults because of these positive social experiences.

Personality characteristics and psychiatric comorbidity— Children who begin to drink at a very early age (before age 12) often share similar personality characteristics that may make them more likely to start drinking. Young people who are disruptive, hyperactive, and aggressive—often referred to as having conduct problems or being antisocial—as well as those who are depressed, withdrawn, or anxious, may be at greatest risk for alcohol problems. Other behavior problems associated with alcohol use include rebelliousness, difficulty avoiding harm or harmful situations, and a host of other traits seen in young people who act out without regard for rules or the feelings of others (i.e., disinhibition).

Hereditary factors—Some of the behavioral and physiological factors that converge to increase or decrease a person's risk for alcohol problems, including tolerance to alcohol's effects, may be directly linked to genetics. For example, being a child of an alcoholic or having several alcoholic family members places a person at greater risk for alcohol problems. Children of alcoholics (COAs) are between 4 and 10 times more likely to become alcoholics themselves than are children who have no close relatives with alcoholism. COAs also are more likely to begin drinking at a young age and to progress to drinking problems more quickly.

Research shows that COAs may have subtle brain differences which could be markers for developing later alcohol problems. For example, using high-tech brain-imaging techniques, scientists have found that COAs have a distinctive feature in one brainwave pattern (called a P300 response) that could be a marker for later alcoholism risk. Researchers also are investigating other brainwave differences in COAs that may be present long before they begin to drink, including brainwave activity recorded during sleep as well as changes in brain structure and function.

Some studies suggest that these brain differences may be particularly evident in people who also have certain behavioral traits, such as signs of conduct disorder, antisocial personality disorder, sensation-seeking, or poor impulse control. Studying how the brain's structure and function translates to behavior will help researchers to better understand how pre-drinking risk factors shape later alcohol use. For example, does a person who is depressed drink to alleviate his or her depression, or does drinking lead to changes in his brain that result in feelings of depression?

Other hereditary factors likely will become evident as scientists work to identify the actual genes involved in addiction. By analyzing the genetic makeup of people and families with alcohol dependence, researchers have found specific regions on chromosomes that correlate with a risk for alcoholism. Candidate genes for alcoholism risk also have been associated with those regions. The goal now is to further refine regions for which a specific gene has not yet been identified and then determine how those genes interact with other genes and gene products as well as with the environment to result in alcohol dependence. Further research also should shed light on the extent to which the same or different genes contribute to alcohol problems, both in adults and in adolescents.

Environmental aspects: Pinpointing a genetic contribution will not tell the whole story, however, as drinking behavior reflects a complex interplay between inherited and environmental factors, the implications of which are only beginning to be explored in adolescents. And what influences drinking at one age may not have the same impact at another. As Rose and colleagues show, genetic factors appear to have more influence on adolescent drinking behavior in late adolescence than in mid-adolescence.

Environmental factors, such as the influence of parents and peers, also play a role in alcohol use. For example, parents who drink more and who view drinking favorably may have children who drink more, and an adolescent girl with an older or adult boyfriend is more likely to use alcohol and other drugs and to engage in delinquent behaviors.

Researchers are examining other environmental influences as well, such as the impact of the media. Today alcohol is widely available and aggressively promoted through television, radio, billboards, and the Internet. Researchers are studying how young people react to these advertisements. In a study of 3rd, 6th, and 9th graders, those who found alcohol ads desirable were more likely to view drinking positively and to want to purchase products with alcohol logos. Research is mixed, however, on whether these positive views of alcohol actually lead to underage drinking.

What Are the Health Risks?

Whatever it is that leads adolescents to begin drinking, once they start they face a number of potential health risks. Although the severe health problems associated with harmful alcohol use are not as common in adolescents as they are in adults, studies show that young people who drink heavily may put themselves at risk for a range of potential health problems.

Brain effects: Scientists currently are examining just how alcohol affects the developing brain, but it's a difficult task. Subtle changes in the brain may be difficult to detect but still have a significant impact on long-term thinking and memory skills. Add to this the fact that adolescent brains are still maturing, and the study of alcohol's effects becomes even more complex. Research has shown that animals fed alcohol during this critical developmental stage continue to show long-lasting impairment from alcohol as they age. It's simply not known how alcohol will affect the long-term memory and learning skills of people who began drinking heavily as adolescents.

Liver effects: Elevated liver enzymes, indicating some degree of liver damage, have been found in some adolescents who drink alcohol. Young drinkers who are overweight or obese showed elevated liver enzymes even with only moderate levels of drinking.

Growth and endocrine effects: In both males and females, puberty is a period associated with marked hormonal changes, including increases in the sex hormones, estrogen and testosterone. These hormones, in turn, increase production of other hormones and growth factors, which are vital for normal organ development. Drinking alcohol during this period of rapid growth and development (i.e., prior to or during puberty) may upset the critical hormonal balance necessary for normal development of organs, muscles, and bones. Studies in animals also show that consuming alcohol during puberty adversely affects the maturation of the reproductive system.

Interventions for Preventing Underage Drinking

Intervention approaches typically fall into two distinct categories: (1) environmental-level interventions, which seek to reduce opportunities for underage drinking, increase penalties for violating minimum legal drinking age (MLDA) and other alcohol use laws, and reduce community tolerance for alcohol use by youth; and (2) individual-level interventions, which seek to change knowledge, expectancies, attitudes, intentions, motivation, and skills so that youth are better able to resist the prodrinking influences and opportunities that surround them. Environmental approaches include the following:

- **Raising the price of alcohol:** A substantial body of research has shown that higher prices or taxes on alcoholic beverages are associated with lower levels of alcohol consumption and alcohol-related problems, especially in young people.

- **Increasing the minimum legal drinking age:** Today all states have set the minimum legal drinking at age 21. Increasing the age at which people can legally purchase and drink alcohol has been the most successful intervention to date in reducing drinking and alcohol-related crashes among people under age 21. NHTSA estimates that a legal drinking age of 21 saves 700 to 1,000 lives annually. Since 1976, these laws have prevented more than 21,000 traffic deaths. Just how much the legal drinking age relates to drinking-related crashes is shown by a recent study in New Zealand. Six years ago that country lowered its minimum legal drinking age to 18. Since then, alcohol-related crashes have risen 12 percent among 18- to 19-year-olds and 14 percent among 15- to 17-year-olds. Clearly a higher minimum drinking age can help to reduce crashes and save lives, especially in very young drivers.

- **Enacting zero-tolerance laws:** All states have zero-tolerance laws that make it illegal for people under age 21 to drive after any drinking. When the first eight states to adopt zero-tolerance laws were compared with nearby sates without such laws, the zero-tolerance states showed a 21-percent greater decline in the proportion of single-vehicle night-time fatal crashes involving drivers under 21, the type of crash most likely to involve alcohol.

- **Stepping up enforcement of laws:** Despite their demonstrated benefits, legal drinking age and zero-tolerance laws generally have not been vigorously enforced. Alcohol purchase laws aimed at sellers and buyers also can be effective, but resources must be made available for enforcing these laws.

Individual-focused interventions include the following:

- **School-based prevention programs:** The first school-based prevention programs were primarily informational and often used scare tactics; it was assumed that if youth understood the dangers of alcohol use, they would choose not to drink. These programs were ineffective. Today, better programs are available and often

449

have a number of elements in common: They follow social influence models and include setting norms, addressing social pressures to drink, and teaching resistance skills. These programs also offer interactive and developmentally appropriate information, include peer-led components, and provide teacher training.

- **Family-based prevention programs:** Parents' ability to influence whether their children drink is well documented and is consistent across racial/ethnic groups. Setting clear rules against drinking, consistently enforcing those rules, and monitoring the child's behavior all help to reduce the likelihood of underage drinking. The Iowa Strengthening Families Program (ISFP), delivered when students were in grade 6, is a program that has shown long-lasting preventive effects on alcohol use.

Section 54.2

Talk to Your Child about Alcohol

Excerpted from text by the National Institute on Alcohol Abuse and Alcoholism (NIAAA, www.niaaa.nih.gov), part of the National Institutes of Health, 2009.

Alcohol is a drug, as surely as cocaine and marijuana are. It's also illegal to drink under the age of 21. And it's dangerous. Kids who drink are more likely to:

- be victims of violent crime;

- have serious problems in school; and

- be involved in drinking-related traffic crashes.

Your child looks to you for guidance and support in making life decisions—including the decision not to use alcohol.

"But my child isn't drinking yet," you may think. "Isn't it a little early to be concerned about drinking?" Not at all. This is the age when some children begin experimenting with alcohol. Even if your child is not yet drinking alcohol, he or she may be receiving pressure to drink.

Act now. Keeping quiet about how you feel about your child's alcohol use may give him or her the impression that alcohol use is OK for kids.

It's not easy. As children approach adolescence, friends exert a lot of influence. Fitting in is a chief priority for teens, and parents often feel shoved aside. Kids will listen, however. Study after study shows that even during the teen years, parents have enormous influence on their children's behavior.

The bottom line is that most young teens don't yet drink. And parents' disapproval of youthful alcohol use is the key reason children choose not to drink. So make no mistake: You can make a difference.

Talking with Your Teen about Alcohol

For many parents, bringing up the subject of alcohol is no easy matter. Your young teen may try to dodge the discussion, and you may feel unsure about how to proceed. To make the most of your conversation, take some time to think about the issues you want to discuss before you talk with your child. Consider too how your child might react and ways you might respond to your youngster's questions and feelings. Then choose a time to talk when both you and your child have some "down time" and are feeling relaxed.

You don't need to cover everything at once. In fact, you're likely to have a greater impact on your child's decisions about drinking by having a number of talks about alcohol use throughout his or her adolescence. Think of this talk with your child as the first part of an ongoing conversation.

And remember, do make it a conversation, not a lecture. You might begin by finding out what your child thinks about alcohol and drinking.

Your Child's Views about Alcohol

Ask your young teen what he or she knows about alcohol and what he or she thinks about teen drinking. Ask your child why he or she thinks kids drink. Listen carefully without interrupting. Not only will this approach help your child to feel heard and respected, but it can serve as a natural "lead-in" to discussing alcohol topics.

Important Facts about Alcohol

Although many kids believe that they already know everything about alcohol, myths and misinformation abound. Here are some important facts to share:

- Alcohol is a powerful drug that slows down the body and mind. It impairs coordination; slows reaction time; and impairs vision, clear thinking, and judgment.

- Beer and wine are not safer than hard liquor. A 12-ounce can of beer, a 5-ounce glass of wine, and 1.5 ounces of hard liquor all contain the same amount of alcohol and have the same effects on the body and mind.

- On average, it takes 2 to 3 hours for a single drink to leave a person's system. Nothing can speed up this process, including drinking coffee, taking a cold shower, or "walking it off."

- People tend to be very bad at judging how seriously alcohol has affected them. That means many individuals who drive after drinking think they can control a car—but actually cannot.

- Anyone can develop a serious alcohol problem, including a teenager.

Good Reasons Not to Drink

In talking with your child about reasons to avoid alcohol, stay away from scare tactics. Most young teens are aware that many people drink without problems, so it is important to discuss the consequences of alcohol use without overstating the case. Some good reasons why teens should not drink:

- **You want your child to avoid alcohol.** Clearly state your own expectations about your child's drinking. Your values and attitudes count with your child, even though he or she may not always show it.

- **It helps maintain self-respect.** Teens say the best way to persuade them to avoid alcohol is to appeal to their self-respect—let them know that they are too smart and have too much going for them to need the crutch of alcohol. Teens also are likely to pay attention to examples of how alcohol might lead to embarrassing situations or events—things that might damage their self-respect or alter important relationships.

- **Drinking is illegal.** Because alcohol use under the age of 21 is illegal, getting caught may mean trouble with the authorities. Even if getting caught doesn't lead to police action, the parents of your child's friends may no longer permit them to associate with your child.

- **Drinking can be dangerous.** One of the leading causes of teen deaths is motor vehicle crashes involving alcohol. Drinking also makes a young person more vulnerable to sexual assault and unprotected sex. And while your teen may believe he or she wouldn't engage in hazardous activities after drinking, point out that because alcohol impairs judgment, a drinker is very likely to think such activities won't be dangerous.

- **You have a family history of alcoholism.** If one or more members of your family has suffered from alcoholism, your child may be somewhat more vulnerable to developing a drinking problem.

- **Alcohol affects young people differently than adults.** Drinking while the brain is still maturing may lead to long-lasting intellectual effects and may even increase the likelihood of developing alcohol dependence later in life.

The "Magic Potion" Myth

The media's glamorous portrayal of alcohol encourages many teens to believe that drinking will make them "cool," popular, attractive, and happy. Research shows that teens who expect such positive effects are more likely to drink at early ages. However, you can help to combat these dangerous myths by watching TV shows and movies with your child and discussing how alcohol is portrayed in them. For example, television advertisements for beer often show young people having an uproariously good time, as though drinking always puts people in a terrific mood. Watching such a commercial with your child can be an opportunity to discuss the many ways that alcohol can affect people—in some cases bringing on feelings of sadness or anger rather than carefree high spirits.

How to Handle Peer Pressure

It's not enough to tell your young teen that he or she should avoid alcohol—you also need to help your child figure out how. What can your daughter say when she goes to a party and a friend offers her a beer? Or what should your son do if he finds himself in a home where kids are passing around a bottle of wine and parents are nowhere in sight? What should their response be if they are offered a ride home with an older friend who has been drinking?

Brainstorm with your teen for ways that he or she might handle these and other difficult situations, and make clear how you are willing to support your child. An example: "If you find yourself at a home

453

where kids are drinking, call me and I'll pick you up—and there will be no scolding or punishment." The more prepared your child is, the better able he or she will be to handle high-pressure situations that involve drinking.

Mom, Dad, Did You Drink When You Were a Kid?

This is the question many parents dread—yet it is highly likely to come up in any family discussion of alcohol. The reality is that many parents did drink before they were old enough to legally do so. So how can one be honest with a child without sounding like a hypocrite who advises, "Do as I say, not as I did"? This is a judgment call. If you believe that your drinking or drug use history should not be part of the discussion, you can simply tell your child that you choose not to share it. Another approach is to admit that you did do some drinking as a teenager, but that it was a mistake—and give your teen an example of an embarrassing or painful moment that occurred because of your drinking. This approach may help your child better understand that youthful alcohol use does have negative consequences.

Warning Signs of a Drinking Problem

Although the following signs may indicate a problem with alcohol or other drugs, some also reflect normal teenage growing pains. Experts believe that a drinking problem is more likely if you notice several of these signs at the same time, if they occur suddenly, and if some of them are extreme in nature.

- Mood changes: flare-ups of temper, irritability, and defensiveness

- School problems: poor attendance, low grades, and/or recent disciplinary action

- Rebelling against family rules

- Switching friends, along with a reluctance to have you get to know the new friends

- A "nothing matters" attitude: sloppy appearance, a lack of involvement in former interests, and general low energy

- Finding alcohol in your child's room or backpack, or smelling alcohol on his or her breath

- Physical or mental problems: memory lapses, poor concentration, bloodshot eyes, lack of coordination, or slurred speech

Chapter 55

Marijuana

Marijuana is a mixture of the dried and shredded leaves, stems, seeds, and flowers of the cannabis sativa plant. The mixture can be green, brown, or gray.

A bunch of leaves seem harmless, right? But think again. Marijuana has a chemical in it called delta-9-tetrahydrocannabinol, better known as THC. A lot of other chemicals are found in marijuana, too—about 400 of them, many of which could affect your health. But THC is the main psychoactive (i.e., mind altering) ingredient. In fact, marijuana's strength or potency is related to the amount of THC it contains. The THC content of marijuana has been increasing since the 1970s. For the year 2007, estimates from confiscated marijuana indicated that it contains almost 10 percent THC on average.

What are the common street names?

There are many slang terms for marijuana that vary from city to city and from neighborhood to neighborhood. Some common names are: pot, grass, herb, weed, Mary Jane, reefer, skunk, boom, gangster, kif, chronic, and ganja.

How is it used?

Marijuana is used in many ways. The most common method is smoking loose marijuana rolled into a cigarette called a joint or nail.

From the National Institute on Drug Abuse (NIDA, teens.drugabuse.gov), part of the National Institutes of Health, January 2010.

Sometimes marijuana is smoked through a water pipe called a bong. Others smoke blunts—cigars hollowed out and filled with the drug. And some users brew it as tea or mix it with food.

How many teens use marijuana?

Some people mistakenly believe that "everybody's doing it" and use that as an excuse to start using marijuana themselves. Well, they need to check the facts, because that's just not true. According to a 2009 survey called Monitoring the Future, about 7 percent of 8th graders, 16 percent of 10th graders, and 21 percent of 12th graders had used marijuana in the month before the survey. In fact, marijuana use declined from the late 1990s through 2007, with a decrease in past-year use of more than 20 percent in all three grades combined from 2000 to 2007. Unfortunately, this trend appears to be slowing, and marijuana use remains at unacceptably high levels, as the most commonly used illegal drug.

What are the short-term effects of marijuana use?

For some people, smoking marijuana makes them feel good. Within minutes of inhaling, a user begins to feel "high," or filled with pleasant sensations. THC triggers brain cells to release the chemical dopamine. Dopamine creates good feelings—for a short time. But that's just one effect.

Imagine this: You're in a ball game, playing out in left field. An easy fly ball comes your way, and you're psyched. When that ball lands in your glove your team will win, and you'll be a hero. But, you're a little off. The ball grazes your glove and hits dirt. So much for your dreams of glory.

Such loss of coordination can be caused by smoking marijuana. And that's just one of its many negative effects. Marijuana affects memory, judgment, and perception. Under the influence of marijuana, you could fail to remember things you just learned, watch your grade point average drop, or crash a car.

Also, since marijuana can affect judgment and decision making, using it can cause you to do things you might not do when you are thinking straight—such as risky sexual behavior, which can result in exposure to sexually transmitted diseases, like HIV [human immunodeficiency virus], the virus that causes AIDS [acquired immunodeficiency syndrome]; or getting in a car with someone who's been drinking or is high on marijuana.

It's also difficult to know how marijuana will affect a specific person at any given time, because its effects vary based on individual factors: a person's genetics, whether they've used marijuana or any other drugs before, how much marijuana is taken, and its potency. Effects can also be unpredictable when marijuana is used in combination with other drugs.

THC impacts brain functioning: THC is up to no good in the brain. THC finds brain cells, or neurons, with specific kinds of receptors called cannabinoid receptors and binds to them.

Certain parts of the brain have high concentrations of cannabinoid receptors. These areas are the hippocampus, the cerebellum, the basal ganglia, and the cerebral cortex. The functions that these brain areas control are the ones most affected by marijuana.

For example, THC interferes with learning and memory—that is because the hippocampus—a part of the brain with a funny name and a big job—plays a critical role in certain types of learning. Disrupting its normal functioning can lead to problems studying, learning new things, and recalling recent events. The difficulty can be a lot more serious than forgetting if you took out the trash this morning, which happens to everyone once in a while.

Do these effects persist? We don't know for sure, but as adolescents your brains are still developing. So is it really worth the risk?

Smoking marijuana can make driving dangerous: The cerebellum is the section of our brain that controls balance and coordination. When THC affects the cerebellum's function, it makes scoring a goal in soccer or hitting a home run pretty tough. THC also affects the basal ganglia, another part of the brain that's involved in movement control.

These THC effects can cause disaster on the road. Research shows that drivers on marijuana have slower reaction times, impaired judgment, and problems responding to signals and sounds. Studies conducted in a number of localities have found that approximately 4 to 14 percent of drivers who sustained injury or death in traffic accidents tested positive for delta-9-tetrahydrocannabinol (THC), the active ingredient in marijuana.

Marijuana use increases heart rate: Within a few minutes after inhaling marijuana smoke, an individual's heart begins beating more rapidly, the bronchial passages relax and become enlarged, and blood vessels in the eyes expand, making the eyes look red. The heart rate, normally 70 to 80 beats per minute, may increase by 20 to 50 beats per minute or, in some cases, even double. This effect can be greater if other drugs are taken with marijuana.

What are the long-term health effects of marijuana use?

The list of negative effects that can arise from using marijuana goes on and on. Here are a few examples.

The brain: When people smoke marijuana for years they can suffer some pretty negative consequences. For example, because marijuana affects brain function, your ability to do complex tasks could be compromised, as well as your pursuit of academic, athletic, or other life goals that require you to be 100 percent focused and alert. In fact, long-term users self-report less life satisfaction, poorer education, and job achievement, and more interpersonal and mental health problems compared to non-users.

Marijuana also may affect your mental health. Studies show that early use may increase your risk of developing psychosis [a severe mental disorder in which there is a loss of contact with reality, including false ideas about what is happening (delusions) and seeing or hearing things that aren't there (hallucinations)], particularly if you carry a genetic vulnerability to the disease. Also, rates of marijuana use are often higher in people with symptoms of depression or anxiety—but it is very difficult to determine which came first, so we don't yet know whether they are causally related.

Lungs and airways: People who abuse marijuana are at risk of injuring their lungs through exposure to respiratory irritants and carcinogens found in marijuana smoke. The smoke from marijuana contains some of the same chemicals found in tobacco smoke; plus, marijuana users tend to inhale more deeply and hold their breath longer, so more smoke enters the lungs. Not surprisingly, marijuana smokers have some of the same breathing problems as tobacco smokers—they are more susceptible to chest colds, coughs, and bronchitis than nonsmokers. And, even though we don't know yet whether or how marijuana use affects the risk for lung and other cancers—why take the risk?

Addiction: Many people don't think of marijuana as addictive—they are wrong. In 2007, the majority of youth (age 17 or younger) entering drug abuse treatment reported marijuana as their primary drug abused. Marijuana increases dopamine, which creates the good feelings or "high" associated with its use. A user may feel the urge to smoke marijuana again, and again, and again to recreate that experience. Repeated use could lead to addiction—a disease where people continue to do something, even when they are aware of the severe negative consequences at the personal, social, academic, and professional levels.

Marijuana users may also experience a withdrawal syndrome when they stop using the drug. It is similar to what happens to tobacco smokers when they quit—people report being irritable, having sleep problems, and weight loss—effects which can last for several days to a few weeks after drug use is stopped. Relapse is common during this period, as users also crave the drug to relieve these symptoms.

Chapter 56

Prescription Medicine Abuse

Prescription drug abuse by teens and young adults is a serious problem in the United States. As reported in the Partnership for a Drug Free America's annual tracking study:

- One in five teens has abused a prescription (Rx) pain medication.

- One in five report abusing prescription stimulants and tranquilizers.

- One in 10 has abused cough medication.

Many teens think these drugs are safe because they have legitimate uses, but taking them without a prescription to get high or self-medicate can be as dangerous—and addictive—as using street narcotics and other illicit drugs.

The Partnership for a Drug-Free America is making sure that parents, young adults, and teens know the very real risks of misusing medicine.

Parents' Questions and Answers

What age are teens abusing prescription drugs?

Kids as young as 12 are trying or using prescription drugs non-medically—to get high or for self-medicating. Pharmaceuticals are often more available to 12-year-olds than illicit drugs because they can be taken from the medicine cabinet at home, rather than marijuana which necessitates knowing someone who uses or sells the drug. Also, pills may have a perception of safety because they are easier to take than smoking pot or drinking alcohol and are professionally manufactured in a lab.

What types of prescription drugs are teens abusing?

The National Survey on Drug Use and Health identifies four types of prescription medications that are commonly abused—pain relievers, stimulants, sedatives, and tranquilizers. Eleven percent of teens (aged 12–17) reported lifetime non-medical use of pain relievers and four percent reported lifetime non-medical use of stimulants.

Do different groups abuse different types of medications?

Yes. Painkillers are the most common pharmaceutical abused by teens, especially by younger teens. Stimulant abuse is more common among older teens and college students than younger teens. Girls are more likely to be current (past month) abusers of prescription medications than boys (4.3 vs. 3.6 percent). [Source: 2002 National Survey on Drug Use and Health]

What can I do to help to prevent my child from misusing prescription drugs?

One easy way to prevent Rx abuse is to keep all prescription medication hidden. Parents and family members whose homes teens visit should keep prescription medications out of teens' reach, rather than in the medicine cabinet. You should also talk to your teen and warn them that taking prescription medications without a doctor's supervision can be just as dangerous and as potentially lethal as taking illicit drugs. For example, painkillers are made from opioids, the same substance as in heroin.

How can I talk to my kids about prescription drug abuse?

Starting a conversation about drugs with your kids is never easy—but it's also not as difficult as you may think. Take advantage of everyday "teachable moments" and, in no time at all, you'll have developed an ongoing dialogue with your child. Teachable moments refer to using everyday events in your life to point out things you'd like your child to know about. When you talk to your kids about drugs make a special point to tell kids how dangerous prescription drug abuse is.

- Pharmaceuticals taken without a prescription or a doctor's supervision can be just as dangerous as taking illicit drugs or alcohol.

- Abusing painkillers is like abusing heroin because their ingredients (both are opioids) are very similar.

- Prescription medications are powerful substances. While sick people taking medication under a doctor's care can benefit enormously, prescription medication can have a very different impact on a well person.

- Many pills look pretty much the same, but depending on the drug and the dosage the effects can vary greatly from mild to lethal.

- Prescription medications, as all drugs, can cause dangerous interactions with other drugs or chemicals in the body.

Chapter 57

Inhalants

Inhalants are a diverse group of volatile substances whose chemical vapors can be inhaled to produce psychoactive (mind-altering) effects. While other abused substances can be inhaled, the term "inhalants" is used to describe substances that are rarely, if ever, taken by any other route of administration. A variety of products common in the home and workplace contain substances that can be inhaled to get high; however, people do not typically think of these products (e.g., spray paints, glues, and cleaning fluids) as drugs because they were never intended to induce intoxicating effects. Yet young children and adolescents can easily obtain these extremely toxic substances and are among those most likely to abuse them.

What types of products are abused as inhalants?

Inhalants generally fall into several categories.

Volatile solvents are liquids that vaporize at room temperature. They include the following:

- Industrial or household products, including paint thinners or removers, degreasers, dry-cleaning fluids, gasoline, and lighter fluid

- Art or office supply solvents, including correction fluids, felt-tip marker fluid, electronic contact cleaners, and glue

From "InfoFacts: Inhalants," by the National Institute on Drug Abuse (NIDA, www.nida.nih.gov), part of the National Institutes of Health, March 2010.

Aerosols are sprays that contain propellants and solvents. They include household aerosol propellants in items such as spray paints, hair or deodorant sprays, fabric protector sprays, aerosol computer cleaning products, and vegetable oil sprays.

Gases are found in household or commercial products and used as medical anesthetics. They include household or commercial products, including butane lighters and propane tanks, whipped cream aerosols or dispensers (whippets), and refrigerant gases, and medical anesthetics, such as ether, chloroform, halothane, and nitrous oxide ("laughing gas").

Inhalants also include nitrites, a special class of inhalants that are used primarily as sexual enhancers. Organic nitrites are volatiles that include cyclohexyl, butyl, and amyl nitrites, commonly known as "poppers." Amyl nitrite is still used in certain diagnostic medical procedures. When marketed for illicit use, organic nitrites are often sold in small brown bottles labeled as "video head cleaner," "room odorizer," "leather cleaner," or "liquid aroma."

These various products contain a wide range of chemicals such as the following:

- Toluene (spray paints, rubber cement, gasoline)
- Chlorinated hydrocarbons (dry-cleaning chemicals, correction fluids)
- Hexane (glues, gasoline)
- Benzene (gasoline)
- Methylene chloride (varnish removers, paint thinners)
- Butane (cigarette lighter refills, air fresheners)
- Nitrous oxide (whipped cream dispensers, gas cylinders)

Adolescents tend to abuse different products at different ages. Among new users ages 12–15, the most commonly abused inhalants are glue, shoe polish, spray paints, gasoline, and lighter fluid. Among new users age 16 or 17, the most commonly abused products are nitrous oxide or whippets. Nitrites are the class of inhalants most commonly abused by adults.

How are inhalants abused?

Inhalants can be breathed in through the nose or mouth in a variety of ways (known as "huffing"), such as sniffing or snorting fumes from a container, spraying aerosols directly into the nose or mouth, or placing an inhalant-soaked rag in the mouth. Users may also inhale fumes from a balloon or a plastic or paper bag that contains an inhalant.

The intoxication produced by inhalants usually lasts just a few minutes; therefore, users often try to extend the "high" by continuing to inhale repeatedly over several hours.

How do inhalants affect the brain?

The effects of inhalants are similar to those of alcohol, including slurred speech, lack of coordination, euphoria, and dizziness. Inhalant abusers may also experience lightheadedness, hallucinations, and delusions. With repeated inhalations, many users feel less inhibited and less in control. Some may feel drowsy for several hours and experience a lingering headache. Chemicals found in different types of inhaled products may produce a variety of additional effects, such as confusion, nausea, or vomiting.

By displacing air in the lungs, inhalants deprive the body of oxygen, a condition known as hypoxia. Hypoxia can damage cells throughout the body, but the cells of the brain are especially sensitive to it. The symptoms of brain hypoxia vary according to which regions of the brain are affected. For example, the hippocampus helps control memory, so someone who repeatedly uses inhalants may lose the ability to learn new things or may have a hard time carrying on simple conversations.

Long-term inhalant abuse can also break down myelin, a fatty tissue that surrounds and protects some nerve fibers. Myelin helps nerve fibers carry their messages quickly and efficiently, and when damaged, can lead to muscle spasms and tremors or even permanent difficulty with basic actions such as walking, bending, and talking.

Although not very common, addiction to inhalants can occur with repeated abuse. According to the 2007 Treatment Episode Data Set, inhalants were reported as the primary substance abused by less than 0.1 percent of all individuals admitted to substance abuse treatment.

What other adverse effects do inhalants have on health?

Lethal effects: Sniffing highly concentrated amounts of the chemicals in solvents or aerosol sprays can directly induce heart failure and death within minutes of a session of repeated inhalation. This syndrome, known as "sudden sniffing death," can result from a single session of inhalant use by an otherwise healthy young person. Sudden sniffing death is particularly associated with the abuse of butane, propane, and chemicals in aerosols.

High concentrations of inhalants may also cause death from suffocation by displacing oxygen in the lungs, causing the user to lose consciousness and stop breathing. Deliberately inhaling from a paper or plastic bag or in a closed area greatly increases the chances of suffocation. Even when using aerosols or volatile products for their legitimate purposes (i.e., painting, cleaning), it is wise to do so in a well-ventilated room or outdoors.

Harmful irreversible effects:

- Hearing loss (spray paints, glues, dewaxers, dry-cleaning chemicals, correction fluids)

- Peripheral neuropathies or limb spasms (glues, gasoline, whipped cream dispensers, gas cylinders)

- Central nervous system or brain damage (spray paints, glues, dewaxers)

- Bone marrow damage (gasoline)

Serious but potentially reversible effects:

- Liver and kidney damage (correction fluids, dry-cleaning fluids)

- Blood oxygen depletion (varnish removers, paint thinners)

HIV/AIDS, hepatitis, and other infectious diseases: Because nitrites are abused to enhance sexual pleasure and performance, they can be associated with unsafe sexual practices that greatly increase the risk of contracting and spreading infectious diseases such as HIV/AIDS [human immunodeficiency virus/acquired immunodeficiency syndrome] and hepatitis.

How widespread is inhalant abuse?

Monitoring the Future Survey:[1] According to the Monitoring the Future survey, a significant increase in past-month inhalant use was measured among 10th graders from 2008 to 2009; prevalence of use rose from 2.1 percent to 2.2 percent among that population. Other prevalence measures remained stable. Lifetime[2] use of inhalants was reported by 14.9 percent of 8th graders, 12.3 percent of 10th graders, and 9.5 percent of 12th graders in 2009; 8.1 percent of 8th graders, 6.1 percent of 10th graders, and 3.4 percent of 12th graders reported use in the past year. However, investigators are concerned that perceived risk associated with inhalant use has been in decline for several years, which may leave young people open to renewed interest.

National Survey on Drug Use and Health (NSDUH):[3] Data from the National Survey on Drug Use and Health show that the primary abusers of most inhalants are adolescents ages 12 to 17; in

2008, 1.1 percent reported using inhalants in the past month. From 2002 to 2008, there were declines in past-month inhalant use among young adults aged 18 to 25 (from 0.5 percent to 0.3 percent). Of the 729,000 persons aged 12 or older who tried inhalants for the first time within the previous year, approximately 67 percent were under age 18 when they first used.

Notes

1. These data are from the 2009 Monitoring the Future survey, funded by the National Institute on Drug Abuse, National Institutes of Health, Department of Health and Human Services, and conducted annually by the University of Michigan's Institute for Social Research. The survey has tracked 12th-graders' illicit drug use and related attitudes since 1975; in 1991, 8th and 10th graders were added to the study. The latest data are on line at www.drugabuse.gov.

2. "Lifetime" refers to use at least once during a respondent's lifetime. "Past year" refers to use at least once during the year preceding an individual's response to the survey. "Past month" refers to use at least once during the 30 days preceding an individual's response to the survey.

3. NSDUH (formerly known as the National Household Survey on Drug Abuse) is an annual survey of Americans aged 12 and older conducted by the Substance Abuse and Mental Health Services Administration, Department of Health and Human Services. This survey is available on line at www.samhsa.gov and can be ordered by phone from NIDA at 877-643-2644.

Part Seven

Adolescent
Safety Concerns

Chapter 58

Driving Safety for Teens

Chapter Contents

Section 58.1

Facts about Teen Drivers

From "Teen Drivers: Fact Sheet," by the Centers for Disease Control and
Prevention (CDC, cdc.gov), January 26, 2009.

Motor vehicle crashes are the leading cause of death for U.S. teens,
accounting for more than one in three deaths in this age group. In 2008,
nine teens ages 16 to 19 died every day from motor vehicle injuries.
Per mile driven, teen drivers ages 16 to 19 are four times more likely
than older drivers to crash. Fortunately, teen motor vehicle crashes
are preventable, and proven strategies can improve the safety of young
drivers on the road.

How big is the problem?

In 2008, about 3,500 teens in the United States aged 15–19 were
killed and more than 350,000 were treated in emergency departments
for injuries suffered in motor-vehicle crashes.

Young people ages 15–24 represent only 14% of the U.S. population.
However, they account for 30% ($19 billion) of the total costs of motor
vehicle injuries among males and 28% ($7 billion) of the total costs of
motor vehicle injuries among females.

Who is most at risk?

The risk of motor vehicle crashes is higher among 16- to 19-year-olds
than among any other age group. In fact, per mile driven, teen drivers
ages 16 to 19 are four times more likely than older drivers to crash.

Among teen drivers, those at especially high risk for motor vehicle
crashes are the following:

- **Males:** In 2006, the motor vehicle death rate for male drivers
  and passengers ages 15 to 19 was almost two times that of their
  female counterparts.

- **Teens driving with teen passengers:** The presence of teen
  passengers increases the crash risk of unsupervised teen drivers.

This risk increases with the number of teen passengers.

- **Newly licensed teens:** Crash risk is particularly high during the first year that teenagers are eligible to drive.

What factors put teen drivers at risk?

- Teens are more likely than older drivers to underestimate dangerous situations or not be able to recognize hazardous situations.

- Teens are more likely than older drivers to speed and allow shorter headways (the distance from the front of one vehicle to the front of the next). The presence of male teenage passengers increases the likelihood of this risky driving behavior.

- Among male drivers between 15 and 20 years of age who were involved in fatal crashes in 2005, 37% were speeding at the time of the crash and 26% had been drinking.

- Compared with other age groups, teens have the lowest rate of seat belt use. In 2005, 10% of high school students reported they rarely or never wear seat belts when riding with someone else.

- Male high school students (12.5%) were more likely than female students (7.8%) to rarely or never wear seat belts.

- African-American students (12%) and Hispanic students (13%) were more likely than white students (10.1%) to rarely or never wear seat belts.

- At all levels of blood alcohol concentration (BAC), the risk of involvement in a motor vehicle crash is greater for teens than for older drivers.

- In 2008, 25% of drivers ages 15 to 20 who died in motor vehicle crashes had a BAC of 0.08 g/dl or higher.

- In a national survey conducted in 2007, nearly three out of ten teens reported that, within the previous month, they had ridden with a driver who had been drinking alcohol. One in 10 reported having driven after drinking alcohol within the same 1-month period.

- In 2008, nearly three out of every four teen drivers killed in motor vehicle crashes after drinking and driving were not wearing a seat belt.

- In 2008, half of teen deaths from motor vehicle crashes occurred between 3 p.m. and midnight and 56% occurred on Friday, Saturday, or Sunday.

How can deaths and injuries resulting from crashes involving teen drivers be prevented?

There are proven methods to helping teens become safer drivers. Research suggests that the most comprehensive graduated driver licensing (GDL) programs are associated with reductions of 38% and 40% in fatal and injury crashes, respectively, among 16-year-old drivers.

Graduated driver licensing systems are designed to delay full licensure while allowing teens to get their initial driving experience under low-risk conditions. When parents know their state's GDL laws, they can help enforce the laws and, in effect, help keep their teen drivers safe.

Section 58.2

Technology and Driving Safety and Risk

"What You Should Know About Technology," © 2007 National Safety Council (www.nsc.org). Reprinted by permission of the National Safety Council, a membership organization dedicated to protecting life and promoting health.

How Does Technology Relate to the Crash Rates and Driving Behaviors of Novice Teen Drivers?

While teenage driver crashes and casualties decreased in the past decade, and in spite of recent attention to the issue, teens are still high risk drivers and unintentional injury from motor vehicle crashes remains the number one cause of death among teens in the United States. In absolute numbers, 3,889 teens aged 16–19—more than 10 every day—died in passenger vehicles driven by a teen in 2005. Per population, teen drivers age 16–19 are involved in about twice as many crashes, fatal and non-fatal, as drivers aged 30–59 (Ferguson, Teoh, & McCartt, 2007).

Technology must be considered for both negative and positive effects on novice teen driving. Factors that cause young drivers to crash more frequently than other drivers amplify the potential risks and benefits of new technology.

Infotainment Technology and Teen Driver Risk

According to Lee, 2007, infotainment technologies include a wide array of devices that enable drivers to perform tasks unrelated to driving and place young drivers at risk, such as making telephone calls, watching videos, managing e-mail, sending and reading instant messages, and selecting and listening to music. Even commonly accepted devices in vehicles, such as a car radio, are changing substantially with satellite radio and MP3 music players, like the iPod. As of 2007, approximately 70% of new cars will include a capability to connect to iPods. All of these systems have the potential to distract drivers, but cell phones have attracted the most attention.

- A focus group study found that teens were more willing than other drivers to use cell phones, text messaging, and PDAs [personal digital assistants] while driving. This study also showed that peer influence may exacerbate the tendency of young drivers to use infotainment technology while driving—passengers in the car increased the use of cell phones.

- A survey of 1,291 college students found that of the respondents that were drivers, 87% owned a cell phone and 86% reported using their phone at least occasionally while driving. The respondents also reported 762 crashes or near-crashes and that 21% of these incidents occurred while using a cell phone.

- Similarly, another survey found that young drivers used a cell phone more often while driving and were more likely to experience a dangerous situation as a result of using a phone compared to experienced drivers.

- New internet services made possible by Wireless Applications Protocol (WAP) may be even more distracting. Text messaging represents one such service that already poses a substantial distraction.

Potential Impact of Emerging Technologies on Driving Safety and Risk

At the same time, emerging technologies such as electronic stability control, collision warning systems, and intelligent speed adaptation that support the driver are recognized by Lee (2007) for the potential to enhance driving safety and may mitigate risks posed by infotainment distractions. Lee notes that:

- Increasingly, cars are being equipped with advanced driver assistance systems (ADAS) that include GPS [global positioning system] and navigation systems, sensor suites, and control systems that can help people drive safely.

- These systems may also use biometric technology to recognize individual drivers and develop a history of driving performance to assess momentary and long-term changes in the driver.

Evidence from Current Research on the Effectiveness of Technology

Young drivers are particularly vulnerable to distractions posed by infotainment systems, but could benefit tremendously from driver support systems. Extending proven approaches to improve teen driving safety, such as GDL, represents the most promising path for implementing new technology. Tailoring technology to teen drivers may have an effect similar to placing an adult passenger in the teen's vehicle (Lee, 2007).

In a pilot study (McGehee, 2007), vehicles with novice teen drivers were equipped with an event-triggered video recording system. As an instructional and monitoring device, the device also recorded seat belt use. Teens and parents received a weekly report which compared their performance to their peers.

Based on the research conducted and presented by McGehee, 2007, the event-triggered video system (with feedback in a weekly graphical report card and video review) can reduce unsafe driving behaviors when reviewed by teens and their parents.

- After 4 weeks of these reports there was a substantial reduction in events due to "coachable" driving errors.

- These results suggest that incorporating both video and parental involvement in driver training can significantly reduce the number of unsafe driving events of newly licensed teens.

- This feedback may help teen drivers, particularly those who experience many incidents, become aware of their unsafe driving behaviors and improve their driving.

Attempts to Increase Effectiveness of Technology and Next Steps

The coming years are likely to bring increasingly complex distractions and vehicles. When paired with novice drivers, this combination has potential to undermine teen driving safety to a greater extent than any one trend alone. However, technology has potential to enhance the safety of young drivers. There is an urgent need for researchers, designers, and policy-makers to consider how to capitalize on the potential benefits of emerging technology.

For example, young drivers might benefit from advanced driver assistance systems developed for the general public, but greater benefits are possible by tuning this technology to the specific needs of young drivers. One promising example is video feedback technology (Lee, 2007).

In regard to video feedback, according to McGehee, 2007:

- One promise of the video feedback intervention is that it could reduce teen fatalities by helping them learn to drive more safely during their first months of unsupervised driving.

- One explanation for the reduction in events is that the teens modified their behavior by learning to slow down for turns, curves and intersections, plan ahead, and look further down the roadway to allow more time to react to traffic situations. If video feedback accomplished only this, it could save many lives.

- A multi-year longitudinal study of the video feedback intervention is needed to assess its long-term effects on teen driver behavior, for example, to find if improvements in teen driver behaviors were sustained.

References

Lee, J.D. (2007). Technology and teen drivers. *Journal of Safety Research,* 38(2), 203–213.

McGehee, D.V. (2007, February). An in-context video feedback intervention pilot on novice drivers: Implications for GDL. In Novice teen driving: GDL and beyond—Research foundations for policy and practice. Symposium conducted in Tucson, AZ.

McGehee D.V., Raby M., Carney C., Lee J.D., Reyes M.L. (2007). Extending parental mentoring using an event-triggered video intervention in rural teen drivers. *Journal of Safety Research,* 38 (2), 215–227.

Note: James Hedlund summarizes information presented and discussed at the Symposium. This summary contains a complete listing of secondary references. See: Hedlund, James. (2007). Novice teen driving: GDL and beyond. *Journal of Safety Research,* 38(2), 259–266.

Section 58.3

Tips for Teen Drivers

Getting a driver's license is one of the most important milestones in a person's life. It means freedom, independence, adventure, and responsibility. Becoming a safe and responsible driver is one of the best things you can do for yourself, your family, and other motorists on the road with you.

Safe, responsible driving all begins with you:

- Buckle up! Make sure you always wear your seat belt and that everyone else in the vehicle is buckled up. This is your best defense against anything that might happen on the road.

- Make sure you get enough sleep. Teens need more sleep than younger children and adults. Teens need at least 9 hours of sleep every night, but most teens are sleep deprived and get less than 7 hours of sleep each night. With school, homework, jobs, sports, and social activities, sleeping for 9 hours can be a challenge, but sleep allows you to stay alert while driving.

- If you are a teen with a motorcycle, make sure you take motorcycle safety training and always wear your safety gear. Motorcycle helmets are required on Virginia roadways and are necessary to protect your head.

- Alcohol use by people under the age of 21 is prohibited in Virginia. Virginia has a "zero tolerance" law regarding teens and alcohol use. Some of the penalties include losing your license, large fines, and maybe jail time. The legal limit for teens is a .02 blood alcohol concentration (BAC), which is the normal alcohol content of the average person. So, even a small amount of alcohol can be too much.

- Single vehicle crashes are the most common type of crash involving teens. Speed, lack of seat belt use, inexperience, and alcohol use are contributing factors to fatalities and serious injuries in these crashes.

- Parents and caregivers have a big role in teen driver safety right from the beginning. Take your teen out to practice their skills, set clear ground rules and stick to them, and most importantly, be a good role model. Always buckle up, obey speed limits, and don't drive aggressively.

- Drive sober. Alcohol and drugs are illegal, slow your reaction time, and distort reality. At the same time, they may make you think you're an awesome driver. Avoid this bad combination. Don't drink and drive.

- Ride with sober drivers. If you're riding with a driver who has been drinking or doing drugs, you're also in danger because 48 percent of teenagers who die in car crashes are passengers.

- Always use your safety belt. These are the facts: Air bags are made to work with safety belts, and most crashes happen close to home. So buckle up for every trip.

- Always drive with your headlights on. See and be seen.

- Don't tailgate. Try to keep 4 seconds of following distance between your car and the vehicle in front of you.

- Focus on your driving. Don't blast the music, talk on the phone, eat, study, or put on makeup while driving.

- Don't load up your car with too many friends. Focus on your driving, and resist distractions and peer pressure.

- Don't get stressed out. Pretend everyone else on the road is a close, personal friend.

- Check the rearview mirror before and after you brake, every time.

- Follow traffic safety rules and don't drive faster than the speed limit. Watch your speed!

- Never let friends drive your car. If your friends drive your car and crash, you could lose money, car privileges, a friendship, and even your life.

Chapter 59

Media, Gaming, and Internet Safety

Chapter Contents

Section 59.1

How Teens Interact Online

Parents planning to ground their teenagers at home for their latest antics might want to consider dropping them off at the mall instead. Being away from the computer may put quite a damper on their social life, according to new research suggesting that teens who use the internet to communicate may have better friendships than those who don't.

Results released in April [2007] from a study by the Pew Research Center show that 89 percent of teens use the Internet at least once a week, and that 61 percent log on at least daily. And private communications, such as instant messaging (IM) and e-mail, eat up most of the time they spend online.

In fact, a 2005 Pew Center report on teens and technology shows that 75 percent of all online teens—about two thirds of teenagers overall—use IM, and that nearly half of teens use it at least once every day.

But how is this popular mode of communication affecting the social development of children and teens? Most teens use the internet to consolidate their existing social networks, not to make new friends, says Patti M. Valkenburg, PhD, professor of child and media research at the University of Amsterdam. And she says all this frequent online communication may help young people develop more intimate friendships by allowing kids to let go of inhibitions.

"The internet exactly meets the needs of teens who would spend their entire day chatting with friends if they could," Valkenburg says.

But this new online candor may also lead some teens—most often those with troubled offline relationships—to make dangerous connections with strangers on the internet, or engage in online harassment, psychologists say. And as internet use continues to grow, teens may end up spending more time cuddling up with a glowing computer screen than flirting at the mall, says developmental psychologist Patricia

Greenfield, PhD, a University of California, Los Angeles (UCLA) psychology professor and co-investigator of the Children's Digital Media Center, which just completed 5 years of research funded by the National Science Foundation.

"As a species, we evolved for face-to-face communication," she says. "The increase in mediated communication makes us freer, but also risks making our social relations less personal and more fleeting."

Sticking Close to Home

Joe712: YT? WAYD?
Steve34: OTP—what's your ETA?
Joe712: 7pm
Steve34: WFM—CUL8R

This may look like a foreign language to some, but to nine out of 10 teenagers, it's merely an IM conversation confirming offline plans between two friends.

Here's the conversation again, decoded:

Joe712: You there? What are you doing?
Steve34: On the phone—what's your estimated time of arrival?
Joe712: 7 p.m.
Steve34: Works for me—see you later!

Such communication makes up the bulk of teens' online talk, as most kids stick to chatting with friends from school, clubs, or other offline social networks, according to a 2004 *Journal of Applied Developmental Psychology* study (Vol. 25, No. 6, pages 633–649). The study shows teens spent about an hour a day conversing online, often about school, friends, and gossip, says study author Elisheva F. Gross, PhD, who works with Greenfield at UCLA. And a 2007 *Developmental Psychology* study (Vol. 43, No. 2, pages 267–277) led by Valkenburg confirms these online teen social habits. The study polled 794 10- to 16-year-olds at six elementary, middle, and high schools in the Netherlands—where teens report similar online habits as youth in the United States, Valkenburg says—and found that 88 percent "often" or "almost always" communicate online with pre-existing, offline friends. The study also reports that respondents who communicated online more often felt closer to their friends, she says.

The reason for this closeness may stem from another one of the study's findings—that nearly one in three adolescents say they're better able to share intimate information about themselves online than offline, especially when it comes to interacting with the opposite sex. It seems that teens, especially those who may be socially anxious in face-to-face situations, view the internet as a relatively low-risk venue for disclosing personal information. Since IM participants can't partake in any passive observations about their IM partners, they're forced to ask more direct questions—questions that might be considered rude in face-to-face settings, says Valkenburg. This, in turn, may stimulate closer friendships she adds.

"[Teens] say they can better talk about secrets such as being in love or things they're ashamed of on the internet than in real-life situations," she says. That sort of "intimate self-disclosure is a main determinant of the quality of friendships."

Dangerous Connections

For some teens, however, rather than serving to further offline friendships, the internet leads to social isolation. In a 2005 *Professional Psychology: Research and Practice* study (Vol. 36, No. 5, pages 498–509) more than 1,000 mental health professionals from 11 professional membership associations, including APA, completed a two-phase mail survey examining the Internet-related problems most reported to them by clients. Cases were categorized in an 11-group inventory of problems, including overuse, risky or inappropriate use, and sexual exploitation and abuse. Participants classified 15 percent of youth clients described in the study as engaging in isolative-avoidant use of the internet. In essence, teens were spending so much time on the internet that they isolated themselves from family and friends, says lead author Kimberly J. Mitchell, PhD, psychology professor at the Crimes Against Children Research Center (CCRC) at the University of New Hampshire.

"The internet was basically their sole means of socialization," she says.

And the same liberating function that often leads to higher-quality offline friendships for most teens can also propel some to make dangerous connections with strangers. In fact, 32 percent of online teens reported that a stranger had contacted them, either through a social networking site such as MySpace.com or other private communication venue or chat room, according to the 2007 Pew study. And a 2003 *Journal of Adolescence* study (Vol. 26, No. 1, pages 105–119) of more than 1,500 youth ages 10 to 17 reveals that 25 percent have formed casual online friendships and 14 percent have formed close online friendships or online romances.

Those at particular risk include teens who are highly troubled—with a history of depression or physical or sexual victimization, for example—and those with high parent-child conflict, says the study's lead author, Janis Wolak, JD, also with CCRC.

"These kids really are looking to escape from their environment," she says. "They may not have a good network of family and friends to bounce things off to determine what's appropriate [online] and what's not."

While some troubled teens may fall into unhealthy romantic relationships online, others suffer from online harassment—ranging from relentless teasing to physical threats, both from people they know offline and from those they meet online, says Mitchell. She says the sheer magnitude of people who may see something posted online about a victim of cyber-bullying sometimes makes it worse than face-to-face schoolyard taunting.

"[The internet] takes the whole writing on the bathroom door [concept] to a completely different perspective," Mitchell says.

For psychologists, the internet may be just one aspect of adolescent social development, but it's one that should be monitored closely as it continues to grow, says Gross. What is for sure, however, is that the internet adds a new dimension to many psychological problems—addiction and social anxiety, for example—that existed well before the internet.

"Ultimately we have to . . . determine how this activity connects with the rest of teenagers' lives and all of the important factors that we already know are affecting their friendships and well-being," says Gross.

Section 59.2

Statistics about Online Sexual Solicitation

Are one in seven youth threatened by online predators?

Articles about online dangers frequently cite statistics from a 2005 University of New Hampshire study that 13% of youth were sexually solicited by online predators. (This statistic is sometimes referenced as coming from the National Center on Missing and Exploited Children, which funded and published the study).

As the authors of the research upon which these numbers are based, we believe these statistics often have been misunderstood. The following points are important caveats that those using or quoting this statistic need to understand in order to avoid further confusion.

- These solicitations did not necessarily come from online predators. They were all unwanted online requests to youth to talk about sex, answer personal questions about sex, or do something sexual. But many could have been from other youth. In most cases, youth did not actually know the ages of solicitors. When they believed they knew, they said about half were other youth.

- These solicitations were not necessarily devious or intended to lure. Most were limited to brief online comments or questions in chatrooms or instant messages. Many were simply rude, vulgar comments like, "What's your bra size?"

- Most recipients did not view the solicitations as serious or threatening. Two thirds were not frightened or upset by what happened.

- Almost all youth handled unwanted solicitations easily and effectively. Most reacted by blocking or ignoring solicitors, leaving sites, or telling solicitors to stop.

- Extremely few youth (only two) were actually sexually victimized by someone they met online. This number was too small to be the basis of a reliable estimate of how many youth in the population get sexually victimized from online meetings.

Nonetheless, we were able to make estimates in the study of some of the more serious types of sexual solicitations. We prefer citing the statistics about these as more representative of threatening or dangerous situations that youth encounter online.

- One in 25 youth (about 4%) got "aggressive" sexual solicitations that included attempts to contact the youth offline. These are the episodes most likely to result in actual victimizations. (About one quarter of these aggressive solicitations came from people the youth knew in person, mostly other youth.)

- One in 25 youth (about 4%) were solicited to take sexual pictures of themselves. In many jurisdictions, these constitute criminal requests to produce child pornography.

- One in 25 youth (about 4%) said they were upset or distressed as a result of an online solicitation. Whether or not the solicitors were online predators, these are the youth most immediately harmed by the solicitations themselves.

We encourage writers and speakers to cite these other estimates as well as mentioning the caveats about the "one in seven" figure.

Reports and papers about this study, information about other research we have done, and contact information for the authors are available at our website www.unh.edu/ccrc. Please feel free to contact us if you have questions about any of our research.

Research funded by the U.S. Department of Justice, OJJDP, and the National Center for Missing & Exploited Children. Program support provided by the Verizon Foundation.

Section 59.3

Computer and Video Game Addiction

Computers, video games, and the internet have become entrenched features of our daily lives. Computer use has reached beyond work and is now a major source of fun and entertainment for many people. For most people, computer use and video game play is integrated into their lives in a balanced healthy manner. For others, time spent on the computer or video game is out of balance, and has displaced work, school, friends, and even family.

What is computer and video game addiction?

When time spent on the computer, playing video games, or cruising the internet reaches a point that it harms a child's or adult's family and social relationships, or disrupts school or work life, that person may be caught in a cycle of addiction. Like other addictions, the computer or video game has replaced friends and family as the source of a person's emotional life. Increasingly, to feel good, the addicted person spends more time playing video games or searching the internet. Time away from the computer or game causes moodiness or withdrawal.

When a person spends up to 10 hours a day or more rearranging or sending files, playing games, surfing the net, visiting chat rooms, instant messaging, and reading e-mails, that easily can reach up to 70 to 80 hours a week online with the computer. Major social, school, or work disruptions will result.

Symptoms of computer or video game addiction for children:

- Most of non-school hours are spent on the computer or playing video games

- Falling asleep in school

- Not keeping up with assignments

- Worsening grades

- Lying about computer or video game use

- Choosing to use the computer or play video games, rather than see friends

- Dropping out of other social groups (clubs or sports)

- Irritable when not playing a video game or on the computer

  For adults:

- Computer or video game use is characterized by intense feelings of pleasure and guilt

- Obsessing and preoccupied about being on the computer, even when not connected

- Hours playing video games or on the computer increasing, seriously disrupting family, social, or even work life

- Lying about computer or video game use

- Experience feelings of withdrawal, anger, or depression when not on the computer or involved with their video game

- May incur large phone or credit bills for online services

- Can't control computer or video game use

- Fantasy life online replaces emotional life with partner

  There are even physical symptoms that may point to addiction:

- Carpal tunnel syndrome

- Sleep disturbances

- Back, neck aches

- Headaches

- Dry eyes

- Failure to eat regularly or neglect personal hygiene

For the computer or video game addicted person, a fantasy world online or in a game has replaced his or her real world. The virtual reality of the computer or game is more inviting than the everyday world of family, school, or work. With the increased access to pornography on the internet and in games, this fantasy world may be highly sexual.

The first step to healing is to recognize the symptoms. Help from a professional is often needed.

Sources

Brenner, Viktor. (1997, June). Parameters of Internet use, abuse, and addiction: The first 90 days of the Internet usage survey. *Psychological Reports,* 80, 879–882.

Brody, Jane E. (2000, May 16). First step is recognizing the signs of Internet abuse. *The New York Times,* pD7(N), pF7(L).

Doten, Patti (1999, October 18). When the Net becomes a trap: On-line addicts may be mired in a virtual world, leaving behind families, friends and real lives. *Boston Globe.*

Dvorak, John C. (1997, June). Net addiction. *PC / Computing,* 10, 85.

Harvard Mental Health Letter (1999, January). Computer addiction: Is it real or virtual? v15, i7.

Hauge, Marney R., Gentile, Douglas A., (2003, April). Video game addiction among adolescents: Associations with academic performance and aggression. Paper presented at a Society for Research in Child Development Conference, Tampa Florida. Accessed at www.psychology. iastate.edu/faculty/dgentile/SRCD%20Video%20Game%20Addiction. pdf (last visited 3/11/05).

Orzack, Dr. Maressa. Licensed clinical psychologist, on the Harvard Medical School faculty, Coordinator of Computer Addiction Services at McLean Hospital. at http://www.computeraddiction.com/ (last visited 3/15/05).

Parents Network Advice about Teenagers—Computer Game Addiction. http://parents.berkeley.edu/advice/teens/gameaddiction.html (last accessed 2/25/05).

Salguero, R. A., Moran, T., Bersabe, R. M. (2002, December). Measuring problem video game playing in adolescents. *Addiction,* 97,12, 1601.

Shaffer, H. J., Hall, M. N., Vander Bilt, J. (2000, April). Computer addiction: A critical consideration. *American Journal of Orthopsychiatry,* 70, 162–168.

Video Games and Public Health (2004, February). *Journal of Adolescence,* 27, 1.

Wright, Carol (2001, Fall). Children and technology: Issues, challenges, and opportunities. *Childhood Education,* 78, 37.

Yang, Dori J. (2000, January 17). Craving your next web fix: Internet addiction is no laughing matter. *U.S. News and World Report,* 128, 41.

Young, Kimberly S. (2004, December). Internet addiction: A new clinical phenomenon and its consequences. *American Behavioral Scientist,* 48,4,402.

Section 59.4

Protecting Teens' Privacy Online

Excerpted from "Kids' Privacy," by the Federal Trade Commission
(www.onguardonline.gov), January 2009.

Your kids' personal information and privacy are valuable—to you, to
them, and to marketers. Here's how to help protect your kids' personal
information when they're online.

Check out sites your kids visit. If a site requires users to register,
see what kind of information it asks for and whether you're comfortable
with what they tell you. If the site allows kids to post information about
themselves, talk to your child about the risks and benefits of disclosing
certain information in a public forum. You also can see whether the site
appears to be following the most basic COPPA (Children's Online Privacy
Protection Act) requirements, like clearly posting its privacy policy for
parents and asking for parental consent before kids can participate.

Take a look at the privacy policy. Just because a site has a
privacy policy doesn't mean it keeps personal information private.
The policy should tell you what the site does with the information it
collects; then, you can decide how you feel about it. Remember, if the
policy says there are no limits to what it collects or who gets to see it,
there are no limits.

Ask questions. If you're not clear on a site's practices or policies,
ask about them. If the site falls under COPPA, the privacy policy has
to include contact information for the site manager.

Be selective with your permission. In many cases, websites need
your OK before they're allowed to collect personal information from your
kids. They may ask for your permission in a number of ways, including
by e-mail or postal mail. Or, you may give your consent by allowing
them to charge your credit card. In addition to considering when to
give your permission, consider how much consent you want to give—in
many cases, it's not all or none. You might be able to give the company
permission to collect some personal information from your child, but say
no to having that information passed along to another marketer.

Know your rights. As a parent, you have the right to have a site delete any personal information it has about your child. Some sites will let you see the information they've collected. But first, they'll need to make sure you really are the parent, either by requiring a signed form or an e-mail with a digital signature, for example, or by verifying a charge made to your credit card. You also have a right to take back your consent and have any information collected from your child deleted.

Report a website. If you think a site has collected or disclosed information from your kids or marketed to them in a way that violates the law, report it to the FTC at ftc.gov/complaint or 877-FTC-HELP (382-4357).

Section 59.5

Social Networking Sites: Safety Tips for Teens

From "Social Networking Sites: Safety Tips for Tweens and Teens," by the Federal Trade Commission (FTC, www.ftc.gov), May 2006.

Try these tips for socializing safely online:

- Think about how different sites work before deciding to join a site. Some sites will allow only a defined community of users to access posted content; others allow anyone and everyone to view postings.

- Think about keeping some control over the information you post. Consider restricting access to your page to a select group of people, for example, your friends from school, your club, your team, your community groups, or your family.

- Keep your information to yourself. Don't post your full name, Social Security number, address, phone number, or bank and credit card account numbers—and don't post other people's information, either. Be cautious about posting information that could be used to identify you or locate you offline. This could include the name of your school, sports team, clubs, and where you work or hang out.

- Make sure your screen name doesn't say too much about you. Don't use your name, your age, or your hometown. Even if you think your screen name makes you anonymous, it doesn't take a genius to combine clues to figure out who you are and where you can be found.

- Post only information that you are comfortable with others seeing—and knowing—about you. Many people can see your page, including your parents, your teachers, the police, the college you might want to apply to next year, or the job you might want to apply for in 5 years.

- Remember that once you post information online, you can't take it back. Even if you delete the information from a site, older versions exist on other people's computers.

- Consider not posting your photo. It can be altered and broadcast in ways you may not be happy about. If you do post one, ask yourself whether it's one your mom would display in the living room.

- Flirting with strangers online could have serious consequences. Because some people lie about who they really are, you never really know who you're dealing with.

- Be wary if a new online friend wants to meet you in person. Before you decide to meet someone, do your research: Ask whether any of your friends know the person, and see what background you can dig up through online search engines.

- If you decide to meet them, be smart about it: Meet in a public place, during the day, with friends you trust. Tell an adult or a responsible sibling where you're going, and when you expect to be back.

- Trust your gut if you have suspicions. If you feel threatened by someone or uncomfortable because of something online, tell an adult you trust and report it to the police and the social networking site. You could end up preventing someone else from becoming a victim.

Section 59.6

Protecting Your Child from Electronic Aggression

From "Technology and Youth: Protecting Your Child from Electronic Aggression," by the Centers for Disease Control and Prevention (CDC, www.cdc.gov), 2009.

Technology and youth seem destined for each other. They are both young, fast paced, and ever changing. In the last 20 years there has been an explosion in new technology. This new technology has been eagerly embraced by young people and has led to expanding knowledge, social networks, and vocabulary that includes instant messaging (IM-ing), blogging, and text messaging.

New technology has many potential benefits for youth. With the help of new technology, young people can interact with others across the United States and throughout the world on a regular basis. Social networking sites like Facebook and MySpace also allow youth to develop new relationships with others, some of whom they have never even met in person. New technology also provides opportunities to make rewarding social connections for those youth who have difficulty developing friendships in traditional social settings or because of limited contact with same-aged peers. In addition, regular Internet access allows teens and preteens to quickly increase their knowledge on a wide variety of topics.

However, the recent explosion in technology does not come without possible risks. Youth can use electronic media to embarrass, harass, or threaten their peers. Increasing numbers of adolescents are becoming victims of this new form of violence—electronic aggression. Research suggests that 9% to 35% of young people report being victims of this type of violence. Like traditional forms of youth violence, electronic aggression is associated with emotional distress and conduct problems at school.

Examples of Electronic Aggression

- Disclosing someone else's personal information in a public area (e.g., website) in order to cause embarrassment

- Posting rumors or lies about someone in a public area (e.g., discussion board)

- Distributing embarrassing pictures of someone by posting them in a public area (e.g., website) or sending them via e-mail

- Assuming another person's electronic identity to post or send messages about others with the intent of causing the other person harm

- Sending mean, embarrassing, or threatening text messages, instant messages, or e-mails

Tips for Parents and Caregivers

Talk to Your Child

Parents and caregivers often ask children where they are going and who they are going with when they leave the house. You should ask these same questions when your child goes on the Internet. Because children are reluctant to disclose victimization for fear of having their Internet and cellular phone privileges revoked, develop solutions to prevent or address victimization that do not punish the child.

Develop Rules

Together with your child, develop rules about acceptable and safe behaviors for all electronic media. Make plans for what they should do if they become a victim of electronic aggression or know someone who is being victimized. The rules should focus on ways to maximize the benefits of technology and decrease its risks.

Explore the Internet

Visit the websites your child frequents, and assess the pros and cons. Remember, most websites and online activities are beneficial. They help young people learn new information, interact with others, and connect with people who have similar interests.

Talk with Other Parents and Caregivers

Talk to other parents and caregivers about how they have discussed technology use with their children. Ask about the rules they have developed and how they stay informed about their child's technology use.

Connect with the School

Parents and caregivers are encouraged to work with their child's school and school district to develop a class for parents and caregivers that educates them about school policies on electronic aggression, recent incidents in the community involving electronic aggression, and resources available to parents and caregivers who have concerns. Work with the school and other partners to develop a collaborative approach to preventing electronic aggression.

Educate Yourself

Stay informed about the new devices and websites your child is using. Technology changes rapidly, and many developers offer information to keep people aware of advances. Continually talk with your child about "where they are going" and explore the technology yourself.

Technology is not going away, and forbidding young people to access electronic media may not be a good long-term solution. Together, parents and children can come up with ways to maximize the benefits of technology and decrease its risks.

Chapter 60

Skin Safety Concerns

Chapter Contents

Section 60.1

Body Piercing: A Guide for Teens

Many different cultures have pierced their bodies for centuries. If you look in a history book, you will find that Egyptians, Greeks, and Romans decorated their bodies with piercings and tattoos. People pierced their bodies to show their importance in a group, or because they thought it protected them from evil. Today, we know much more about the risks of body piercing. Body piercing is a serious decision. Before you decide what you want to do, ask your friends, parents, and trusted adults what they think.

What are teens saying about body piercing today?

Ask other teens who have been pierced what they thought of the whole experience. How much did it cost? Was it painful? How long did it take to heal? If they had the chance to do it over again, would they?

Some tips teens have passed along to us:

• You do not have to pierce your body to belong.

• You can always change your mind or wait if you are not sure.

• If you do decide to have your body pierced, never pierce your own body or let a friend do it because you can run into very serious health problems.

Are there any medical reasons why I should not get a piercing?

Yes. There are medical conditions (see the list in the following text) that could interfere with the natural healing process after a piercing, which makes getting a piercing under these circumstances not only a bad decision, but a risky one.

The Association of Professional Piercers feels that you should not consider getting pierced if:

- you have a skin irritation or an unusual lesion or a rash, lump, cut, moles, or lots of freckles (where you want to get pierced);

- you have diabetes, hemophilia, an autoimmune disorder, certain heart conditions, or another medical condition that might interfere with the healing process;

- if you have plans to become pregnant and want a nipple or navel piercing;

- if you are already pregnant; or

- if a licensed professional piercer feels that it would be a bad idea.

Bottom line, if you are wondering if it is safe for you to have an oral or body piercing, you should talk to your health care provider.

What are the risks of body piercing?

The most serious risks are infections, allergic reactions, bleeding, and damage to nerves or teeth. Infections may be caused by hepatitis, HIV [human immunodeficiency virus], tetanus, bacteria, and yeast. If the piercer washes his/her hands and uses gloves and sterile equipment and you take good care of your piercing, the risk of infection is lowered (but still exists).

Did you know that:

- you can get and/or spread a serious infection (including HIV), if the piercing equipment hasn't been sterilized properly;

- infections caused by bacteria getting into the puncture of the piercing may also happen later, even after the piercing has healed; and

- if the studio uses a piercing gun to do body piercings, leave! Piercing guns cannot be sterilized and should not be used for body piercing.

Another cause of problems from piercings is using wrong kind of jewelry for the area pierced. If the jewelry is too small, it can actually cut off the blood supply to the tissue, causing swelling and pain. If the jewelry is either too thin or too heavy, or if you are allergic to the metal, your body may reject the jewelry. This means that your body reacts against the jewelry because it is a foreign object.

Know the risks before you have your body pierced:

- Bacterial infection (where you had the piercing)

- Excessive (a lot of) bleeding

- Allergic reactions (to certain kinds of jewelry)

- Damage to nerves (for example, you may lose feeling at the area that gets pierced)

- Keloids (thick scarring at the piercing site)

- Dental damage (swelling and infection of the tongue, chipped/broken teeth, choking on loose jewelry)

Is the healing time the same for all body parts?

Healing time (see Table 60.1) is different depending on the part of your body that you get pierced. Some parts are more likely to get infected or have problems. Piercings on your earlobes usually take about 6–8 weeks to heal. However, piercings on the side of your ear (cartilage) can take anywhere from 4 months to 1 year to heal. The reason for this is that the type of tissue in each area is different, and the amount of pressure placed on the pierced area while you are sleeping is different too.

Tongue piercings swell a lot at first, but heal fairly quickly if the right type of jewelry is used. However, metal jewelry in the tongue may damage your gums and chip the enamel surface of your teeth. In fact, the ADA (American Dental Association—a group of dentists that set professional standards for dentists in the United States) is against any type of oral piercings because of all the risks.

In some cases, nipple piercings can damage some of the milk-producing glands in a young woman's breasts. This can cause infections or problems later on if the woman decides to breast-feed her baby. Some pierced areas, such as the navel (belly button), are more likely to become infected because of irritation from tight clothing. A pierced site needs air to help the healing process.

If I decide that a piercing is important to me, where should I go?

You should ask friends and relatives with piercings where they went and if they liked the place. Look for a place that does a lot of piercings and that only employs piercers with piercing licenses. Some states make piercers get a license, while other states do not. So there are actually people who are doing body piercings with very little training.

As you can imagine, this can be very dangerous for you. However, the APP (Association of Professional Piercers—a professional organization of piercers) makes safety rules for people who do piercings, and has a list of piercers who comply with the standards of their organization. Go to http://www.safepiercing.org/locate-a-member/searchable-member-database to search for registered members of the APP.

Table 60.1. Body Piercings and Healing Times

Pierced Body Part	Healing Time
Earlobe	6 to 8 weeks
Ear cartilage	4 months to 1 year
Eyebrow	6 to 8 weeks
Nostril	2 to 4 months
Nasal septum	6 to 8 months
Nasal bridge	8 to 10 weeks
Tongue	4 weeks
Lip	2 to 3 months
Nipple	3 to 6 months
Navel (belly button)	4 months to 1 year
Female genitalia	4 to 10 weeks
Male genitalia	4 weeks to 6 months

What should I look for in a piercing salon?

When you go into a salon, look around. Make sure that there is a certificate on the wall that says the piercer is registered with the APP. Is the place clean?

The shop should be kept clean and sanitary. The lighting should be good so that the piercers can see well while working. Does the staff wash their hands and use sterile gloves and instruments? All the instruments should either be brand new and disposable (meant to be thrown away after one use) or be sterilized in pouches. If the piercer uses disposable needles, you should see him/her open sealed packages of the needles. The piercers should throw away the needles in a biohazard container after using them.

What do I need to bring to the piercing salon?

You may need to bring a copy of your birth certificate. If you are under 18 years old, you will need your parents' or guardians' permission. Your parent/guardian will need to go with you to the piercing salon and sign a consent form. Since the law is different from state to state, you will need to find out what the law in your area says about whether or not you need parental permission to have a piercing.

What kind of jewelry should I buy?

Implant grade stainless steel jewelry is generally reasonably priced and safe to use for new piercings. Both 316L and 316LVM types of stainless steel meet the standards for "implant grade" that has been approved by the American Society of Testing and Materials (ASTM), an organization that is not related to the government, but sets high standards for all kinds of materials that are manufactured in the United States. The European organization that is similar to the ASTM is called the ISO.

Implant grade stainless steel is least likely to produce a foreign body reaction or infection in the skin. Other safe choices for new piercings are metals such as gold (at least 18 karat), titanium, or niobium. All of these cost more than implant grade stainless steel.

Silver is not a good choice for new piercings because the tarnish from silver gets deposited into the skin. The deposits often darken the skin around the piercing, which can be permanent. Sterling silver jewelry can be safely worn on most healed piercings, but it should not be worn in the mouth or genital area where the skin is moist.

Gold jewelry should be at least 18 karat (75% gold) for new piercings and at least 14k gold for healed piercings. Gold-filled or gold-plated jewelry should never be used in any piercings because the metal is very thin. The finish wears away easily and it chips with slightest contact of the body. Some people have difficulty with white gold because it contains nickel—a metal that many people are allergic to.

Titanium is used for jewelry and for surgical implants in the body. For example, titanium implants are used for shoulder replacement surgery because they are lightweight and porous. There are actually tiny pores in the metal that allow tissue in the body to attach to it. For this reason, it is recommended that titanium jewelry be highly polished to reduce the porosity (pores or very tiny holes in the metal).

For people who are extremely sensitive to metal, Teflon or nylon piercings may be used.

Look for a salon that has a large choice of jewelry. The salon should not tell you to use a certain type of jewelry just because it's the only kind they have.

What's up with all the different kinds of jewelry?

- Bars, which are the type of jewelry used in some piercings like the tongue, are measured in length (how long the bar is). When the piercing is first done, a longer bar will be used. When the piercing heals, a shorter bar is used.

- Ring jewelry is measured by diameter, or how wide the ring is.

- Gauge means the thickness of the jewelry. The smaller the gauge number, the thicker the jewelry. The APP says that jewelry no greater than 14 gauge should be used below the neck. This is because of the risk of a foreign body reaction and the possibility of the ring cutting the skin.

How are piercings done?

An experienced piercer uses a hollow needle to create a hole by passing the needle through the body part you want pierced. The jewelry is then inserted through the hole. Sometimes there can be a small amount of bleeding. You should not take aspirin or any pain medication that contains aspirin the week before any piercing is done, since these medicines may cause you to bleed a little bit more than usual. Remember, piercing guns should never be used since they can damage tissue and cause infection.

How much will a piercing cost?

There are actually two costs with piercings—the site cost and the jewelry cost. The site cost depends on where on your body you get pierced. For example, ear and nose piercings usually cost less than tongue, nipple, or genital piercings. Gold jewelry costs more than stainless steel or another metal. You should shop around and check prices at different piercing salons before you decide on where to have your piercing done.

How should I clean my new piercing?

Follow these steps to prevent infection:

1. First, wash your hands with soap and water before touching or cleaning the pierced area. (Don't let anyone else touch the pierced area until it is healed.)

2. Remove any crusty material from the site and from the jewelry with warm water.

3. Gently wash the area around the piercing with a fragrance free saline solution or a non-iodized sea salt mixture (your licensed piercer may give you a sample). Follow the instructions on the package.

4. When showering, use a drop of fragrance-free antibacterial liquid soap to clean the jewelry and the piercing. Do not leave it on the piercing for more than 30 seconds.

5. Gently rinse all of the soap and any crusty scabs, leaving no suds or residue. Do not rub or pull the crusty material as the skin around it may bleed. As the piercing heals, the material will dry and fall off on its own.

6. Gently dry the area with a paper towel or plain white napkin. Do not use towels as bacteria can be a problem. Also jewelry tends to get caught on towels but won't on disposable paper products.

7. Repeat steps 1–6 twice a day until the skin heals. (Over-washing or over-scrubbing can irritate the area.)

8. Avoid over cleaning. This will likely break down your skin and delay healing.

9. Do not use antibacterial ointments because they don't allow air to get to the area and they trap bacteria.

How can I prevent infections after I get pierced?

Preventing infections isn't hard. It shouldn't take a lot of your time to keep your piercing clean, and if you keep it clean you won't have complications. The following recommendations are especially important during the healing process. However, you can also follow these safety measures even after your piercing has healed completely.

• Do not use alcohol, peroxide, or other strong soaps to clean the area. These products are harsh and will irritate and dry out your skin. Other strong solutions such as Betadine® will discolor gold jewelry.

• Rinse the pierced skin after exercising, since sweat may irritate the piercing.

- Keep the pierced area from coming in contact with other people's body fluids, such as saliva and sweat. Do not have oral sexual contact for 4–6 weeks if you have a tongue, lip, or genital piercing.

- Do not let anyone touch, kiss, or lick the piercing (for example, the earlobe) while it is still healing.

- Keep things clean that come in contact with the body part that has been pierced. For example, keep your phone clean if you have an ear piercing, keep your glasses clean for ear and eyebrow piercings, cover your earlobe with a tissue if you use hairspray, and try not to apply makeup close to piercing sites.

- Wear clean clothing with soft fabric for navel piercings. Avoid wearing jeans because the material can be irritating.

- Don't wear pantyhose, leotards, belts, or tight clothing while a navel piercing is healing.

- Wear loose-fitting clothing with a navel piercing to let the air help with healing. Constant and rough friction can cause scarring and longer healing time.

- Stop or at least limit the amount of caffeine and alcohol you consume as they can slow healing.

- Do not smoke, chew tobacco, or eat spicy foods while your oral piercing is healing.

- Avoid using cosmetics, lotions, hairspray, or other kinds of beauty products around your piercing.

- Check your jewelry many times during the day to see if any parts have become loose, especially if you have a tongue piercing. If a bar becomes loose, you can accidentally swallow it or damage a permanent tooth. Do not hang charms or pendants from any piercing that's healing.

- Do not use a hot tub or swim in public pools until your piercing has healed. If you must swim, cover the piercing with a waterproof Band-Aid®.

- Avoid direct sunlight, tanning beds, sand, tanning oils, and lotions as they can burn and irritate the piercing (which can cause scarring).

- Rinse tongue or lip piercings after every meal or snack. Rinse for 30 to 60 seconds after eating with an antibacterial, alcohol-free mouthwash, or a warm salt-water rinse. Or, alternately, make a mix with one part water, and one part hydrogen peroxide, and apply it directly to the piercing site with a cotton swab. The bubbling peroxide can help remove food stuck in the site.

- Throw out your old toothbrush and get a new, soft-bristled toothbrush if you have a tongue or lip piercing. This is to avoid exposure to bacteria from your old toothbrush.

- See your dentist for regular checkups and if you think you have a problem. Studies have shown that people who have piercings in their mouth are much more likely to have injuries to their teeth and gums.

- Eat healthy foods. Foods rich in vitamins and minerals help your body heal.

- Take a multi-vitamin with vitamin C and zinc to speed up the healing process and boost tissue regeneration.

Be on the lookout for signs of infection that may include one or more of the following: redness, swelling, discharge, bad smell, a rash at or around the piercing site, or a fever. If you think you have an infection, don't try to take care of it by yourself. Make an appointment to see your health care provider.

Body piercing is a big decision. We hope that this helps you understand the risks, and that the information will help you make a decision that's best for you. If you do decide to get a body piercing, we hope that you will follow the guidelines here. Go to a reliable salon/piercer, buy the right kind of jewelry, keep the site clean and away from irritating materials, and see your health care provider if you have symptoms of an infection.

Section 60.2

Cosmetics: Frequently Asked Questions

Excerpted from "Cosmetics and Your Health," by the Office on Women's Health (www.womenshealth.gov), part of the U.S. Department of Health and Human Services, November 1, 2004. Reviewed by David A. Cooke, MD, FACP, May 13, 2010.

What are cosmetics? How are they different from over-the-counter (OTC) drugs?

Cosmetics are products people use to cleanse or change the look of the face or body. Cosmetic products include the following:

- Skin creams
- Lotions
- Perfumes
- Lipsticks
- Fingernail polishes
- Eye and face makeup products
- Permanent waves
- Hair dyes
- Toothpastes
- Deodorants

Unlike drugs, which are used to treat or prevent disease in the body, cosmetics do not change or affect the body's structure or functions.

Are cosmetics safe?

Yes, for the most part. Serious problems from cosmetics are rare. But sometimes problems can happen. The most common injury from cosmetics is from scratching the eye with a mascara wand. Eye infections can result if the scratches go untreated. These infections can lead to ulcers on the cornea (clear covering of the eye), loss of lashes, or even blindness. To play it safe, never try to apply mascara while riding in a car, bus, train, or plane.

Sharing makeup can also lead to serious problems. Cosmetic brushes and sponges pick up bacteria from the skin. And if you moisten brushes with saliva, the problem can be worse. Washing your hands before using makeup will help prevent this problem.

Sleeping while wearing eye makeup can cause problems too. If mascara flakes into your eyes while you sleep, you might wake up with itching, bloodshot eyes, infections, or eye scratches. So be sure to remove all makeup before going to bed.

Cosmetic products that come in aerosol containers also can be a hazard. For example, it is dangerous to use aerosol hairspray near heat, fire, or while smoking. Until hairspray is fully dry, it can catch on fire and cause serious burns. Fires related to hairsprays have caused injuries and death. Aerosol sprays or powders also can cause lung damage if they are deeply inhaled into the lungs.

How can I protect myself against the dangers of cosmetics?

- Never drive and put on makeup. Not only does this make driving a danger, hitting a bump in the road and scratching your eyeball can cause serious eye injury.

- Never share makeup. Always use a new sponge when trying products at a store. Insist that salespersons clean container openings with alcohol before applying to your skin.

- Keep makeup containers closed tight when not in use.

- Keep makeup out of the sun and heat. Light and heat can kill the preservatives that help to fight bacteria. Don't keep cosmetics in a hot car for a long time.

- Don't use cosmetics if you have an eye infection, such as pinkeye. Throw away any makeup you were using when you first found the problem.

- Never add liquid to a product unless the label tells you to do so.

- Throw away any makeup if the color changes or it starts to smell.

- Never use aerosol sprays near heat or while smoking because they can catch on fire.

- Don't deeply inhale hairsprays or powders. This can cause lung damage.

- Avoid color additives that are not approved for use in the eye area, such as permanent eyelash tints and kohl (color additive that contains lead salts and is still used in eye cosmetics in other countries). Be sure to keep kohl away from children. It may cause lead poisoning.

What are hypoallergenic cosmetics?

Hypoallergenic cosmetics are products that makers claim cause fewer allergic reactions than other products. Women with sensitive skin, and even those with "normal" skin, may think these products will be gentler. But there are no federal standards for using the term hypoallergenic. The term can mean whatever a company wants it to mean. Cosmetic makers do not have to prove their claims to the FDA.

Some products that have natural ingredients can cause allergic reactions. If you have an allergy to certain plants or animals, you could have an allergic reaction to cosmetics with those things in them. For example, lanolin from sheep wool is found in many lotions. But it's a common cause of allergies, too.

Can cosmetics cause acne?

Some skin and hair care products can cause acne. To help prevent and control acne flare-ups, take good care of your skin. For example, use a mild soap or cleanser to gently wash your face twice a day.

Choose noncomedogenic makeup and hair care products. This means that they don't close up the pores.

Are tattoos and permanent makeup safe?

FDA is looking into the safety of tattoos and permanent makeup since they are now more popular. The inks, or dyes, used for tattoos are color additives. Right now, no color additives have been approved for tattoos, including those used in permanent makeup.

You should be aware of these risks of tattoos and permanent makeup:

- Tattoo needles and supplies can transmit diseases, such as hepatitis C and HIV [human immunodeficiency virus]. Be sure all needles and supplies are sterile before they are used on you.

- Tattoos and permanent makeup are not easy to take off. Removal may cause a permanent change in color.

- Think carefully before getting a tattoo. You could have an allergic reaction.

- You cannot make blood donations for a year after getting a tattoo or permanent makeup.

Are hair dyes safe?

The decision to change your hair color may be a hard one. Some studies have linked hair dyes with a higher risk of certain cancers, while other studies have not found this link. Most hair dyes also don't have to go through safety testing that other cosmetic color additives do before hitting store shelves. Women are often on their own trying to figure out whether hair dyes are safe.

When hair dyes first came out, the main ingredient in coal-tar hair dye caused allergic reactions in some people. Most hair dyes are now made from petroleum sources. But FDA still considers them to be coal-tar dyes. This is because they have some of the same compounds found in these older dyes.

Cosmetic makers have stopped using things known to cause cancer in animals. For example, 4-methoxy-m-phenylenediamine (4MMPD) or 4-methoxy-m-phenylenediamine sulfate (4MMPD sulfate) are no longer used. But chemicals made almost the same way have replaced some of the cancer-causing compounds. Some experts feel that these newer ingredients aren't very different from the things they're replacing.

Experts suggest that you may reduce your risk of cancer by using less hair dye over time.

Section 60.3

Safe Hair Removal

Excerpted from "Skin and Hair Health," by the Office on Women's Health (www.womenshealth.gov), part of the U.S. Department of Health and Human Services, 2008.

Your hair is one of the first things that others notice about you. The shape and structure of your hair depend on your race. For instance, African hair is typically flat with tight curls. Asian hair is typically round and thick. Caucasian hair may be fine and straight or thick and wavy. Natural oils from hair glands also affect the look and feel of your hair.

Basic hair care involves a healthy lifestyle and proper care. Wash oily hair daily and limit how much you touch your hair. For dry hair, keep blow-drying time short and avoid overstyling, which can lead to dryness and breakage. Protecting your hair from wind, sun, and chlorine in water also will help to keep it from drying out and breaking.

If you color or relax your hair, carefully read the product label. Hair dyes and relaxers can harm both your skin and hair. Talk with your doctor if your skin or scalp swells or gets itchy after using any hair product. Even natural products, such as henna dye, can cause an allergic reaction.

Cultural norms often affect a woman's choice to remove body hair. Many women shave their legs and underarms. Wet hair first, then shave in the direction that your hair grows. Chemicals called depilatories dissolve unwanted hair. Depilatories can irritate, so always test on a small area of skin before using. Never use chemicals around your eyes or on broken skin. For laser, epilator (electrolysis), waxing, sugaring, or threading treatments, find a licensed technician. Serious side effects of hair removal can include swelling, blistering, scarring, and infection.

Section 60.4

The Risks of Tanning

Excerpted from "The Risks of Tanning," by the U.S. Food and Drug Administration (FDA, www.fda.gov), May 5, 2009.

UV (ultraviolet) radiation, whether from natural or artificial sources, damages the skin. Here are some of the short- and long-term side effects of UV exposure.

Sunburn

Sunburn, also called erythema, is one of the most obvious signs of UV exposure and skin damage. Often marked by redness and peeling (usually after a few days), sunburn is a form of short-term skin damage.

Sunburn can be a very painful effect of UV exposure. Studies have shown a link between severe sunburn and melanoma, the deadliest form of skin cancer. Pay careful attention to protecting yourself from UV rays.

Suntan

There is no such thing as a safe tan. The increase in skin pigment, called melanin, which causes the tan color change in your skin is a sign of damage.

Once skin is exposed to UV radiation, it increases the production of melanin in an attempt to protect the skin from further damage. Melanin is the same pigment that colors your hair, eyes, and skin. The increase in melanin may cause your skin tone to darken over the next 48 hours.

Evidence suggests that tanning greatly increases your risk of developing skin cancer. And, contrary to popular belief, getting a tan will not protect your skin from sunburn or other skin damage. The extra melanin in tanned skin provides a sun protection factor (SPF) of about 2 to 4; far below the minimum recommended SPF of 15.

Premature Aging

Sometimes referred to as "photoaging," premature aging is the result of unprotected UV exposure. It takes the form of leathery, wrinkled skin, and dark spots.

Skin Cancer

There are two main types of skin cancer:

- Melanoma

- Non-melanoma

Melanoma is the less common, but more dangerous form of skin cancer, and accounts for most of the deaths due to skin cancer each year. Melanoma is cancer that begins in the epidermal cells that produce melanin (melanocytes). According to the American Cancer Society (ACS) melanoma is almost always curable when detected in its early stages.

Non-melanomas (basal cell and squamous cell carcinomas) occur in the basal or squamous cells located at the base of the epidermis, both inside and outside the body. Non-melanomas often develop in sun-exposed areas of the body, including the face, ears, neck, lips, and the backs of the hands.

Predisposition to skin cancer can be hereditary, meaning it is passed through the generations of a family through genes. There is also strong evidence suggesting that exposure to UV rays, both UVA and UVB, can cause skin cancer.

UV radiation may promote skin cancer in two different ways:

- By damaging the DNA in skin cells, causing the skin to grow abnormally and develop benign or malignant growths

- By weakening the immune system and compromising the body's natural defenses against aggressive cancer cells

Actinic or Solar Keratoses

A fourth type of growth, actinic or solar keratoses, is a concern because it can progress into cancer. Actinic keratoses are considered the earliest stage in the development of skin cancer and are caused by long-term exposure to sunlight.

They are the most common premalignant skin condition, occurring in more than a million Americans each year.

Eye Damage (Photokeratitis)

Photokeratitis can be thought of as a sunburn of the cornea. It is caused by intense UVC/UVB exposure of the eye. Photokeratitis is also called "snow blindness" because many people develop this condition at high altitudes in a snowy environment where the reflections of UVB are high. This condition can also be produced by exposure to intense artificial sources of UVC/UVB, like broken mercury vapor lamps, or certain types of tanning lamps.

Eye Damage (Cataracts)

Cataracts are one form of eye damage that research has shown may increase with UV exposure. Clouding of the natural lens of the eye causing decreased vision and possible blindness are all effects of cataracts.

Other types of eye damage include cancer around the eyes, macular degeneration, and irregular tissue growth that can block vision (pterygium).

Immune System Suppression

According to the World Health Organization (WHO), all people, regardless of skin color, are vulnerable to the effects of immune suppression. Overexposure to UV radiation may suppress proper functioning of the body's immune system and the skin's natural defenses, increasing sensitivity to sunlight, diminishing the effects of immunizations, or causing reactions to certain medications.

In people who have been treated for an infection of the Herpes simplex virus, sun exposure can weaken the immune system so that it can no longer keep the virus under control. This results in reactivation of the infection and recurring cold sores.

Section 60.5

Tattoos and Teens

"Tattoos: The Hidden Dangers," by Roberta Renicker, RN, BN, MSA. © 2003 Children's Mercy Hospital Section of Adolescent Medicine (www.childrens-mercy.org). Reprinted with permission. Reviewed by David A. Cooke, MD, FACP, May 13, 2010.

What do Eminem, Mike Tyson, and P. Diddy all have in common? For one thing, some teens look up to them. For another, they all have tattoos, and sooner or later an adolescent you know will want to be 'N Sync with the latest body art.

It can be called self-expression, right of passage, or even disfigurement, but the real issue is larger than style or independence. There is a real health danger that health providers, parents, caretakers, and teens need to know more about in order to make responsible choices.

People with tattoos are nine times more likely to be infected with hepatitis C according to a recent study by Robert Haley, MD, Chief of Epidemiology at the University of Texas Southwestern Medical Center in Dallas.

Hepatitis C can develop into a chronic disease that attacks the liver, leading to liver failure and liver cancer at an early age. It is spread by infected blood and infected needles, which is the virus' connection with tattooing. Tattoos involve many needles and the making of many tiny punctures in the skin. Each puncture carries the potential for contamination—not just from hepatitis, but also HIV [human immunodeficiency virus] and other communicable diseases.

Hepatitis C is considered the silent killer as frequently there are no symptoms. People can have the virus for 10 or more years and not be aware they have it until they have reached end-stage liver failure. Treatment is available, but it is costly. The best prevention is not putting oneself at risk for exposure to the virus.

There is a major epidemic of hepatitis C in this country. Parents and teens need to be educated that a tattoo is not just a neat picture on their skin. Tattoos can result in life-long infections.

Young people can see the rock stars with tattoos, yet they go into a tattoo parlor and they do not see viruses or the potential health risks.

Adolescents are also buying tattoo kits (advertised on the back of tattoo magazines). They are having tattoo parties and giving each other tattoos. Some may get tattoos at flea markets or fly-by-night shops that want to make easy money. It is doubtful they are concerned about hepatitis C.

Many people are trying their best to provide safe tattooing, but this industry has a lot of nonconformists. There are some tattoo shops and reputable artists that try to use good health practices. They believe it is important to enforce infection control procedures in their shops. There are, however, many who do not care. Health departments officials find it difficult to catch up with the flea market artist ready to make a fast buck and drive to the next town.

Regardless of risk, regulation, and cost, if an adolescent wants a tattoo he/she will probably get one. Health care providers and parents can help our kids make responsible decisions. We can help them become informed consumers. We need to keep them informed of the risks. Parents and caretakers can be encouraged to talk with their teens about the risk of infections from tattoos and other risk issues.

Health providers can advocate for teens to become informed consumers. Here are a few points for teens to keep in mind before they allow a tattoo to be placed on them. Remind them that this may have a major health impact later in their lives.

• Ask if the artist uses an autoclave to sterilize equipment.

• Make sure the artist wears disposable gloves.

• Ask what training the artist has taken. Is there a certificate available?

• Find out if your state has requirements for cleanliness inspections.

• Make sure that your hepatitis B vaccine is complete.

• Individual containers of ink, ointment, and water should be used for one client and then discarded.

• New sterile needles must always be removed from a sterile wrapper and opened in front of the teen. If this is not happening, empower them to leave.

• Are used needles discarded into a special container?

• Ask yourself—"Is my life worth the risk of a homemade job?" Don't settle for second rate. You're worth it!

Section 60.6

Tinea Infections:
Athlete's Foot, Jock Itch, and Ringworm

This section includes text excerpted from "Athlete's Foot (*Tinea Pedis*)," by the Centers for Disease Control and Prevention (CDC, www.cdc.gov), December 24, 2009; and excerpted from "Dermatophytes (Ringworm)," by the CDC, National Center for Zoonotic, Vector-Borne, and Enteric Diseases, December 27, 2008.

Athlete's Foot (Tinea Pedis)

Athlete's foot, or *tinea pedis*, is an infection of the skin and feet that can be caused by a variety of different fungi. Although *tinea pedis* can affect any portion of the foot, the infection most often affects the space between the toes. Athlete's foot is typically characterized by skin fissures or scales that can be red and itchy.

Tinea pedis is spread through contact with infected skin scales or contact with fungi in damp areas (for example, showers, locker rooms, or swimming pools). *Tinea pedis* can be a chronic infection that recurs frequently. Treatment may include topical creams (applied to the surface of the skin) or oral medications.

Appropriate hygiene techniques may help to prevent or control *tinea pedis*.

- Nails should be clipped short and kept clean. Nails can house and spread the infection.

- Avoid walking barefoot in locker rooms or public showers (wear sandals).

For control of athlete's foot infection, persons with active tinea pedis infection should do the following:

- Keep feet clean, dry, and cool.

- Avoid using swimming pools, public showers, or foot baths.

- Wear sandals when possible or air shoes out by alternating them every 2–3 days.

517

- Avoid wearing closed shoes and wearing socks made from fabric that doesn't dry easily (for example, nylon).

- Treat the infection with recommended medication.

Ringworm

Dermatophytes are types of fungi that cause common skin, hair, and nail infections. Infections caused by these fungi are also known by the names tinea and ringworm. It is important to emphasize that ringworm is not caused by a worm, but rather by a type of fungus called a dermatophyte. One example of a very common dermatophyte infection is athlete's foot, which is also called tinea pedis. Another common dermatophyte infection affecting the groin area is jock itch, also known as tinea cruris.

Trichophyton rubrum and *Trichophyton tonsurans* are two common dermatophytes. These two species are usually transmitted from person to person. Another common dermatophyte is *Microsporum canis*, which is transmitted from animals such as cats and dogs to people. Dermatophytes like to live on moist areas of the skin, such as places where there are skin folds. They can also contaminate items in the environment, such as clothing, towels, and bedding.

Who gets dermatophyte infections?

Dermatophyte infections are very common. They can affect anyone, including people who are otherwise healthy. Dermatophyte infections may be more common among people with suppressed immune systems, people who use communal baths, and people who are involved in contact sports such as wrestling. Outbreaks of infections can occur in schools, households, and institutional settings.

The dermatophyte infection that affects the scalp and hair is known as tinea capitis. It is especially common among school-aged children. For reasons that are not well understood, tinea capitis does not usually occur after puberty.

Other kinds of dermatophyte infections tend to be more common in adolescents and adults.

How are dermatophyte infections spread?

Spread usually occurs through direct contact with an infected person or animal. Clothing, bedding, and towels can also become contaminated and spread the infection.

What are the symptoms of a dermatophyte infection?

Dermatophyte infections can affect the skin on almost any area of the body, such as the scalp, legs, arms, feet, groin, and nails. These infections are usually itchy. Redness, scaling, or fissuring of the skin, or a ring with irregular borders and a cleared central area may occur. If the infection involves the scalp, an area of hair loss may result. More aggressive infections may lead to an abscess or cellulitis. Areas infected by dermatophytes may become secondarily infected by bacteria.

How soon do symptoms appear?

Symptoms typically appear between 4 and 14 days following exposure.

If I have symptoms, should I see my doctor?

Yes. Most of the time these infections can be successfully treated with medication prescribed by your doctor.

How is a dermatophyte infection diagnosed?

Your doctor may make a presumptive diagnosis based on your symptoms and physical examination. To confirm the diagnosis your doctor may obtain scrapings of affected skin or clippings of affected nails. These may be examined under a microscope and may be sent to the laboratory for a fungal culture. Keep in mind that the results of the fungal culture may not be available for 2–4 weeks.

How can dermatophyte infections be treated?

The particular medication and duration of treatment is based on the location of the infection. Scalp infections usually require treatment with an oral antifungal medication. Infections of other areas of skin are usually treated with topical antifungal medications. Nail infections can be challenging to treat, and may be treated with oral and/or topical antifungal medications.

How can dermatophyte infections be prevented?

Good hygiene, such as regular handwashing, is important. People should avoid sharing hairbrushes, hats, and other articles of clothing that may come into contact with infected areas. Pets with signs of skin disease should be evaluated by a veterinarian. Beauty salons and barbershops should disinfect instruments with approved disinfectants after each use. Contact your local and/or state health department for specific guidelines and regulations in your area.

Chapter 61

Work Safety for Teens

Are You a Working Teen?

Every year about 70 teens die from work injuries in the United States. Another 70,000 get hurt badly enough that they go to a hospital emergency room. Teens are often injured on the job due to unsafe equipment and stressful conditions. Also teens may not receive adequate safety training and supervision. As a teen, you are much more likely to be injured when working on jobs that you are not allowed to do by law.

What are my rights on the job?

By law, your employer must provide the following:

- A safe and healthful workplace

- Safety and health training, in many situations, including providing information on chemicals that could be harmful to your health

- For many jobs, payment for medical care (and maybe lost wages) if you get hurt or sick because of your job

- At least the federal minimum wage

This chapter contains text excerpted from "Are You a Working Teen?" by the National Institute for Occupational Safety and Health (NIOSH, www.cdc.gov/niosh), part of the Centers for Disease Control and Prevention, 1997, and excerpted from "Promoting Safe Work for Young Workers," by NIOSH, November 1999. Both documents were reviewed by David A. Cooke, MD, FACP, May 13, 2010.

521

Many states have minimum wages that may be higher than the federal wage, and lower wages may be allowed when workers receive tips from customers.

You also have a right to the following:

- Report safety problems to OSHA (Occupational Safety and Health Administration)

- Work without racial or sexual harassment

- Refuse to work if the job is immediately dangerous to your life or health

- Join or organize a union

What hazards should I watch out for?

- If you're a janitor or do cleanup work, look out for toxic chemicals in cleaning products or blood on discarded needles.

- If you're in food service, look out for slippery floors, hot cooking equipment, or sharp objects.

- If you're in retail or sales positions, hazards may include violent crimes and heavy lifting.

- If you do office or clerical work, hazards may include stress, harassment, or poor computer workstation design.

Is it OK to do any kind of work?

No. There are laws that protect teens from doing dangerous work. No worker under 18 may do the following:

- Drive a motor vehicle as a regular part of the job or operate a forklift at any time

- Operate many types of powered equipment like a circular saw, box crusher, meat slicer, or bakery machine

- Work in wrecking, demolition, excavation, or roofing

- Work in mining, logging, or a sawmill

- Work in meatpacking or slaughtering

- Work where there is exposure to radiation

- Work where explosives are manufactured or stored

Also, no one 14 or 15 years old may do the following:

- Bake or cook on the job (except at a serving counter)
- Operate power-driven machinery, except certain types which pose little hazard such as those used in offices
- Work on a ladder or scaffold
- Work in warehouses
- Work in construction, building, or manufacturing
- Load or unload a truck, railroad car, or conveyor

There are many other restrictions regarding the type of work you can and cannot do. If you are under 14, there are even stricter laws to protect your health and safety. States have their own child labor laws that may be stricter than the federal laws. Check with your school counselor, job placement coordinator, or state Department of Labor to make sure the job you are doing is allowed.

What are my safety responsibilities on the job?

To work safely you should do the following:

- Follow all safety rules and instructions.
- Use safety equipment and protective clothing when needed.
- Look out for coworkers.
- Keep work areas clean and neat.
- Know what to do in an emergency.
- Report any health and safety hazard to your supervisor.

Should I be working this late or this long?

Federal child labor laws protect younger teens from working too long, too late, or too early. Some states have laws on the hours that older teens may work. If you have questions on working hours, call your local or state Department of Labor office, or go to www.dol.gov.

What if I need help?

- Talk to your boss about the problem.
- Talk to your parents or teachers.

- For more information on working safe, visit the Department of Labor website at www.dol.gov or call your local Wage and Hour Office (under Department of Labor in the blue pages of your local telephone book).

You have a right to speak up. It is illegal for your employer to fire or punish you for reporting a workplace problem.

Promoting Safe Work for Young Workers

Through part-time employment, school-to-work programs, apprenticeships, and internships, teens are a vital and an increasing part of our labor force. For adolescents, employment can be a valuable experience: In addition to its financial benefits, work gives adolescents the opportunity to learn important job skills, explore future careers, and, in some cases, enhance their academic education.

But employment also can have negative consequences for young workers. Far too often, working teens suffer injuries that can have devastating effects on their physical well-being. And working too many hours can jeopardize an adolescent's academic and social development.

Although increased prevention efforts are needed to reduce occupational injuries among all workers, young workers warrant special attention for the following reasons.

Do most teens in the United States work?

In 1996, approximately 42% of 16- and 17-year-old teens were in the labor force at any single time. An estimated 80% of youths are employed at some point before they leave high school.

Teens aged 16 and 17 worked an average of 21 hours per week, 23 weeks of the year in 1988.

Teens typically work at part-time, temporary, or low-paying jobs, often after already putting in a day of work at school. Twenty hours of employment per week during the school year combined with a full class schedule adds up to a 50-hour workweek, not including homework or extracurricular activities.

Teens work predominantly in retail and service industries. Typical places of employment include restaurants, grocery stores, department stores, gas stations, and offices.

Do many working teens get injured?

The National Institute for Occupational Safety and Health (NIOSH) estimates that in the United States, 200,000 teens aged 14 to 17 are injured on the job every year. Among the most common injuries suffered by working teens are lacerations, contusions, abrasions, sprains and strains, burns, and fractures or dislocations. Not surprisingly, most injuries occur in the workplaces that employ the most teens—retail shops, restaurants, and grocery stores. What may be surprising is the fact that teens are injured at a higher rate than are adult workers, even though youths are prohibited from holding the most dangerous types of jobs, such as mining, manufacturing, and construction.

Do many occupational injuries are serious enough to require medical treatment?

Approximately 100,000 teens aged 15 to 17 visit emergency departments each year for work-related injuries. This figure compares with 322,000 teens aged 15 to 17 who visit emergency departments for all motor vehicle traffic-related injuries, including vehicle occupants, pedestrians, bicyclists, and motorcyclists.

Approximately 70 teens died as a result of occupational injuries each year between 1980 and 1989.

Work-related injuries can have long-term consequences. Common occupational injuries such as burns, back sprains, and eye damage can cause permanent disability. In addition to injury, workplace hazards such as chemical exposure, noise, extreme temperatures, repetitive motions, and infectious agents can pose long-term health risks for adolescents.

Teens are injured doing legal jobs as well as doing jobs that are prohibited by child labor laws.

Federal child labor laws restrict the types of jobs teens can do and the hours they can work; some state laws are stricter than federal laws. Working in illegal jobs puts youth at particular risk for injuries. According to one study, 19% of all injuries to young workers treated in emergency rooms involved working in illegal jobs; this figure is 41% according to another study. However, laws alone provide insufficient protection: Most injuries occur when teens are working in compliance with child labor laws.

Is working too many hours associated with social and academic problems?

Teens who work more than 20 hours per week are at risk for increased drug and alcohol use and decreased academic performance.

Teachers report that students who work many hours outside of school are often sleepy and unresponsive in class.

Are young workers are at risk because they lack experience?

As inexperienced workers, adolescents are not likely to be familiar with job tasks, workplace hazards, ways to avoid injury, and their rights as workers.

Although a common perception is that teens get injured because they are reckless, teens injured on the job often have a very different profile. The positive characteristics of adolescents—their energy, enthusiasm, and desire for increased challenge and responsibility—combined with a reluctance to ask questions or make demands, can result in their assuming tasks for which they are either unprepared or incapable of performing safely.

The physical characteristics of teens also make them vulnerable to workplace injury. Adolescents between the ages of 14 and 17, especially boys, grow at very different rates. Small teens may not be able to reach machine parts and may lack the strength required for certain tasks. Large boys may be given adult tasks simply because of their size without regard for their lack of experience and maturity.

Chapter 62

Other Teen Safety Concerns

Chapter Contents

Section 62.1

Adolescent Sports Injuries

The number of adolescents who participate in organized sports has increased over the last few decades. In particular, the number of young women participating in sports has grown very rapidly. With this increase has come a corresponding increase in sports injuries. Forty percent of all pediatric injuries are sports related. Estimates put this number at 4.4 million injuries per year. Overall, male and female injury rates are becoming equal.

Injuries related to sports participation fall into two types of trauma: micro (due to repetitive trauma) and macro (due to a single traumatic event). Often these injuries are trivialized and the young athlete is asked or encouraged to "toughen up and play through the pain." This approach is not in the young athlete's best interest for the following reasons:

- It often leads to delayed healing and return to sports.

- It can turn an easily treatable injury into one that becomes difficult to treat.

- In some cases, it can result in a prominent injury that precludes sports participation.

The adolescent is still growing. The growth plates (physis) are cartilaginous (strong connective tissue) areas of the bones from which the bones elongate or enlarge. Repetitive stress or sudden large forces can cause injury to these areas. In the adolescent knee, such injuries include:

- **Fracture:** Breaking of the growth plates. A fracture through the growth plate can be a very serious injury that can stop the bone from growing properly. These fractures should be treated by an orthopedist, as some will require surgery.

- **Osgood-Schlatter's disease:** Pain at the knob just below the kneecap (tibia tubercle). Overuse injury may occur because of year-round sports participation. This type of injury responds to rest and activity modification. Adolescents will outgrow Osgood-Schlatter's.

- **Sinding-Larsen-Johansson disease:** Pain at the lower pole of the kneecap (patella). Sinding-Larsen-Johansson disease is caused by overuse and is treated with rest. Adolescents will outgrow it.

- **Osteochondritis dissecans:** Separation of a piece of bone from its bed in the knee joint. This injury is usually due to one major macro event, with repetitive macro trauma that prevents complete healing. This injury is potentially very serious. Treatment varies from rest to surgery.

- **Bipartite/multipartite patella:** Results from failure of a bone growth center to fuse normally. Rest is the first line of treatment, but if pain persists, surgery may be required.

- **Anterior knee pain:** Anterior knee pain, or patella femoral syndrome, is often passed off as growing pains. Causes of this pain include overuse, muscle imbalance, poor flexibility, poor alignment, or, more commonly, a combination of these. Anterior knee pain is one of the most difficult adolescent knee injuries to sort out and treat. Accurate diagnosis and treatment depend on finding a musculoskeletal specialist with a special interest and expertise in this difficult area.

- **Patellar instability:** Patellar (kneecap) instability can range from partial dislocation (subluxation) to dislocation with fracture. Partial dislocation can often be treated conservatively. Dislocation with or without fracture is a much more serious injury and usually will require surgery.

- **Knee ligaments and the menisci** (cartilage between the leg bones) have greater blood supply and are more elastic in adolescents than in adults. As adolescents near the end of bone growth, their injuries become more adult-like, and adolescents become more susceptible to meniscal and anterior cruciate ligament (ACL) injuries.

- **Medial collateral ligament (MCL) injury:** This injury results from a lateral blow to the knee. Pain is felt on inner side (medially) of the knee. MCL injuries respond well to protective bracing and conservative treatment.

- **Anterior cruciate ligament (ACL) injury:** This injury is most commonly caused by a non-contact twisting or deceleration mechanism, which results in excessive hyperextension or interval rotation forces on the anterior cruciate ligament. Non-contact injuries of the ACL are becoming more common than contact injuries. Adolescent females are at high risk. Combination injuries with MCL or menisci are common. Surgical reconstruction is needed if the adolescent wishes to continue participating in "stop-and-start" sports.

- **Meniscal injury:** An injury to the meniscus, the crescent-shaped cartilage between the thighbone (femur) and lower leg bone (tibia). These injuries usually result from twisting. Swelling, catching, and locking of the knee are common. Nearly all of these types of injuries will require arthroscopic surgery.

Making the Diagnosis

In most cases, the physician can make the diagnosis by taking the patient's medical history and performing a physical exam. The adolescent's age, sex, and level of participation in sports are important. A description of how the injury occurred is valuable. The physician will want to know if there was a "pop," swelling, history of previous injury, family history of similar injury, locking or giving way of the knee, or other signs or symptoms. While special tests can be helpful, in certain circumstances an accurate diagnosis can be made 90 percent of the time by taking a good history and performing a systematic exam of the knee.

Conclusion

- Adolescent sports injuries continue to rise.

- Certain injuries tend to occur to certain age groups and sexes.

- In most cases, a good history and physical exam by an adolescent sports medicine expert will provide an accurate diagnosis.

- Knee swelling, pain, and loss of function are not normal.

- Remember, not all serious knee injuries result from major trauma.

- Injuries that appear minor can have serious consequences.

- Adolescents have a lot of enjoyable sporting years ahead of them. It would be a shame to see this enjoyment end too soon.

- When in doubt, seek expert medical advice. It's better to be safe than sorry.

Section 62.2

Noise and Hearing Damage

This section includes text excerpted from "Noise-Induced Hearing Loss," by the National Institute on Deafness and Other Communication Disorders (NIDCD, nidcd.nih.gov), part of the National Institutes of Health, October 2008; and from "How Loud Is Too Loud?" by the NICHD, October 2008.

Noise-Induced Hearing Loss

Every day, we experience sound in our environment, such as the sounds from television and radio, household appliances, and traffic. Normally, we hear these sounds at safe levels that do not affect our hearing. However, when we are exposed to harmful noise—sounds that are too loud or loud sounds that last a long time—sensitive structures in our inner ear can be damaged, causing noise-induced hearing loss (NIHL). These sensitive structures, called hair cells, are small sensory cells that convert sound energy into electrical signals that travel to the brain. Once damaged, our hair cells cannot grow back.

NIHL can be caused by a one-time exposure to an intense impulse sound, such as an explosion, or by continuous exposure to loud sounds over an extended period of time, such as noise generated in a wood-working shop.

Sound is measured in units called decibels. On the decibel scale, an increase of 10 means that a sound is 10 times more intense, or powerful. To your ears, it sounds twice as loud. The humming of a refrigerator is 45 decibels, normal conversation is approximately 60 decibels, and the noise from heavy city traffic can reach 85 decibels. Sources of noise that can cause NIHL include motorcycles, firecrackers, and small firearms, all emitting sounds from 120 to 150 decibels. Long or repeated exposure to sounds at or above 85 decibels can cause hearing loss. The louder the sound, the shorter the time period before NIHL can occur. Sounds of less than 75 decibels, even after long exposure, are unlikely to cause hearing loss.

Although being aware of decibel levels is an important factor in protecting one's hearing, distance from the source of the sound and duration of exposure to the sound are equally important. A good rule of thumb is to avoid noises that are too loud and too close or that last too long.

To protect your hearing:

- Know which noises can cause damage (those at or above 85 decibels).

- Wear earplugs or other hearing protective devices when involved in a loud activity (special earplugs and earmuffs are available at hardware and sporting goods stores).

- Be alert to hazardous noise in the environment.

- Protect the ears of children who are too young to protect their own.

- Make family, friends, and colleagues aware of the hazards of noise.

- If you suspect hearing loss, have a medical examination by an otolaryngologist (a physician who specializes in diseases of the ears, nose, throat, head, and neck) and a hearing test by an audiologist (a health professional trained to measure and help individuals deal with hearing loss).

How Loud Is Too Loud?

Noise-induced hearing loss (NIHL) occurs when tiny sensory hair cells in our inner ears are damaged by sounds that are too loud and that last for too long. But how loud is too loud, and how much time is too long? The answers are related: The louder the sound, the shorter the time before damage can occur.

How is sound measured?

Sound is measured in units called decibels. Decibel levels begin at zero, which is near total silence and the weakest sound our ears can hear. By comparison, a whisper is 30 decibels and a normal conversation is 60 decibels. An increase of 10 means that a sound is 10 times more intense, or powerful. To your ears, it sounds twice as loud. The sound of an ambulance siren at 120 decibels is about 1 trillion times more intense than the weakest sound our ears can hear. Sounds that reach 120 decibels are painful to our ears at close distances.

Scientists believe that, depending upon the type of sound, the pure force of its vibrations at high decibel levels can cause hearing loss. Recent studies also show that exposure to sounds at harmful decibel levels triggers the formation of molecules inside the ear that damage hair cells. These destructive molecules play an important role in hearing loss in children and adults who listen to loud noise for too long.

How does time multiply the danger of NIHL?

NIHL is related both to the decibel level of a sound and to the amount of time you are exposed to it. The distance you are from the sound also matters. A sound gets louder as you move closer to the source and softer as you move away from it. If you are far away from the sound, its intensity and its potential to cause damage are much lower. In addition, the impact of noise adds up over a lifetime. If you are exposed to loud sounds on a regular basis, your risk for permanent damage adds up as you age.

NIHL is also related to a person's genes. Some people are more likely than others to develop NIHL when they listen to certain sounds. Scientists are working to determine which people are more at risk for NIHL and which are less at risk. For this reason, we all need to protect our hearing when we are exposed to loud noise.

Researchers who study hearing loss in the workplace have found that a person who is exposed to noise levels at 85 decibels or higher for a prolonged period of time is at risk for hearing loss. For this reason, these workers are required to wear hearing protectors, such as earplugs or earmuffs, while they are on the job. Many devices that children use today have noise levels much higher than 85 decibels. For example, an MP3 player at maximum level is roughly 105 decibels. That's 100 times more intense than 85 decibels! Scientists recommend no more than 15 minutes of unprotected exposure to sounds that are 100 decibels. In addition, regular exposure to sounds at 110 decibels for more than 1 minute risks permanent hearing loss.

How can I reduce the possibility of NIHL?

Your ears can be your warning system for potentially dangerous noises. The noise is too loud when the following are true:

- You have to raise your voice to be understood by someone standing nearby.
- The noise hurts your ears.
- You develop a buzzing or ringing sound in your ears, even temporarily.
- You don't hear as well as you normally do until several hours after you get away from the noise.

If you are around noises at this level, take protective action. To avoid NIHL, do the following:

- Block the noise (wear earplugs or earmuffs).

- Avoid the noise (walk away).

- Turn down the sound.

Section 62.3

Repetitive Stress Injuries in Teens

"Repetitive Stress Injuries," November 2009, reprinted with permission from www.kidshealth.org. Copyright © 2009 The Nemours Foundation. This information was provided by KidsHealth, one of the largest resources online for medically reviewed health information written for parents, kids, and teens. For more articles like this one, visit www.KidsHealth.org, or www.TeensHealth.org.

Michael started running track freshman year, gradually working up to longer and longer distances. Now a senior, he recently took up trail running and dreams of running the Marine Corps Marathon someday.

Michael's love for his chosen sport made it really hard when he started having some shin pain during his sophomore year. His doctor told him to take a break from running for 6 weeks because he had developed a stress fracture. But after a few weeks of rest, Michael went back to running as if nothing had happened and he hasn't had any problems since.

What Are Repetitive Stress Injuries?

Repetitive stress injuries (RSIs) are injuries that happen when too much stress is placed on a part of the body, resulting in inflammation (pain and swelling), muscle strain, or tissue damage. This stress generally occurs from repeating the same movements over and over again.

RSIs are common work-related injuries, often affecting people who spend a lot of time using computer keyboards.

While most common in adults, RSIs are becoming more prevalent in teens because they spend more time than ever using computers.

Playing sports like tennis that involve repetitive motions can also lead to RSIs. You may hear sports-related RSIs referred to as overuse injuries. Teens who spend a lot of time playing musical instruments or video games are also at risk for RSIs.

In general, RSIs include more than 100 different kinds of injuries and illnesses resulting from repetitive wear and tear on the body. These injuries vary from person to person in type and severity.

In teens, overuse injuries most often occur at growth plates (areas at the ends of bones where bone cells multiply rapidly, making bones longer as someone grows). Areas most affected by RSIs are the elbows, shoulders, knees, and heels.

What Causes Repetitive Stress Injuries?

Most RSI conditions found in teens are linked to the stress of repetitive motions at the computer or in sports. When stress occurs repeatedly over time, the body's joints don't have the chance to recover, and the joints and surrounding tendons and muscles become irritated and inflamed.

Certain jobs that involve repetitive tasks—such as scanning items as a supermarket checker or carrying heavy trays as a waiter—can lead to RSIs. Sometimes, playing musical instruments can cause problems from overuse of certain hand or arm movements. Any repetitive movement can cause an injury—even text messaging.

Using improper equipment while playing sports is another important factor in RSIs. For example, running in athletic shoes that don't provide enough support can lead to shin splits and foot and ankle problems. Improperly fitted tennis rackets can contribute to a condition called tennis elbow.

Teens may be susceptible to RSIs because of the significant physical growth that occurs in the teen years. The growth spurt (the rapid growth period during puberty) can create extra tightness and tension in muscles and tendons, making teens more prone to injury.

Nutritional factors also come into play in RSIs. Proper nutrition is essential for developing and maintaining strong muscles and bones—and to keep up the energy levels needed to play sports and perform other physical activities well.

What Happens When Teens Have RSIs?

Symptoms of RSIs include:

- tingling, numbness, or pain in the affected area;

- stiffness or soreness in the neck or back;
- feelings of weakness or fatigue in the hands or arms;
- popping or clicking sensation.

If you notice any of these warning signs of RSIs, make an appointment to see a doctor. Even if your symptoms seem to come and go, don't ignore them or they may lead to more serious problems.

Without treatment, RSIs can become more severe and prevent you from doing simple everyday tasks and participating in sports, music, and other favorite activities.

What Kinds of Repetitive Stress Injuries Can Teens Get?

RSIs that can develop in teens include [the following]:

- **Bursitis:** Inflammation of a bursa, which is a fluid-filled sac that acts as a cushion for a joint, is known as bursitis (pronounced: bur-sye-tis). Signs of bursitis include pain and swelling. It is associated with frequent overhead reaching, carrying overloaded backpacks, and overusing certain joints during sports, such as the knee or shoulder.

- **Carpal tunnel syndrome:** In carpal tunnel syndrome, swelling occurs inside a narrow "tunnel" formed by bone and ligament in the wrist. This tunnel surrounds nerves that conduct sensory and motor impulses to and from the hand, causing pain, tingling, numbness, and weakness. Carpal tunnel syndrome is caused by repeated motion that can happen during activities like typing or playing video games (using joysticks). It's rare in teens and more common in adults, especially those in computer-related jobs.

- **Epicondylitis:** This condition is characterized by pain and swelling at the point where the bones join at the elbow. Epicondylitis (pronounced: eh-pih-kon-dih-lye-tis) is nicknamed "tennis elbow" because it frequently occurs in tennis players.

- **Osgood-Schlatter disease:** This is a common cause of knee pain in teens, especially teen athletes who are undergoing a growth spurt. Frequent use and physical stress (such as running long distances) can cause inflammation at the area where the tendon from the kneecap attaches to the shinbone.

- **Patellar femoral syndrome:** This is a softening or breaking down of kneecap cartilage. Squatting, kneeling, and climbing stairs and hills can aggravate pain around the knee.

- **Shin splints:** This term refers to pain along the shin or front of the lower leg. Shin splints are commonly found in runners and are usually harmless, although they can be quite painful. They can be difficult to tell apart from stress fractures.

- **Stress fractures:** Stress fractures are tiny cracks in the bone's surface caused by rhythmic, repetitive overloading. These injuries can occur when a bone comes under repeated stress from running, marching, walking, or jumping, or from stress on the body like when a person changes running surfaces or runs in worn-out sneakers.

- **Tendonitis:** In tendonitis, tearing and inflammation occur in the tendons, rope-like bands of tissue that connect muscles to bones. Tendonitis is associated with repetitive overstretching of tendons from overuse of certain muscles.

Preventing Repetitive Stress Injuries

Preventing Computer-Related Injuries

To prevent injuries from computer use, make sure your computer equipment and furniture fit you properly and that you use correct typing and sitting positions. If your parents are shopping for new computer furniture, suggest that they buy pieces that can be adjusted for each family member.

Here are some tips:

- Make sure the top of your computer screen is aligned with your forehead.

- Sit up straight with your back touching the back of your seat. Chairs that provide extra support, especially lumbar (lower back) support are helpful. Avoid slouching over your keyboard or tensing your shoulders, which can place unnecessary stress on your neck, back, and spine.

- Let your legs rest comfortably with your feet flat on the floor or on a footrest. (To test whether your legs are in a good position, try placing a pencil on your knee—the pencil should roll toward your waist, not off of your knee.)

- Use a light touch when typing. Place the keyboard close to you so that you don't have to reach for it.

- Fingers and wrists should remain level while typing. Try a wrist rest for extra support. Your wrists and forearms should be at a 90-degree angle to the upper part of your arms. Elbows should be placed close to the side of the body to prevent bending the wrists side to side.

- It's easy to lose track of time when you're surfing the internet or immersed in a homework assignment. Be sure to take breaks (to stretch or walk around) about every 30 minutes—even if you don't feel tired or feel any pain. (If you lose track of time, use a timer so you know when you're due for a break.)

- Try an ergonomic ("ergonomic" means specially designed for comfort) keyboard that has a curved design, and use a trackball instead of a mouse.

Preventing Sports-Related Injuries

Begin any sports season with a full physical exam from your doctor so that any problems or concerns can be addressed before you begin workouts and competitions. More tips [include the following]:

- Always warm up and cool down with appropriate stretching exercises before and after playing.

- Wear the proper clothing and equipment for your sport. For example, tennis players should be fitted for rackets that allow for a good grip on the handle. Wear appropriate safety gear for your sport, such as kneepads and wrist supports.

- Drink plenty of water before, during, and after your workouts. Listen to your body and rest when you feel tired.

- Vary your day-to-day activities. Alternate distance running with bicycling or swimming, for example.

- If you are experiencing symptoms such as pain, swelling, numbness, or stiffness while playing your sport, stop playing right away and see your doctor as soon as possible.

What Do Doctors Do?

The sooner an RSI is diagnosed, the sooner your body can heal, so be sure to see your doctor if you have symptoms.

The doctor will try to assess how the injury occurred and what motions cause pain. Your doctor may perform x-rays, blood tests, or other tests to make sure there are no other health problems. In addition to doing a physical examination, the doctor may ask you about any concerns and symptoms you have, your past health, your family's health, any medications you're taking, any allergies you may have, and other issues. This is called the medical history.

If you are diagnosed with an RSI, resting the affected area is the key to getting better. Your doctor may recommend that you take anti-inflammatory medication (such as ibuprofen) for a period of time. Ice packs are sometimes recommended to reduce pain and swelling.

After the swelling and pain have gone away, your doctor may suggest a rehabilitation program with a physical therapist to exercise your muscles and prevent loss of joint movement.

Taking Care of Yourself

Prevention is the best medicine when it comes to RSIs. Overall flexibility and strength can help to prevent RSIs, so exercise regularly and stay active (remembering warm-ups, cool-downs, and stretching, of course).

To avoid overusing muscles and joints, be sensible about the amount of time you spend doing any repeated motions. If an activity is repetitive, take breaks and do something different every 30 minutes or so.

Part Eight

Violence against Adolescents

Chapter 63

Youth Violence: A Public Health Problem

Chapter Contents

Section 63.1

Statistics on Youth Violence

Excerpted from "Youth Violence," by the Centers for Disease Control and Prevention (CDC, www.cdc.gov), 2009. Full reference information available at http://www.cdc.gov/ViolencePrevention/pdf/yv-datasheet-a.pdf.

- In 2006, 5,958 young people ages 10 to 24 were murdered—an average of 16 each day.

- Homicide was the second leading cause of death for young people ages 10 to 24 years old.

- Among 10- to 24-year-olds, 87% (5,159) of homicide victims were male and 13% (799) were female.

- Among homicide victims ages 10 to 24 years old, 84% were killed with a firearm.

Health Disparities

- Among 10- to 24-year-olds, homicide is the leading cause of death for African Americans; the second leading cause of death for Hispanics; and the third leading cause of death for Asian/ Pacific Islanders and American Indians and Alaska Natives.

- Homicide rates among non-Hispanic, African-American males 10–24 years of age (62.2 per 100,000) exceed those of Hispanic males (21.5 per 100,000) and non-Hispanic, White males in the same age group (3.4 per 100,000).

Nonfatal Injuries due to Violence

- In 2007, more than 668,000 young people ages 10 to 24were treated in emergency departments for injuries sustained from violence.

- In 2007, of a nationally representative sample of students in grades 9–12, 4.2% reported being in a physical fight one or more times in the previous 12 months that resulted in injuries that had to be treated by a doctor or nurse.

Violence-Related Behaviors

In a 2007 nationally representative sample of youth in grades 9–12, researchers found the following:

- 35.5% reported being in a physical fight in the 12 months preceding the survey; the prevalence was higher among males (44.4%) than females (26.5%).

- 18.0% reported carrying a weapon (gun, knife, or club) on 1 or more days in the 30 days preceding the survey.

- 5.2% carried a gun on 1 or more days in the 30 days preceding the survey.

- Males were more likely than females to carry a weapon (28.5% versus 7.5%) on 1 or more days in the 30 days preceding the survey.

- Males were also more likely than females to carry a gun on 1 or more days in the 30 days preceding the survey (9.0% versus 1.2%).

School Violence

In a 2007 nationally representative sample of youth in grades 9–12, researchers found the following:

- 12.4% reported being in a physical fight on school property in the 12 months preceding the survey.

- 16.3% of male students and 8.5% of female students reported being in a physical fight on school property in the 12 months preceding the survey.

- 27.1% of students reported having property stolen or deliberately damaged on school property.

- 5.5% did not go to school on 1 or more days in the 30days preceding the survey because they felt unsafe at school or on their way to or from school.

- 5.9% reported carrying a weapon (gun, knife, or club) on school property on 1 or more days in the 30 days preceding the survey.

- 7.8% reported being threatened or injured with a weapon on school property one or more times in the 12 months preceding the survey.

Bullying

An estimated 30% of 6th to 10th graders in the United States were either a bully, a target of bullying, or both.

School-Associated Violent Deaths

- Less than 1% of all homicides and suicides among school-age youth occur on school grounds, on the way to or from school, or on the way to or from school-sponsored events.

- From 1992 to 1999, perpetrators of school-associated homicides were nine times as likely as victims to have exhibited some form of suicidal behavior before the event, and were more than twice as likely as victims to have been bullied by their peers.

- More than half of the incidents over this period were preceded by some signal, such as threats, notes, or journal entries that indicated the potential for the coming event.

- Most of the events occurred during the transition times around the start of the school day, the lunch period, and at the end of the school day.

- During the past 7 years, 116 students were killed in 109 separate incidents—an average of 16.5 student homicides each year.

- Rates of school-associated student homicides decreased between 1992 and 2006. However, they remained relatively stable in recent years. Rates were significantly higher for males, students in secondary schools, and students in central cities.

- From 1999 to 2006, most school-associated homicides included gunshot wounds (65%), stabbing or cutting (27%), and beating (12%).

Juvenile Arrests

- Juveniles accounted for 16% of all violent crime arrests and 26% of all property crime arrests in 2007.

- In 2007, 1,350 juveniles were arrested for murder, 3,580 for forcible rape, and 57,650 for aggravated assault.

Section 63.2

Youth Violence Risk and Protective Factors

From "Youth Violence: Risk and Protective Factors," by the Centers for Disease Control and Prevention (CDC, www.cdc.gov), August 11, 2008.

Risk Factors for the Perpetration of Youth Violence

Research on youth violence has increased our understanding of factors that make some populations more vulnerable to victimization and perpetration. Risk factors increase the likelihood that a young person will become violent. However, risk factors are not direct causes of youth violence; instead, risk factors contribute to youth violence.

Research associates the following risk factors with perpetration of youth violence.

Individual Risk Factors

- History of violent victimization
- Attention deficits, hyperactivity, or learning disorders
- History of early aggressive behavior
- Involvement with drugs, alcohol, or tobacco
- Low IQ
- Poor behavioral control
- Deficits in social cognitive or information-processing abilities
- High emotional distress
- History of treatment for emotional problems
- Antisocial beliefs and attitudes
- Exposure to violence and conflict in the family

Family Risk Factors

- Authoritarian childrearing attitudes
- Harsh, lax, or inconsistent disciplinary practices

- Low parental involvement
- Low emotional attachment to parents or caregivers
- Low parental education and income
- Parental substance abuse or criminality
- Poor family functioning
- Poor monitoring and supervision of children

Peer/Social Risk Factors

- Association with delinquent peers
- Involvement in gangs
- Social rejection by peers
- Lack of involvement in conventional activities
- Poor academic performance
- Low commitment to school and school failure

Community Risk Factors

- Diminished economic opportunities
- High concentrations of poor residents
- High level of transiency
- High level of family disruption
- Low levels of community participation
- Socially disorganized neighborhoods

Protective Factors for the Perpetration of Youth Violence

Protective factors buffer young people from the risks of becoming violent. These factors exist at various levels. To date, protective factors have not been studied as extensively or rigorously as risk factors. However, identifying and understanding protective factors are equally as important as researching risk factors.

Individual/Family Protective Factors

- Intolerant attitude toward deviance
- High IQ

- High grade point average

- Positive social orientation

- Religiosity

- Connectedness to family or adults outside the family

- Ability to discuss problems with parents

- Perceived parental expectations about school performance are high

- Frequent shared activities with parents

- Consistent presence of parent during at least one of the following: when awakening, when arriving home from school, at evening mealtime, or going to bed

- Involvement in social activities

Peer/Social Protective Factors

- Commitment to school

- Involvement in social activities

Section 63.3

Warning Signs of Youth Violence

Introduction

Violence. It's the act of purposefully hurting someone. And it's a major issue facing today's young adults. One in 12 high schoolers is threatened or injured with a weapon each year. If you're between the ages of 12 and 24, you face the highest risk of being the victim of violence.

At the same time, statistics show that by the early 1990s the incidence of violence caused by young people reached unparalleled levels in American society.

There is no single explanation for the overall rise in youth violence. Many different factors cause violent behavior. The more these factors are present in your life, the more likely you are to commit an act of violence.

Reasons for Violence

What causes someone to punch, kick, stab, or fire a gun at someone else or even him/herself?

There is never a simple answer to that question. But people often commit violence because of one or more of the following:

Expression: Some people use violence to release feelings of anger or frustration. They think there are no answers to their problems and turn to violence to express their out of control emotions.

Manipulation: Violence is used as a way to control others or get something they want.

Retaliation: Violence is used to retaliate against those who have hurt them or someone they care about.

Violence is a learned behavior: Like all learned behaviors, it can be changed. This isn't easy, though. Since there is no single cause of violence, there is no one simple solution. The best you can do is learn to recognize the warning signs of violence and to get help when you see them in your friends or yourself.

Factors that contribute to violent behavior include:

- peer pressure;
- need for attention or respect;
- feelings of low self-worth;
- early childhood abuse or neglect;
- witnessing violence at home, in the community, or in the media; and
- easy access to weapons.

Recognizing Violence Warning Signs in Others

Often people who act violently have trouble controlling their feelings. They may have been hurt by others. Some think that making people fear them through violence or threats of violence will solve their problems or earn them respect. This isn't true.

People who behave violently lose respect. They find themselves isolated or disliked, and they still feel angry and frustrated.

If you see these immediate warning signs, violence is a serious possibility:

- Loss of temper on a daily basis
- Frequent physical fighting
- Significant vandalism or property damage
- Increase in use of drugs or alcohol
- Increase in risk-taking behavior
- Detailed plans to commit acts of violence
- Announcing threats or plans for hurting others
- Enjoying hurting animals
- Carrying a weapon

If you notice the following signs over a period of time, the potential for violence exists:

- A history of violent or aggressive behavior
- Serious drug or alcohol use
- Gang membership or strong desire to be in a gang
- Access to or fascination with weapons, especially guns
- Threatening others regularly
- Trouble controlling feelings like anger
- Withdrawal from friends and usual activities
- Feeling rejected or alone
- Having been a victim of bullying
- Poor school performance
- History of discipline problems or frequent run-ins with authority
- Feeling constantly disrespected
- Failing to acknowledge the feelings or rights of others

What You Can Do If Someone You Know Shows Violence Warning Signs

When you recognize violence warning signs in someone else, there are things you can do. Hoping that someone else will deal with the situation is the easy way out.

Above all, be safe. Don't spend time alone with people who show warning signs. If possible without putting yourself in danger, remove the person from the situation that's setting them off.

Tell someone you trust and respect about your concerns and ask for help. This could be a family member, guidance counselor, teacher, school psychologist, coach, clergy, school resource officer, or friend.

If you are worried about being a victim of violence, get someone in authority to protect you. Do not resort to violence or use a weapon to protect yourself.

The key to really preventing violent behavior is asking an experienced professional for help. The most important thing to remember is don't go it alone.

Dealing with Anger

It's normal to feel angry or frustrated when you've been let down or betrayed. But anger and frustration don't justify violent action. Anger is a strong emotion that can be difficult to keep in check, but the right response is always stay cool.

Here are some ways to deal with anger without resorting to violence:

- Learn to talk about your feelings. If you're afraid to talk or if you can't find the right words to describe what you're going through, find a trusted friend or adult to help you one-on-one.

- Express yourself calmly. Express criticism, disappointment, anger, or displeasure without losing your temper or fighting. Ask yourself if your response is safe and reasonable.

- Listen to others. Listen carefully and respond without getting upset when someone gives you negative feedback. Ask yourself if you can really see the other person's point of view.

- Negotiate. Work out your problems with someone else by looking at alternative solutions and compromises.

Anger is part of life, but you can free yourself from the cycle of violence by learning to talk about your feelings. Be strong. Be safe. Be cool.

Are You at Risk for Violent Behavior?

If you recognize any of the warning signs for violent behavior in yourself, get help.

You don't have to live with the guilt, sadness, and frustration that comes from hurting others.

Admitting you have a concern about hurting others is the first step. The second is to talk to a trusted adult such as a school counselor or psychologist, teacher, family member, friend, or clergy. They can get you in touch with a licensed mental health professional who cares and can help.

Controlling Your Own Risk for Violent Behavior

Everyone feels anger in his or her own way. Start managing it by recognizing how anger feels to you.

When you are angry, you probably feel:

- muscle tension;
- accelerated heartbeat;
- a "knot" or "butterflies" in your stomach;
- changes in your breathing;

- trembling;

- goose bumps; or

- flushed in the face.

You can reduce the rush of adrenaline that's responsible for your heart beating faster, your voice sounding louder, and your fists clenching if you:

- take a few slow, deep breaths and concentrate on your breathing;

- imagine yourself at the beach, by a lake, or anywhere that makes you feel calm and peaceful; or

- try other thoughts or actions that have helped you relax in the past.

Keep telling yourself:

- "Calm down."

- "I don't need to prove myself."

- "I'm not going to let him/her get to me."

Stop. Consider the consequences. Think before you act. Try to find positive or neutral explanations for what that person did that provoked you. Don't argue in front of other people. Make your goal to defeat the problem, not the other person. Learn to recognize what sets you off and how anger feels to you. Learn to think through the benefits of controlling your anger and the consequences of losing control. Most of all, stay cool and think. Only you have the power to control your own violent behavior; don't let anger control you.

Violence against Self

Some people who have trouble dealing with their feelings don't react by lashing out at others. Instead, they direct violence toward themselves. The most final and devastating expression of this kind of violence is suicide.

Like people who are violent toward others, potential suicide victims often behave in recognizable ways before they try to end their lives. Suicide, like other forms of violence, is preventable. The two most important steps in prevention are recognizing warning signs and getting help. Warning signs of potential self-violence include:

- previous suicide attempts;

- significant alcohol or drug use;

- threatening or communicating thoughts of suicide, death, dying, or the afterlife;

- sudden increase in moodiness, withdrawal, or isolation;

- major change in eating or sleeping habits;

- feelings of hopelessness, guilt, or worthlessness;

- poor control over behavior;

- impulsive, aggressive behavior;

- drop in quality of school performance or interest;

- lack of interest in usual activity;

- getting into trouble with authority figures;

- perfectionism;

- giving away important possessions; or

- hinting at not being around in the future or saying good-bye.
  These warning signs are especially noteworthy in the context of:

- a recent death or suicide of a friend or family member;

- a recent break-up with a boyfriend or girlfriend, or conflict with parents; or

- news reports of other suicides by young people in the same school or community.

Often, suicidal thinking comes from a wish to end deep psychological pain. Death seems like the only way out. But it isn't.

If a friend mentions suicide, take it seriously. Listen carefully, then seek help immediately. Never keep their talk of suicide a secret, even if they ask you to. Remember, you risk losing that person. Forever.

When you recognize the warning signs for suicidal behavior, do something about it. Tell a trusted adult what you have seen or heard. Get help from a licensed mental health professional as soon as possible. They can help work out the problems that seem so unsolvable but, in fact, are not.

Take a stand against violence.

Chapter 64

Bullying and Hazing

Chapter Contents

Section 64.1

Facts and Statistics on Bullying

From "Bullying Facts and Statistics," by the National Youth Violence
Prevention Resource Center (www.safeyouth.org), December 27, 2007.

Prevalence

Almost 30% of youth in the United States (or over 5.7 million) are
estimated to be involved in bullying as either a bully, a target of bullying, or both. In a recent national survey of students in grades 6–10, 13%
reported bullying others, 11% reported being the target of bullies, and
another 6% said that they bullied others and were bullied themselves.

Male vs. Female

Bullying takes on different forms in male and female youth. While
both male and female youth say that others bully them by making
fun of the way they look or talk, males are more likely to report being
hit, slapped, or pushed. Female youth are more likely than males to
report being the targets of rumors and sexual comments. While male
youth target both boys and girls, female youth most often bully other
girls, using more subtle and indirect forms of aggression than boys. For
example, instead of physically harming others, they are more likely to
spread gossip or encourage others to reject or exclude another girl.

Risk Factors for Bullying Behavior

While many people believe that bullies act tough in order to hide
feelings of insecurity and self-loathing, in fact, bullies tend to be confident, with high self-esteem. They are generally physically aggressive,
with pro-violence attitudes, and are typically hot-tempered, easily
angered, and impulsive, with a low tolerance for frustration. Bullies
have a strong need to dominate others and usually have little empathy
for their targets. Male bullies are often physically bigger and stronger
than their peers. Bullies tend to get in trouble more often, and to dislike
and do more poorly in school, than teens who do not bully others. They
are also more likely to fight, drink, and smoke than their peers.

Children and teens that come from homes where parents provide little emotional support for their children, fail to monitor their activities, or have little involvement in their lives, are at greater risk for engaging in bullying behavior. Parents' discipline styles are also related to bullying behavior: an extremely permissive or excessively harsh approach to discipline can increase the risk of teenage bullying.

Surprisingly, bullies appear to have little difficulty in making friends. Their friends typically share their pro-violence attitudes and problem behaviors (such as drinking and smoking) and may be involved in bullying as well. These friends are often followers that do not initiate bullying, but participate in it.

Risk Factors for Being Targeted by Bullies

Children and youth who are bullied are typically anxious, insecure, and cautious and suffer from low self-esteem, rarely defending themselves or retaliating when confronted by students who bully them. They are often socially isolated and lack social skills. One study found that the most frequent reason cited by youth for persons being bullied is that they "didn't fit in." Males who are bullied tend to be physically weaker than their peers.

Long-Term Impact on Youth

There appears to be a strong relationship between bullying other students and experiencing later legal and criminal problems as an adult. In one study, 60% of those characterized as bullies in grades 6–9 had at least one criminal conviction by age 24. Chronic bullies seem to maintain their behaviors into adulthood, negatively influencing their ability to develop and maintain positive relationships.

Bullying can lead the children and youth that are the target of bullying to feel tense, anxious, and afraid. It can affect their concentration in school, and can lead them to avoid school in some cases. If bullying continues for some time, it can begin to affect children and youth's self-esteem and feelings of self-worth.

It also can increase their social isolation, leading them to become withdrawn and depressed, anxious and insecure. In extreme cases, bullying can be devastating for children and youth, with long-term consequences. Researchers have found that years later, long after the bullying has stopped, adults who were bullied as youth have higher levels of depression and poorer self-esteem than other adults.

Effective Programs

Effective programs have been developed to reduce bullying in schools. Research has found that bullying is most likely to occur in schools where there is a lack of adult supervision during breaks, where teachers and students are indifferent to or accept bullying behavior, and where rules against bullying are not consistently enforced.

While approaches that simply crack down on individual bullies are seldom effective, when there is a school-wide commitment to end bullying, it can be reduced by up to 50%. One approach that has been shown to be effective focuses on changing school and classroom climates by: raising awareness about bullying, increasing teacher and parent involvement and supervision, forming clear rules and strong social norms against bullying, and providing support and protection for all students. This approach involves teachers, principals, students, and everyone associated with the school, including janitors, cafeteria workers, and crossing guards. Adults become aware of the extent of bullying at the school, and they involve themselves in changing the situation, rather than looking the other way. Students pledge not to bully other students, to help students who are bullied, and to make a point to include students who are left out.

Section 64.2

Effects of Bullying and What Teens Can Do to Stop It

Excerpted from "What Is Bullying?" by the Health Resources and Services Administration (www.stopbullyingnow.hrsa.gov), 2006.

A lot of young people have a good idea of what bullying is because they see it every day. Bullying happens when someone hurts or scares another person on purpose and the person being bullied has a hard time defending himself or herself. Usually, bullying happens over and over. Bullying can include the following:

- Punching, shoving, and other acts that hurt people physically
- Spreading bad rumors about people
- Keeping certain people out of a group
- Teasing people in a mean way
- Getting certain people to gang up on others

Bullying also can happen online or electronically. Cyberbullying is when teens bully each other using the Internet, mobile phones, or other cyber technology. This can include the following:

- Sending mean text, e-mail, or instant messages
- Posting nasty pictures or messages about others in blogs or on websites
- Using someone else's user name to spread rumors or lies about someone

There are many ways that young people bully each other, even if they don't realize it at the time. Unfortunately, not everyone takes bullying seriously, including adults.

Why Do Kids Bully?

There are all kinds of reasons why young people bully others, either occasionally or often. Do any of these reasons sound familiar to you?

- Because I see others doing it

- Because it's what you do if you want to hang out with the right crowd

- Because it makes me feel, stronger, smarter, or better than the person I'm bullying

- Because it's one of the best ways to keep others from bullying me

Whatever the reason, bullying is something we all need to think about. Whether we've done it ourselves—or whether friends or other people we know are doing it—we all need to recognize that bullying has a terrible effect on the lives of young people. It may not be happening to you today, but it could tomorrow. Working together, we can make the lives of young people better.

Do You Bully?

If you're not sure if what you're doing is really bullying, here's a hint: If you are hurting or threatening others in some way and using your size, strength, or popularity to do it, you're probably bullying someone.

Hurting and making others feel bad is never cool. Just admitting that you are doing things to harm others takes some guts. But that's not enough. Trying to find out what you should do to change the way you're acting—now that's a step in the right direction. So check out these tips; they'll help you to start treating others with the respect they deserve.

Think about what you're doing and how it affects others. If you think calling others names is really harmless, or if you think pushing, hitting or stealing from other kids is funny, you've forgotten what it feels like to be hurt yourself. Teasing, hitting, keeping others out of a group—all of these things harm someone. All of us have been hurt at one time or another and we all know how it feels—awful. So the next time you are about to bully someone:

- put yourself in their shoes;

- think about how it must make them feel;

- and just don't do it.

Talk to an adult. Making other people feel badly should never make you feel good. If it does, or if you're not really sure why you bully other kids, you need to talk to an adult about it.

Even though you might think an adult won't understand, or that you'll get yourself into trouble, he or she can help. Whether it is your parent, a teacher, or another trusted grown-up, you should tell an adult how you've been acting so that he or she can help you deal with it. School counselors are also great people to talk to about how you feel and how to change the way you treat others.

Effects of Bullying

If you've ever heard an adult—or anyone else—say that bullying is "just a fact of life" or "no big deal," you're not alone. Too often, people just don't take bullying seriously—or until the sad and sometimes scary stories are revealed.

- It happens a lot more than some people think. Studies show that between 15–25% of U.S. students are bullied with some frequency, while 15–20% report they bully others with some frequency.

- It can mess up a kid's future. Young people who bully are more likely than those who don't bully to skip school and drop out of school. They are also more likely to smoke, drink alcohol, and get into fights.

- It scares some people so much that they skip school. As many as 160,000 students may stay home on any given day because they're afraid of being bullied.

- It can lead to huge problems later in life. Children who bully are more likely to get into fights, vandalize property, and drop out of school. And 60% of boys who were bullies in middle school had at least one criminal conviction by the age of 24.

Section 64.3

What Is Hazing?

This section contains text from "What Is Hazing?" reprinted with permission from HazingPrevention.org, © 2010; and from "Hazing in View—High School Students at Risk," by Elizabeth Allan, PhD, and Mary Madden, PhD © 2008. Reprinted with permission from the National Collaborative for Hazing Research and Prevention (www.hazingstudy.org).

What Is Hazing?

Hazing is any action taken or situation created intentionally that causes embarrassment, harassment, or ridicule, risks emotional and/or physical harm to members of an organization or team, whether new or not, regardless of the person's willingness to participate.

Still confused? Ask yourself these questions:

- Would I feel comfortable participating in this activity if my parents were watching?

- Would we get in trouble if the Dean of Students walked by?

- Am I being asked to keep these activities a secret?

- Am I doing anything illegal?

- Does participation violate my values or those of my organization?

- Is it causing emotional distress or stress of any kind to myself or others?

Every college/university, national governing body, athletic department, and fraternity/sorority has an anti-hazing policy.

If you don't know what yours is or how to report hazing, ask. Forty-four states have laws against hazing. Find out if yours is one of them [http://www.chaptertools.net/site_files/file_1204602480.doc].

Hazing Statutes

The difference between hazing and bullying is subtle. The same power dynamics are involved. The same intimidation tactics are used.

564

The same second-class citizenship issues arise. The only real difference between bullying and hazing is that bullying can happen to anyone, any time; and hazing is done to a person or group of people in order to gain entrance into a club, organization, team, or formal group.

Hazing in View: High School Students at Risk
Background

These findings are derived from the National Study on Student Hazing (Allan & Madden, 2008). The analysis is based on survey responses from 11,482 post-secondary students on 53 campuses across the United States and more than 300 interviews with staff and students from 18 of those campuses. Data gathering focused on the nature and prevalence of hazing among students in both secondary and postsecondary settings. Data on high school hazing are derived from college students reflecting back on their high school experiences.

It is not uncommon to find the term hazing used synonymously with bullying. While similarities exist between hazing and bullying, hazing is a term that carries a particular meaning pertaining to certain types of behaviors that occur in the context of groups. More specifically, the term "hazing" refers to any activity expected of someone joining a group (or to maintain full status in a group) that humiliates, degrades, or risks emotional and/or physical harm, regardless of the person's willingness to participate.

Key Findings

1. Forty-seven percent of students say they were hazed while in high school. This mirrors the results of a 2000 study conducted by Nadine Hoover and Norm Pollard that showed that 48% of high school students belonging to groups experienced hazing.

2. Hazing occurs in range of co-curricular high school activities including: athletics, ROTC, performing arts, band, and others school activities. Additionally, 16% experienced class hazing—meaning an initiation into the high school itself.

3. Hazing behaviors in high school range in nature and can include dangerous and illegal activities. The most frequently reported behaviors were:

    -   28%—associate with specific people and not others;

    -   21%—sing or chant by self or selected group members/not related to a game or event;

565

- 19%—be yelled, screamed, or cursed at by other members of the group;

- 12%—participate in a drinking game;

- 12%—deprive self of sleep;

- 12%—get a tattoo or body piercing;

- 11%—drink large amounts of a non-alcoholic beverage;

- 11%—endure harsh weather conditions without proper clothing;

- 9%—be awakened by other members during the night;

- 8%—make prank telephone calls or harass others;

- 8%—drink alcoholic beverages until the point of getting sick or passing out.

4. The mean number of hazing behaviors experienced by males (M = 2.4) was significantly higher than females (M = 1.5).

5. A gap exists between student experiences of hazing and their recognition of specific behaviors as hazing and/or their willingness to label it as such. Eight out of ten individuals who reported experiencing a specific hazing behavior while in high school do not consider her/himself to be have been hazed.

6. Much hazing appears to occur "in view" of adults both in school and in the community—for example, class hazing of new students.

Recommendations

Assess school policies to ensure that hazing is recognized as a behavior that is differentiated from bullying and has consequences: Most public schools have policies that address bullying and of course these policies are essential. High schools also need to ensure that they have clear policies that accurately define and effectively prohibit hazing. Policies should make clear that hazing can occur regardless of a student's consent.

Reduce the extent to which upperclass students are privileged within the school environment including within student organizations and on athletic teams: The research shows that students are at risk for hazing as a new member of the school or of a team or organization. Those who perpetuate the hazing are upperclass students. Their actions, whether real or perceived, tend to be justified by their seniority status, which is often unintentionally reinforced by special privileges, either formal or informal, given to them within a school, team, or student organization. If upperclass students are afforded privileges, it should also be clear that the privileges come with responsibilities. In the case of hazing, it should be made clear that it is a responsibility of all upperclass students to do their part to ensure that hazing does not occur.

Educate all teachers, administrators, coaches, organizational advisors, and other school personnel, as well as parents, and community members about hazing: Hazing is not the well-kept secret many believe it to be. This study shows that hazing happens in view of adults in the school and in the community. Adults may be inclined to dismiss hazing as nothing more than silly pranks or harmless antics, yet data from this investigation indicate hazing can involve high-risk behaviors that are dangerous, abusive, and illegal. Aside from the fact that hazing itself is illegal in 44 states, hazing is also likely to violate the law through underage drinking and sexual activities where consent is questionable due to the coercive dynamics and peer pressure inherent in hazing. These same dynamics contribute to a group context where embarrassment, humiliation, and degradation can take an emotional toll and lead to what is called the hidden harm of hazing—the emotional scars that can result from the humiliating and degrading aspects of hazing.

Involve all students in hazing prevention efforts. Introduce these efforts in middle school or earlier and continue the education into and through high school: This study shows that students are at risk for hazing as a new member of the school. Therefore, it is important that all students be educated about hazing. Also, some respondents in this study report being hazed prior to high school in association with either a middle school or community activity.

Design prevention efforts to be more comprehensive than simply one-time presentations or distribution of anti-hazing policies: Focus on helping all students:

- develop an understanding of the power dynamics in order to identify hazing regardless of context;
- understand the role coercion and groupthink can play in hazing;
- recognize the potential for harm even in activities they consider to be "low level";

- generate strategies for building group unity and sense of accomplishment that do not involve hazing;

- align group membership behavior with the purpose and values espoused by the school and its associated activities;

- develop leadership skills students need to intervene on behalf of their peers if hazing behaviors are practiced in their group;

- develop critical thinking skills needed to make ethical judgments in the face of moral dilemmas.

Findings from this investigation highlight some of the complexities related to hazing. It is clear that students continue to have a limited understanding of the definition of hazing and risks associated with it. This is highlighted by the fact that nearly half of high school students report experiencing a hazing behavior, but eight out of 10 of these do not consider themselves to have been hazed. In addition, students who have been hazed tend to dismiss institutional and legal definitions of hazing and minimize the potential harm that can result.

Focus additional hazing prevention efforts on team coaches, group advisors, and students involved in student groups and athletic teams: Students involved in athletics and other co-curricular activities are at highest risk for hazing. Therefore, it is important that they receive additional education about what constitutes hazing. As well, students belonging to groups should receive additional guidance and education on how to implement non-hazing traditions and initiations to welcome new members to their groups. Coaches and group advisors need to be educated about signs that may indicate a group is engaging in hazing.

Send a clear message that hazing will not be tolerated and those engaging in hazing behaviors will be held accountable: School administrators need to convey the message that hazing is considered a serious issue and will not be dismissed, minimized, or trivialized as silly pranks, antics, or as a normal part of the school climate. If a hazing event occurs, it is important the consequences are not perceived to be simply a "slap on the wrist" and that the resulting consequences for the group or organization be made public. This reinforces the message that hazing is not tolerated. When students have knowledge of a group caught hazing but fail to hear of consequences, they interpret the silence to mean hazing is not taken seriously.

Chapter 65

Choking Games

Teens experiment with attitudes, appearances, and behaviors. While most of it is harmless, some experiments can have tragic results.

One experiment that backfires involves young people trying to get high by choking themselves or their friends. Teens—usually in middle school and early high school—try it alone or with others. They do it for the perceived high that occurs as oxygen rushes back to the brain—putting the player at high risk for nerve damage, even death.

Sound dangerous?

It is. The challenge of losing consciousness and reviving is known by many names, including: pass-out, tingling, blackout, choking game, suffocation roulette, and other names in different areas of the country.

The Game That Kills

The United States began tracking the choking deaths of youths between the ages of 6 and 19 in 1995. An accurate count is difficult because many of these deaths are reported as suicides. Some estimates place the number of choking deaths between 250 and 1,000 each year. Most players who die alone are male, with an average age of 13. More than 90 percent of those who died had parents who were unaware of the game.

From "Risky Business: The Choking Game," by the Substance Abuse and Mental Health Services Administration (SAMHSA, family.samhsa.gov), part of the U.S. Department of Health and Human Services, July 23, 2008.

A yearly Canadian survey of Ontario school districts found that 7 percent of kids in grades 7 to 12, or 79,000 kids, have played the game.

How the Game Kills

The game usually involves two children. When the child being choked starts to lose consciousness due to lack of oxygen, the second releases the pressure, allowing the blood to rush to the brain. Keeping oxygen from the brain can cause permanent loss of brain functions such as concentration, memory, and death.

Kids Don't Know It Kills

Some kids play because of peer pressure. Others receive a dare, a challenge, or a defined rite of passage that allows them into a social group. Some youths play for the quick, 5- to 10-second feelings that choking is believed to create. Still others are trying to find a cheap high. But it's not.

What is clear is that most children who play the game do not understand the risk to their health or the possibility of death. Even when a person survives, thousands of brain cells have been killed.

The children who play are, more often than not, well-adjusted, high-achieving students looking to have a sensational experience.

Look for the Warning Signs

The following signs may indicate your child or his or her friends are thinking about or playing the choking game.

Signs of your child playing the choking game may include the following:

- Questions about the effects, sensations, or dangers of strangulation

- Changes in personality, such as being angry or irritated or unusual demands for privacy

- Complaints of headaches (sometimes very bad ones), loss of concentration, a flushed face, or tiny red dots on the face

- Bloodshot eyes or any other noticeable signs of stress on the eyes

- Any suspicious mark on the side of the neck, sometimes hidden by a turtleneck, a scarf, or a turned-up collar

If you notice the following, it may be a sign your child is playing the choking game:

- Any kind of strap (including bed sheets, belts, t-shirts, ropes) tied in strange knots and/or found in unusual places, or laying near the child without any reason—and a child avoids answering questions about such objects

- A thud in the bedroom or against a wall—which could mean a fall if a child is alone and choking himself

- Locked or blocked bedroom/bathroom doors

- Wear marks on furniture such as bunk beds or closet rods

- Your child's internet history of websites or chat rooms that mention asphyxiation or choking

If you suspect your child or a friend is playing the choking game, supervise him or her very closely. Dispose of items that could be used for this purpose. Seek professional counseling and support for your child and your family.

Learn the Facts

Teens are often curious about risky behaviors. They may wrongly think that the choking game is a safe alternative to drinking or trying other substances such as pot or prescription drugs.

Your teen might hear about classmates who play the choking game or even know some friends who play. When your child talks about it with you, listen and take time to give your teen the facts to counter any myths.

One myth is that choking provides a harmless high. In actuality, the "high" is the cells of the brain seizing and beginning the process of permanent cell death. When a person becomes unconscious, pressure is released and the secondary "high" of the oxygen/blood rushing to the brain is achieved. The fact is that pressure on the neck cuts off blood to the brain and causes unconsciousness and possibly death.

Make Sure Your Loved Ones Understand

Talk to the children in your life. Make sure they understand why the game is so dangerous. Pointing out the dangers—as well as your concern for his or her safety—may help your child avoid experimenting with choking.

If you have difficulty speaking to your teen about it, you may want to bring up the subject as part of a more comprehensive discussion about drinking alcohol or using mood changing substances.

You also may want to talk to your child's school about choking to make sure they're watching for warning signs among students. School systems across the country are increasingly more aware of the problem and developing public education for counselors, teachers, parents, and students. Don't wait for the school to take action; your child's safety is your responsibility. Become an educated and involved parent by helping your children to understand the dangers of choking.

Children may be indicted and prosecuted by the law for their involvement in a death or injury of another person from choking.

Chapter 66

Dating Violence and Abusive Relationships

Most teenagers do not experience physical aggression when they date. However, for one in 10 teens, abuse is a very real part of dating relationships.

According to the 2007 Youth Risk Behavior Survey, approximately 10 percent of adolescents nationwide reported being the victim of physical violence at the hands of a romantic partner during the previous year. The rate of psychological victimization is even higher: Between two and three in 10 reported being verbally or psychologically abused in the previous year, according to the National Longitudinal Study of Adolescent Health.

As for perpetration rates, there are currently no nationwide estimates for who does the abusing, and state estimates vary significantly. In South Carolina, for example, nearly 8 percent of adolescents reported being physically violent to a romantic partner. Interestingly, the rates of reported victimization versus perpetration in the state were similar for boys and girls. However, when it comes to severe teen dating violence—including sexual and physical assault—girls were disproportionately the victims.

At a workshop on teen dating violence, co-sponsored by the U.S. Departments of Justice (DOJ) and Health and Human Services (HHS), researchers presented findings from several studies that found that

From "Teen Dating Violence: A Closer Look at Adolescent Romantic Relationships," by Carrie Mulford, PhD, and Peggy C. Giordano, PhD, by the National Institute of Justice (www.ojp.usdoj.gov/nij), October 27, 2008.

girls and boys perpetrate the same frequency of physical aggression in romantic relationships. This finding was at odds with what practitioners attending the workshop said they encounter in their professional experience. Most of the practitioners in attendance—representing national organizations, schools and victim service community-based agencies—said that they primarily see female victims, and when they discuss teen dating violence with students, they hear that boys are the primary perpetrators.

So what is the reality?

Because teen dating violence has only recently been recognized as a significant public health problem, the complex nature of this phenomenon is not fully understood. Although research on rates of perpetration and victimization exists, research that examines the problem from a longitudinal perspective and considers the dynamics of teen romantic relationships is lacking. Consequently, those in the field have to rely on an adult framework to examine the problem of teen dating violence.

However, we find that this adult framework does not take into account key differences between adolescent and adult romantic relationships. And so, to help further the discussion, this article offers a gender-based analysis of teen dating violence with a developmental perspective. We look at what we know—and what we don't know—about who is the perpetrator and who is the victim in teen dating violence. We also discuss how adult and adolescent romantic relationships differ in the hope that an examination of existing research will help us better understand the problem and move the field toward the creation of developmentally appropriate prevention programs and effective interventions for teenagers.

Victims and Perpetrators: What the Research Says

In 2001–2005, Peggy Giordano and her colleagues at Bowling Green State University interviewed more than 1,300 seventh, ninth, and 11th graders in Toledo, Ohio. [Editor's Note: Giordano is one of the authors of this article.]

More than half of the girls in physically aggressive relationships said both they and their dating partner committed aggressive acts during the relationship. About a third of the girls said they were the sole perpetrators, and 13 percent reported that they were the sole victims. Almost half of the boys in physically aggressive relationships reported mutual aggression, nearly half reported they were the sole victim, and 6 percent reported that they were the sole perpetrator.

These findings are generally consistent with another study that looked at more than 1,200 Long Island, NY, high school students who were currently dating. In that 2007 survey, 66 percent of boys and 65 percent of girls who were involved in physically aggressive relationships reported mutual aggression. Twenty-eight percent of the girls said that they were the sole perpetrator; 5 percent said they were the sole victim. These numbers were reversed for the boys: 5 percent said they were the sole perpetrator; 27 percent the sole victim.

Who Perpetrates Teen Dating Violence?

In a third study, teen couples were videotaped while performing a problem-solving task. Researchers later reviewed the tapes and identified acts of physical aggression that occurred between the boys and girls during the exercise. They found that 30 percent of all the participating couples demonstrated physical aggression by both partners. In 17 percent of the participating couples, only the girls perpetrated physical aggression, and in 4 percent, only the boys were perpetrators. The findings suggest that boys are less likely to be physically aggressive with a girl when someone else can observe their behavior.

Considered together, the findings from these three studies reveal that frequently there is mutual physical aggression by girls and boys in romantic relationships. However, when it comes to motivations for using violence and the consequences of being a victim of teen dating violence, the differences between the sexes are pronounced. Although both boys and girls report that anger is the primary motivating factor for using violence, girls also commonly report self-defense as a motivating factor, and boys also commonly cite the need to exert control. Boys are also more likely to react with laughter when their partner is physically aggressive. Girls experiencing teen dating violence are more likely than boys to suffer long-term negative behavioral and health consequences, including suicide attempts, depression, cigarette smoking, and marijuana use.

Applying Adult Perspectives to Teen Dating Violence

Why do teenagers commit violence against each other in romantic relationships? We have already touched on the existing body of research on perpetration and victimization rates. Yet there is not a great deal of research that uses a longitudinal perspective or that considers the dynamics of teen romantic relationships. As a result, practitioners and researchers in the field tend to apply an adult intimate partner violence framework when examining the problem of teen dating violence.

A split currently exists, however, among experts in the adult intimate partner violence arena.

Some experts hold that men and women are mutually combative and that this behavior should be seen as part of a larger pattern of family conflict. Supporters of this view generally cite studies that use "act" scales, which measure the number of times a person perpetrates or experiences certain acts, such as pushing, slapping, or hitting. These studies tend to show that women report perpetrating slightly more physical violence than men. It is interesting to note that most studies on teen dating violence that have been conducted to date have relied primarily on "act" scales.

Another group of experts holds that men generally perpetrate serious intimate partner violence against women. They contend that men in patriarchal societies use violence to exert and maintain power and control over women. These experts also maintain that "act" scales do not accurately reflect the nature of violence in intimate relationships because they do not consider the degree of injury inflicted, coercive and controlling behaviors, the fear induced, or the context in which the acts occurred. Studies using "act" scales, they contend, lack information on power and control and emphasize the more common and relatively minor forms of aggression rather than more severe, relatively rare forms of violence in dating and intimate partner relationships. Instead, supporters of this perspective use data on injuries and in-depth interviews with victims and perpetrators.

We believe, however, that applying either of these adult perspectives to adolescents is problematic. Although both views of adult intimate partner violence can help inform our understanding of teen dating violence, it is important to consider how adolescent romantic relationships differ from adult romantic relationships in several key areas.

How Teen Dating Violence Differs: Equal Power

One difference between adolescent and adult relationships is the absence of elements traditionally associated with greater male power in adult relationships. Adolescent girls are not typically dependent on romantic partners for financial stability, and they are less likely to have children to provide for and protect.

The study of seventh, ninth, and 11th graders in Toledo, for example, found that a majority of the boys and girls who were interviewed said they had a relatively "equal say" in their romantic relationships. In cases in which there was a power imbalance, they were more likely to say that the female had more power in the relationship. Overall, the study found that the boys perceived that they had less power in the relationship than the girls did. Interestingly, males involved in relationships in which one or both partners reported physical aggression had a perception of less power than males in relationships without physical aggression. Meanwhile, the girls reported no perceived difference in power regardless of whether their relationships included physical aggression.

It is interesting to note that adults who perpetrate violence against family members often see themselves as powerless in their relationships. This dynamic has yet to be adequately explored among teen dating partners.

Lack of Relationship Experience

A second key factor that distinguishes violence in adult relationships from violence in adolescent relationships is the lack of experience teens have in negotiating romantic relationships. Inexperience in communicating and relating to a romantic partner may lead to the use of poor coping strategies, including verbal and physical aggression. A teen who has difficulty expressing himself or herself may turn to aggressive behaviors (sometimes in play) to show affection, frustration, or jealousy. A recent study in which boys and girls participated in focus groups on dating found that physical aggression sometimes stemmed from an inability to communicate feelings and a lack of constructive ways to deal with frustration.

As adolescents develop into young adults, they become more realistic and less idealistic about romantic relationships. They have a greater capacity for closeness and intimacy. Holding idealistic beliefs about romantic relationships can lead to disillusionment and ineffective coping mechanisms when conflict emerges. It also seems reasonable to expect that physical aggression may be more common when adolescents have not fully developed their capacity for intimacy, including their ability to communicate.

The Influence of Peers

We would be remiss to try to understand teen behavior and not consider the profound influence of friends. Peers exert more influence on each other during their adolescent years than at any other time. Research has confirmed that peer attitudes and behaviors are critical influences on teens' attitudes and behaviors related to dating violence.

Not only are friends more influential in adolescence than in adulthood, but they are also more likely to be "on the scene" and a key element in a couple's social life. In fact, roughly half of adolescent dating violence occurs when a third party is present. Relationship dynamics often play out in a very public way because teens spend a large portion of their time in school and in groups. For various reasons, a boyfriend or girlfriend may act very differently when in the presence of peers, a behavior viewed by adolescents as characteristic of an unhealthy relationship. For example, boys in one focus group study said that if a girl hit them in front of their friends, they would need to hit her back to "save face."

Conflict over how much time is spent with each other versus with friends, jealousies stemming from too much time spent with a friend of the opposite sex, and new romantic possibilities are all part of the social fabric of adolescence. Although "normal" from a developmental perspective, navigating such issues can cause conflict and, for some adolescents, lead to aggressive responses and problematic coping strategies, such as stalking, psychological, or verbal abuse, and efforts to gain control.

Where Do We Go from Here?

Adult relationships differ substantially from adolescent dating in their power dynamics, social skill development, and peer influence. These factors are critical to understanding physical violence and psychological abuse in early romantic relationships and may help explain the similar perpetration rates among boys and girls suggested by current statistics.

All of this points to important implications for teen dating violence prevention and intervention strategies. Because girls engage in high levels of physical aggression and psychological abuse and most abusive relationships are characterized by mutual aggression, prevention efforts must be directed toward both males and females, and interventions for victims should include services and programming for boys and girls. Interventions must also distinguish between severe forms of violence that produce injury and fear and other more common abuse, and they must respond with appropriate safety planning, mental health services, and criminal or juvenile justice involvement.

More research on traditionally gendered relationship dynamics—and the links to relationship violence—is also needed. For instance, some male behavior may stem from an attempt to emulate other males who they believe (not always accurately, as data show) are confident and "in charge." Further, nearly one in five adolescent girls reports having sex with a partner 3 or more years older. These girls are at increased risk of acquiring a sexually transmitted disease because they are less likely to use a condom—possibly a result of unequal power dynamics in these relationships. This power imbalance might also increase their risk for violent victimization by older partners.

And finally, research on the extent to which teens involved in abusive relationships become involved in adult abusive relationships—whether as victims or perpetrators—is sorely needed. Many delinquent youth, for example, have a well-documented path of illegal behavior; this behavior peaks in adolescence and dramatically declines in early adulthood. A similar look at aggressive adolescent romantic relationships may help us better understand the possible progression from teen dating violence to adult intimate partner violence.

Chapter 67

Sexual Assault

What is sexual assault?

Sexual assault and abuse is any type of sexual activity that you do not agree to, including the following:

- Inappropriate touching

- Vaginal, anal, or oral penetration

- Sexual intercourse that you say no to

- Rape

- Attempted rape

- Child molestation

Sexual assault can be verbal, visual, or anything that forces a person to join in unwanted sexual contact or attention. Examples of this are voyeurism (when someone watches private sexual acts), exhibitionism (when someone exposes him/herself in public), incest (sexual contact between family members), and sexual harassment. It can happen in different situations: in the home by someone you know, on a date, or by a stranger in an isolated place.

From "Sexual Assault," by the Office on Women's Health (www.womens health.gov), part of the U.S. Department of Health and Human Services, July 16, 2009.

Rape is a common form of sexual assault. It is committed in many situations—on a date, by a friend or an acquaintance, or when you think you are alone. Educate yourself on date rape drugs. They can be slipped into a drink when a victim is not looking. Never leave your drink unattended—no matter where you are. Attackers use date rape drugs to make a person unable to resist assault. These drugs can also cause memory loss so the victim doesn't know what happened.

Rape and sexual assault are never the victim's fault—no matter where or how it happens.

What do I do if I've been sexually assaulted?

These are important steps to take right away after an assault:

- Get away from the attacker to a safe place as fast as you can. Then call 911 or the police.

- Call a friend or family member you trust. You also can call a crisis center or a hotline to talk with a counselor. One hotline is the National Sexual Assault Hotline at 800-656-HOPE (656-4673). Feelings of shame, guilt, fear, and shock are normal. It is important to get counseling from a trusted professional.

- Do not wash, comb, or clean any part of your body. Do not change clothes if possible, so the hospital staff can collect evidence.

- Do not touch or change anything at the scene of the assault. Go to your nearest hospital emergency room as soon as possible. You need to be examined, treated for any injuries, and screened for possible sexually transmitted infections (STIs) or pregnancy. The doctor will collect evidence using a rape kit for fibers, hairs, saliva, semen, or clothing that the attacker may have left behind.

While at the hospital, you may take the following steps:

- If you decide you want to file a police report, you or the hospital staff can call the police from the emergency room.

- Ask the hospital staff to connect you with the local rape crisis center. The center staff can help you make choices about reporting the attack and getting help through counseling and support groups.

Where else can I go for help?

If you are sexually assaulted, it is not your fault. Don't be afraid to ask for help or support. Help is available. You can call these organizations:

- National Domestic Violence Hotline—800-799-SAFE (799-7233) or 800-787-3224 (TDD)

- National Sexual Assault Hotline—800-656-HOPE (656-4673)

There are many organizations and hotlines in every state and territory. These crisis centers and agencies work hard to stop assaults and help victims. You can find contact information for these organizations at www.womenshealth.gov/violence/state. You also can obtain the numbers of shelters, counseling services, and legal assistance in your phone book or online.

How can I lower my risk of sexual assault?

There are things you can do to reduce your chances of being sexually assaulted. Follow these tips from the National Crime Prevention Council.

- Be aware of your surroundings—who's out there and what's going on.

- Walk with confidence. The more confident you look, the stronger you appear.

- Know your limits when it comes to using alcohol.

- Be assertive—don't let anyone violate your space.

- Trust your instincts. If you feel uncomfortable in your surroundings, leave.

- Don't prop open self-locking doors.

- Lock your door and your windows, even if you leave for just a few minutes.

- Watch your keys. Don't lend them. Don't leave them. Don't lose them. And don't put your name and address on the key ring.

- Watch out for unwanted visitors. Know who's on the other side of the door before you open it.

- Be wary of isolated spots, like underground garages, offices after business hours, and apartment laundry rooms.

- Avoid walking or jogging alone, especially at night. Vary your route. Stay in well-traveled, well-lit areas.

- Have your key ready to use before you reach the door—home, car, or work.

- Park in well-lit areas and lock the car, even if you'll only be gone a few minutes.

- Drive on well-traveled streets, with doors and windows locked.

- Never hitchhike or pick up a hitchhiker.

- Keep your car in good shape with plenty of gas in the tank.

- In case of car trouble, call for help on your cellular phone. If you don't have a phone, put the hood up, lock the doors, and put a banner in the rear mirror that says, "Help. Call police."

How can I help someone who has been sexually assaulted?

You can help someone who is abused or who has been assaulted by listening and offering comfort. Go with her or him to the police, the hospital, or to counseling. Reinforce the message that she or he is not at fault and that it is natural to feel angry and ashamed.

Chapter 68

Youth Gangs and Violence

Although once thought to be an inner-city problem, gang violence has spread to communities throughout the United States. At last count, there were more than 24,500 different youth gangs around the country, and more than 772,500 teens and young adults were members of gangs.

Teens join gangs for a variety of reasons. Some are seeking excitement; others are looking for prestige, protection, a chance to make money, or a sense of belonging. Few teens are forced to join gangs; in most cases, teens can refuse to join without fear of retaliation.

Membership on the Rise

There has been a dramatic increase in gang activity in the United States since the 1970s. In the 1970s, gangs were active in less than half the states, but now every state reports youth gang activity. And, while many people think of gangs as just an inner-city problem, that is clearly no longer the case. In the past few decades we have seen a dramatic increase in the growth of gang problems in smaller cities, towns, and rural areas.

Since 1996, the overall number of gangs and gang members in the United States has decreased. However, in cities with a population over 25,000, gang involvement still remains near peak levels.

Excerpted from "Youth Gangs and Violence," by the National Youth Violence Prevention Resource Center (safeyouth.org), January 4, 2008.

Age of Members

Most youth gang members are between the ages of 12 and 24, and the average age is about 17 to 18 years. Around half of youth gang members are 18 or older, and they are much more likely to be involved in serious and violent crimes than younger gang members. Only about one in four youth gang members are ages 15 to 17.

For most teens, gang membership is a brief phase. Three studies that tracked teens over time found that one half to two thirds of youth gang members leave the gang by the 1-year mark.

Girls in Gangs

Male youth are much more likely to join gangs than female youth. It is hard to get a good estimate of the number of female gangs and gang members, however, because many police jurisdictions do not count girls as gang members. While the national estimates based on police reports indicate that only about 8 percent of gang members are female, one 11-city survey of eighth graders found that 38 percent of gang members are female. Female gangs are somewhat more likely to be found in small cities and rural areas than in large cities, and female gang members tend to be younger, on average, than male gang members.

Female gang members are involved in less delinquent or criminal activity than male gang members, and they commit fewer violent crimes. However, female gang members are still an important concern. In one survey, 78 percent of female gang members reported being involved in gang fights, 65 percent reported carrying a weapon for protection, and 39 percent reported attacking someone with a weapon.

Not Just an Inner-City Problem

Although many people think of gangs as a problem confined to the inner-city neighborhoods, that is clearly no longer the case. In the past few decades there has been a dramatic increase in the growth of gang problems in smaller cities, towns, and villages. When surveyed in 1999, 66 percent of large cities, 47 percent of suburban counties, 27 percent of small cities, and 18 percent of rural counties reported active youth gangs.

Gangs in suburban, small town, and rural areas are different than gangs in large cities. They include more females, white, and younger youth, and are more likely to have ethnically and racially mixed memberships.

Gangs at School

Youth gangs are linked with serious crime problems in elementary and secondary schools in the United States. Students report much higher drug availability when gangs are active at their school. Schools with gangs have nearly double the likelihood of violent victimization at school than those without a gang presence. Teens that are gang members are much more likely than other teens to commit serious and violent crimes. For example, a survey in Denver found that while only 14 percent of teens were gang members, they were responsible for committing 89 percent of the serious violent crimes.

Chapter 69

Coping with Violence and Trauma

Disasters cause major damage. Hurricanes Katrina and Rita were examples. They occurred in 2005. Many homes were destroyed. Whole communities were damaged. Many survivors were displaced. There were also many deaths.

Trauma is also caused by major acts of violence. The September 11, 2001, terrorist attacks were examples. Another example was the 1999 shootings at Columbine High School in Colorado. The Oklahoma City bombing in 1995 was also an example. These acts claim lives. They also threaten our sense of security.

Beyond these events, teens face many other traumas. Each year, they are injured. They see others harmed by violence. They suffer sexual abuse. They lose loved ones. Or, they witness other tragic events.

Teens are very sensitive. They struggle to make sense of trauma. They also respond differently to traumas. They may have emotional reactions. They may hurt deeply. They may find it hard to recover from frightening experiences. They need support. Adult helpers can provide this support. This may help children resolve emotional problems.

What Is Trauma?

There are two types of trauma—physical and mental. Physical trauma includes the body's response to serious injury and threat. Mental trauma

Excerpted from "Helping Children and Adolescents Cope with Violence and Disasters: What Parents Can Do," by the National Institute of Mental Health (NIMH, www.nimh.nih.gov), part of the National Institutes of Health, January 27, 2009.

includes frightening thoughts and painful feelings. They are the mind's response to serious injury. Mental trauma can produce strong feelings. It can also produce extreme behavior; such as intense fear or helplessness, withdrawal or detachment, lack of concentration, irritability, sleep disturbance, aggression, hyper vigilance (intensely watching for more distressing events), or flashbacks (sense that event is reoccurring).

A response could be fear. It could be fear that a loved one will be hurt or killed. It is believed that more direct exposures to traumatic events causes greater harm. For instance, in a school shooting, an injured student will probably be more severely affected emotionally than a student who was in another part of the building. However, secondhand exposure to violence can also be traumatic. This includes witnessing violence such as seeing or hearing about death and destruction after a building is bombed or a plane crashes.

Helping Young Trauma Survivors

Helping teens begins at the scene of the event. It may need to continue for weeks or months. Most teens recover within a few weeks. Some need help longer. Grief (a deep emotional response to loss) may take months to resolve. It could be for a loved one or a teacher. It could be for a friend or pet. Grief may be re-experienced or worsened by news reports or the event's anniversary.

Some teens may need help from a mental health professional. Some people may seek other kinds of help. They may turn to religious leaders. They may turn to community leaders.

How Parents Can Help

After violence or a disaster parents and family should do the following:

- Identify and address their own feelings—this will allow them to help others.

- Explain to teens what happened.

- Let teens know the following:

  - You love them.

  - The event was not their fault.

  - You will take care of them, but only if you can; be honest.

  - It's okay for them to feel upset.

Do:

- Allow teens to cry.
- Allow sadness.
- Let teens talk about feelings.
- Let them write about feelings.
- Let them draw pictures.

Don't:

- Expect teens to be brave or tough.
- Make teens discuss the event before they are ready.
- Get angry if teens show strong emotions.

Try to keep normal routines (such routines may not be normal for some teens), such as the following:

- Eating dinner together
- Watching TV together
- Reading books, exercising, playing games

If you can't keep normal routines, make new ones together.

How Teens React to Trauma

Teens' reactions to trauma can be immediate. Reactions may also appear much later. Reactions differ in severity. They also cover a range of behaviors. People from different cultures may have their own ways of reacting. Other reactions vary according to age.

One common response is loss of trust. Another is fear of the event reoccurring. Some teens are more vulnerable to trauma's effects. Teens with existing mental health problems may be more affected. Teens who have experienced other traumatic events may be more affected.

Children between 12 and 17 have various reactions:

- Flashbacks to the traumatic event (flashbacks are the mind re-living the event)
- Avoiding reminders of the event
- Drug, alcohol, tobacco use and abuse
- Antisocial behavior—i.e., disruptive, disrespectful, or destructive behavior

591

- Physical complaints
- Nightmares or other sleep problems
- Isolation or confusion
- Depression
- Suicidal thoughts

Adolescents may feel guilty about the event. They may feel guilt for not preventing injury or deaths. They may also have thoughts of revenge.

Some teens will have prolonged problems after a traumatic event. These may include grief, depression, anxiety, and posttraumatic stress disorder (PTSD). They may show a range of symptoms, such as the following:

- Re-experiencing the event
  - Through trauma-specific nightmares/ dreams
  - In flashbacks and unwanted memories
  - By distress over events that remind them of the trauma
- Avoidance of reminders of the event
- Lack of responsiveness
- Lack of interest in things that used to interest them
- A sense of having "no future"
- Increased sleep disturbances
- Irritability
- Poor concentration
- Be easily startled

Teens experience trauma differently. It is difficult to tell how many will develop mental health problems. Some trauma survivors get better with only good support. Others need counseling by a mental health professional. If, after a month in a safe environment, teens are not able to perform normal routines or new symptoms develop, then contact a health professional.

Some people are more sensitive to trauma. Factors that may influence how someone may respond include the following:

- Being directly involved in the trauma, especially as a victim

- Severe and/or prolonged exposure to the event
- Personal history of prior trauma
- Family or personal history of mental illness and severe behavioral problems
- Lack of social support
- Lack of caring family and friends
- Ongoing life stressors such as moving to a new home or new school, divorce, job change, or financial troubles

Some symptoms may require immediate attention. Contact a mental health professional if these symptoms occur:

- Flashbacks
- Racing heart and sweating
- Being easily startled
- Being emotionally numb
- Being very sad or depressed
- Thoughts or actions to end life

Part Nine

Additional Help and Information

Chapter 70

Glossary of Terms about Adolescent Health

abstinence: Not having sex of any kind.[1]

acne: Pimples on the skin often caused by hormone changes during puberty.[1]

addiction: A chronic, relapsing disease characterized by compulsive drug-seeking and abuse and by long-lasting chemical changes in the brain.[2]

adolescence: The period of life from puberty to adulthood when a young person grows up.[1]

aggression: Behavior, physical or verbal, that is intended to harm another person.[3]

alcoholic: Someone who is addicted to alcohol.[1]

alcoholism: Alcoholism means that someone often drinks too much alcohol (such as beer, wine, or liquor) and can't stop.[1]

allergy: A sensitivity to things that are usually not harmful, such as certain foods or animals.[1]

Definitions in this chapter were compiled from documents published by several public domain sources. Terms marked 1 are from publications by the Office on Women's Health (www.womenshealth.gov); terms marked 2 are from the National Institute on Drug Abuse (www.nida.nih.gov); terms marked 3 are from the Office of the Surgeon General (www.surgeongeneral.gov); terms marked 4 are from the National Institute of Mental Health (www.nimh.nih.gov); and terms marked 5 are from the Health Resources and Services Administration (www.hrsa.gov).

amenorrhea: When a woman does not have periods either ever (after age 16) or when periods stop as a result of pregnancy, too much exercise, extreme obesity or not enough body fat, or emotional distress.[1]

anal sex: Sex that involves putting the penis in the anus, or butt.[1]

anemia: When the total amount of red blood cells or hemoglobin is below normal. Anemia can cause severe fatigue and other health problems. There are many different types of anemia.[1]

anorexia nervosa: An illness in which people don't eat enough and therefore can't stay at a healthy body weight.[1]

anxiety disorder: Any of a group of illnesses that fill people's lives with overwhelming anxieties and fears that are chronic and unremitting.[4]

asthma: A lung disorder that affects your airways. When the airways are inflamed, a person may wheeze, feel short of breath, cough, and feel tightness in the chest.[1]

attention deficit hyperactivity disorder (ADHD): A mental illness characterized by an impaired ability to regulate activity level (hyperactivity), attend to tasks (inattention), and inhibit behavior (impulsivity).[4]

behavioral therapy: A kind of therapy used by a psychologist or a psychiatrist that helps people to change the way they behave and act.[1]

binge-eating disorder: A condition marked by periods of out-of-control eating. Unlike bulimia nervosa, binge-eating disorder usually does not involve purging (throwing up or doing other things to get rid of the food).[1]

bipolar disorder: A depressive disorder in which a person alternates between episodes of major depression and mania (periods of abnormally and persistently elevated mood). Also referred to as manic-depression.[4]

birth control pill: A kind of medicine that women can take daily to prevent pregnancy. It is sometimes called the pill or oral contraception.[1]

body mass index: A mathematical formula to assess relative body weight. The measure correlates highly with body fat. Calculated as weight in kilograms divided by the square of the height in meters (kg/m^2).[5]

bulimia nervosa: An illness defined by uncontrollable overeating, usually followed by making oneself throw up or purge (get rid of food) in other ways.[1]

clitoris: A female sex organ located near the top of the vagina.[1]

condom: A type of birth control used to prevent pregnancy and the spread of some sexually transmitted diseases (STDs). The male condom is a thin rubber-like sheath put on the penis before sex. The female condom is a pouch put into the vagina before sex to prevent pregnancy.[1]

conduct disorder: A personality disorder of children and adolescents involving persistent antisocial behavior. Individuals with conduct disorder frequently participate in activities such as stealing, lying, truancy, vandalism, and substance abuse.[4]

date rape: When you are forced to have sex by someone you know.[1]

depression: An illness that involves the body, mood, and thoughts. It affects the way a person functions, eats and sleeps, feels about herself, and thinks about things. It is more than just feeling "down in the dumps" or "blue" for a short time.[1]

diabetes: A disease in which your blood sugar levels are above normal.[1]

douching: Rinsing or cleaning out the vagina, usually with a prepackaged mix of fluids.[1]

drug abuse: The use of illegal drugs or the inappropriate use of legal drugs. The repeated use of drugs to produce pleasure, to alleviate stress, or to alter or avoid reality (or all three).[2]

drug: A chemical compound or substance that can alter the structure and function of the body. Psychoactive drugs affect the function of the brain, and some of these may be illegal to use and possess.[2]

dysmenorrhea: Painful menstrual periods that can also go along with nausea and vomiting and either constipation or diarrhea. Dysmenorrhea is common among teenagers.[1]

eating disorder: An illness that involves serious problems with normal eating behaviors, such as feelings of distress and concern about body shape or weight, severe overeating, or starving oneself.[1]

ejaculation: The release of semen (whitish fluid that contains sperm) from a man's penis.[1]

endometriosis: A condition where tissue that normally lines the uterus grows in other areas of the body. This can cause pain, irregular menstrual bleeding, and infertility for some women.[1]

fallopian tube: One of a pair of organs that connect the ovaries to the uterus. There is a fallopian tube on each side of the uterus. When one of the ovaries releases an egg, it travels through the fallopian tube toward the uterus. Fertilization (when a man's sperm and a woman's egg join together) usually happens in the fallopian tube.[1]

genital area: The area around the vagina, penis, scrotum, anus, and thigh.[1]

gland: A cell, group of cells, or organ that makes chemicals and releases them for use by other parts of the body or to be excreted.[1]

gynecological examination: When a doctor checks inside the vagina to make sure organs are healthy.[1]

gynecologist: A doctor who has special training in caring for a women's reproductive organs and system.[1]

hazing: A humiliating or degrading act expected of someone joining a group. It may cause physical or emotional harm, even if the person wants to participate. Hazing occurs with sports teams, social groups, and fraternities or sororities.[1]

hormone: A chemical substance formed in glands in the body and carried in the blood to organs and tissues, where it influences function, structure, and behavior.[2]

immunization: A treatment that protects your body against infection from certain diseases, such as the measles, whooping cough, and chicken pox.[1]

menarche: The first menstrual period or beginning of menstruation.[1]

meningitis: A dangerous infection that affects the brain and spinal cord.[1]

menstruation: The blood flow from the uterus that happens about every 28 days in women of childbearing age who are not pregnant. Commonly called a woman's period.[1]

mental illness: A health condition that changes a person's thinking, feelings, or behavior (or all three) and that causes the person distress and difficulty in functioning.[4]

nicotine: The addictive drug in tobacco. Nicotine activates a specific type of acetylcholine receptor.[2]

obesity: Having too much body fat. Obesity is more extreme than being overweight, which means weighing too much. Obesity is measured using body mass index.[1]

obsessive-compulsive disorder (OCD): An anxiety disorder in which a person experiences recurrent unwanted thoughts or rituals that the individual cannot control.[4]

oppositional defiant disorder: A disruptive pattern of behavior of children and adolescents that is characterized by defiant, disobedient, and hostile behaviors directed toward adults in positions of authority.[4]

oral sex: Sucking and/or licking a partner's sex organ.[1]

ovary: One of a pair of the female reproductive organs on each side of the uterus that contain eggs and make female hormones. An ovary is about the size of an almond or grape.[1]

ovulation: When an ovary releases an egg, about once each month, as part of the menstrual cycle.[1]

panic disorder: An anxiety disorder in which people have feelings of terror, rapid heartbeat, and rapid breathing that strike suddenly and repeatedly with no warning.[4]

Pap test: A test done on a sample of cells collected from the cervix to look for cell changes that could be cancer or that could turn into cancer.[1]

peer pressure: Social pressure on somebody to act or dress a certain way to be accepted as part of a group.[1]

penis: A male sex organ.[1]

phobia: An intense fear of something that poses little or no actual danger.[4]

posttraumatic stress disorder (PTSD): Disorder in which a stressful experience is traumatic and produces severe, recurring symptoms.[3]

psychotherapy: A treatment method for mental illness in which a mental health professional and a patient discuss problems and feelings to find solutions. Psychotherapy can help individuals change their thought or behavior patterns or understand how past experiences affect current behaviors.[4]

puberty: The process of developing from a child to sexual maturity, when a person becomes capable of having children. In a girl, puberty includes a growth spurt, development of breasts and hips, growth of body hair, and the beginning of menstruation (having periods).[1]

pubic area: On and around the genitals.[1]

reproductive organ: A body part involved in producing a baby. In a female, they include the uterus, ovaries, fallopian tubes, and vagina. In a male, they include the testicles and penis.[1]

schizophrenia: A chronic, severe, and disabling brain disease. People with schizophrenia often suffer terrifying symptoms such as hearing internal voices or believing that other people are reading their minds, controlling their thoughts, or plotting to harm them.[4]

scoliosis: When the spine curves away from the middle of the body to the side.[1]

semen: Whitish fluid containing sperm that comes out of the male's penis. Also known as cum.[1]

sex hormones: Hormones that are found in higher quantities in one sex than in the other. Male sex hormones are the androgens, which include testosterone; and the female sex hormones are the estrogens and progesterone.[2]

sexual assault: Any type of sexual activity that you do not agree to, including touching you, forcing you to touch someone, and forcing a body part into your vagina, rectum (bottom), or mouth. Another term for this can be molestation.[1]

sexual contact: Any type of touching during sexual activity between two people, including sexual intercourse, oral sex, and skin-to-skin contact in the genital area (around the vagina, penis, scrotum, anus, and thigh).[1]

sexual intercourse: When a man's penis is put into a woman's vagina.[1]

sexually transmitted disease (STD): Infection that is spread from person to person through sexual contact. Also called sexually transmitted infection.[1]

sperm: Cell found in semen that can unite with a female's egg after having sexual intercourse and lead to pregnancy.[1]

symptom: Something that indicates the presence of a disease.[4]

syphilis: A sexually transmitted disease caused by bacteria that progresses in stages. Without treatment, the infection can cause damage throughout the body and even death.[1]

testosterone: A male hormone that controls many of the changes males go through during puberty—deeper voice, body and facial hair, and the making of sperm.[1]

tobacco: A plant widely cultivated for its leaves, which are used primarily for smoking.[2]

uterus: A pear-shaped, hollow organ in a female's pelvis where a baby develops during pregnancy.[1]

vagina: A muscular passage that leads down from the cervix to the outside of a female's body. During menstruation, menstrual blood flows from the uterus through the cervix and out of the body through the vagina. Also called the birth canal.[1]

virgin: Someone who has never had sexual intercourse.[1]

virus: A kind of germ that can infect cells and cause disease.[1]

vulva: The external female reproductive organ, which covers the entrance to the vagina.[1]

withdrawal: Pulling the penis out of the vagina during sexual intercourse, before ejaculation.[1]

Chapter 71

Directory of Adolescent Health Organizations for Parents and Teens

Government Agencies That Provide Information about Adolescent Health

Agency for Healthcare Research and Quality (AHRQ)

Office of Communications and Knowledge Transfer
540 Gaither Road
Suite 2000
Rockville, MD 20850
Phone: 301-427-1364
Fax: 301-427-1873
Website: www.ahrq.gov

Centers for Disease Control and Prevention (CDC)

1600 Clifton Road
Atlanta, GA 30333
Toll-Free: 800-CDC-INFO
(232-4636)
Toll-Free TTY: 888-232-6348
Phone: 404-639-3311
Websites: www.cdc.gov; www.cdc
.gov/HealthyYouth
E-mail: cdcinfo@cdc.gov

Child Welfare Information Gateway

Children's Bureau/ACYF
1250 Maryland Avenue, SW
Eighth Floor
Washington, DC 20024
Toll-Free: 800-394-3366
Website: www.childwelfare.gov
E-mail: info@childwelfare.gov

Resources in this chapter were compiled from several sources deemed reliable; all contact information was verified and updated in May 2010.

Federal Interagency Forum on Child and Family Statistics
Website: www.childstats.gov

Federal Trade Commission (FTC)
600 Pennsylvania Avenue, NW
Washington, DC 20580
Phone: 202-326-2222
Website: www.ftc.gov

Health Resources and Services Administration (HRSA)
5600 Fishers Lane
Rockville, MD 20857
Toll-Free: 888-ASK-HRSA
(275-4772)
Toll-Free TTY: 877-489-4772
Website: www.hrsa.gov
E-mail: ask@hrsa.gov

Healthfinder®
National Health Information
Center
P.O. Box 1133
Washington, DC 20013-1133
Toll-Free: 800-336-4797
Phone: 301-565-4167
Fax: 301-984-4256
Website: www.healthfinder.gov
E-mail: healthfinder@nhic.org

National Cancer Institute (NCI)
NCI Office of Communications
and Education
Public Inquiries Office
6116 Executive Boulevard
Suite 300
Bethesda, MD 20892-8322
Toll-Free: 800-4-CANCER
(422-6237)
TTY: 800-332-8615
Website: www.cancer.gov
E-mail: cancergovstaff@mail.nih
.gov

National Diabetes Education Program (NDEP)
One Diabetes Way
Bethesda, MD 20814-9692
Phone: 301-496-3583
Toll-Free: 888-693-NDEP
(693-6337)
Website: ndep.nih.gov

National Highway Traffic Safety Administration (NHTSA)
1200 New Jersey Avenue, SE
West Building
Washington, DC 20590
Toll-Free: 888-327-4236 (Hotline)
Toll-Free TTY: 800-424-9153
Website: www.nhtsa.dot.gov

National Institute of Arthritis and Musculoskeletal and Skin Diseases (NIAMS)
Information Clearinghouse
National Institutes of Health
1 AMS Circle
Bethesda, MD 20892-3675
Toll Free: 877-22-NIAMS
(226-4267)
Phone: 301-495-4484
TTY: 301–565–2966
Fax: 301-718-6366
Website: www.niams.nih.gov
E-mail: NIAMSinfo@mail.nih.gov

National Institute of Diabetes, Digestive and Kidney Diseases (NIDDK)
Office of Communications &
Public Liaison
NIDDK, NIH
Building 31
Room 9A06
31 Center Drive
MSC 2560
Bethesda, MD 20892-2560
Phone: 301-496-3583
Website: www.niddk.nih.gov

National Institute of Neurological Disorders and Stroke (NINDS)
NIH Neurological Institute
P.O. Box 5801
Bethesda, MD 20824
Toll-Free: 800-352-9424
Phone: 301-496-5751
TTY: 301-468-5981
Website: www.ninds.nih.gov
E-mail: braininfo@ninds.nih.gov

National Institute on Alcohol Abuse and Alcoholism (NIAAA)
5635 Fishers Lane
MSC 9304
Bethesda, MD 20892-9304
Phone: 301-443-3860
Website: www.niaaa.nih.gov
E-mail: niaaaweb-r@exchange
.nih.gov

National Institute on Child Health and Human Development (NICHD)
P.O. Box 3006
Rockville, MD 20847
Toll-Free: 800-370-2943
Toll-Free TTY: 888-320-6942
Toll-Free Fax: 866-760-5947
Website: www.nichd.nih.gov
E-mail: NICHDInformation
ResourceCenter@mail.nih.gov

National Institute on Deafness and Other Communication Disorders (NIDCD)
National Institutes of Health
31 Center Drive
MSC 2320
Bethesda, MD 20892-2320
Website: www.nidcd.nih.gov
E-mail: nidcdinfo@nidcd.nih.gov

National Institute on Drug Abuse (NIDA)

6001 Executive Boulevard
Room 5213
Bethesda, MD 20892-9561
Phone: 301-443-1124
Phone: 240-221-4007 (Spanish)
Website: www.drugabuse.gov
E-mail: information@nida.nih.gov

National Institute on Mental Health (NIMH)

Science Writing, Press, and
Dissemination Branch
6001 Executive Boulevard
Room 8184
MSC 9663
Bethesda, MD 20892-9663
Toll-Free: 866-615-6464
Toll-Free TTY: 866-415-8051
Phone: 301-443-4513
TTY: 301-443-8431
Fax: 301-443-4279
Website: www.nimh.nih.gov
E-mail: nimhinfo@nih.gov

National Institutes of Health (NIH)

9000 Rockville Pike
Bethesda, MD 20892
Phone: 301-496-4000
TTY: 301-402-9612
Website: www.nih.gov
E-mail: NIHinfo@od.nih.gov

National Women's Health Information Center (NWHIC)

Office on Women's Health
200 Independence Avenue, SW
Washington, DC 20201
Toll-Free: 800-994-9662
Toll-Free TTY: 888-220-5446
Website: www.womenshealth.gov

National Youth Anti-Drug Media Campaign

White House Office of National
Drug Control Policy
P.O. Box 6000
Rockville, MD 20849-6000
Toll-Free: 800-666–3332
Toll-Free: 800-662-HELP
(662-4357) (Helpline)
Fax: 301-519-5212
Website: www.theantidrug.com

National Youth Violence Prevention Resource Center (NYVPRC)

Website: www.safeyouth.org

Substance Abuse and Mental Health Services Administration (SAMHSA)

SAMHSA's Health Information
Network
P.O. Box 2345
Rockville, MD 20847-2345
Toll-Free: 877-SAMHSA-7
(726-4727)
Toll-Free: TTY: 800-487-4889
Fax: 240-221-4292
Website: www.samhsa.gov
E-mail: SHIN@samhsa.hhs.gov

U.S. Department of Education (DOE)
400 Maryland Avenue, SW
Washington, DC 20202
Toll-Free: 800-USA-LEARN
(872-5327)
Toll-Free TTY: 800-437-0833
Website: www.ed.gov

U.S. Department of Health and Human Services (HHS)
200 Independent Avenue, SW
Washington, DC 20201
Toll-Free: 877-696-6775 (Hotline)
Website: www.hhs.gov

U.S. Department of Labor (DOL)
200 Constitution Avenue, NW
Washington, DC 20210
Toll-Free: 866-4-USA-DOL
(487-2365)
Toll-Free TTY: 877-889-5627
Website: www.dol.gov

U.S. Food and Drug Administration (FDA)
10903 New Hampshire Avenue
Silver Spring, MD 20993
Toll-Free: 888-INFO-FDA
(463-6332)
Website: www.fda.gov

U.S. National Library of Medicine (NLM)
8600 Rockville Pike
Bethesda, MD 20894
Toll-Free: 888-FIND-NLM
(346-3656)
Toll-Free TDD: 800-735-2258
Phone: 301-594-5983
Fax: 301-402-1384
Website: www.nlm.nih.gov
E-mail: custserv@nlm.nih.gov

Private Agencies That Provide Information about Adolescent Health

AAA Foundation for Traffic Safety
607 14th Street, NW
Suite 201
Washington, DC 20005
Phone: 202-638-5944
Fax: 202-638-5943
Website: www.aaafoundation.org
E-mail: info@aaafoundation.org

American Academy of Child and Adolescent Psychiatry
3615 Wisconsin Avenue, NW
Washington, DC 20016-3007
Phone: 202-966-7300
Fax: 202-966-2891
Website: www.aacap.org

American Academy of Dermatology
P.O. Box 4014
Schaumburg, IL 60168
Toll-Free: 866-503-SKIN
(503-7546)
Phone: 847-330-0230
Fax: 847-240-1859
Website: www.aad.org

American Academy of Family Physicians
P.O. Box 11210
Shawnee Mission, KS 66207-1210
Toll-Free: 800-274-2237
Phone: 913-906-6000
Fax: 913-906-6075
Website: www.aafp.org

American Academy of Pediatrics
141 Northwest Point Boulevard
Elk Grove Village, IL 60007-1098
Phone: 847-434-4000
Fax: 847-434-8000
Website: www.aap.org
E-mail: kidsdocs@aap.org

American Association of Diabetes Educators
200 W. Madison Street
Suite 800
Chicago, IL 60606
Toll-Free: 800-338-3633
Website: www.diabeteseducator
.org
E-mail: aade@aadenet.org

American Association of Suicidology
5221 Wisconsin Avenue, NW
Washington, DC 20015
Phone: 202-237-2280
Fax: 202-237-2282
Website: www.suicidology.org

American College of Sports Medicine
P.O. Box 1440
Indianapolis, IN 46206-1440
Phone: 317-637-9200
Fax: 317-634-7817
Website: www.acsm.org

American College of Obstetricians and Gynecologists
P.O. Box 96920
Washington, DC 20090-6920
Phone: 202-638-5577
Website: www.acog.org

American Diabetes Association
National Call Center
1701 North Beauregard Street
Alexandria, VA 22311
Toll-Free: 800-DIABETES
(342-2383)
Website: www.diabetes.org
E-mail: AskADA@diabetes.org

American Heart Association
National Center
7272 Greenville Avenue
Dallas, TX 75231
Toll-Free: 800-AHA-USA-1
(242-8721)
Website: www.americanheart.org

American Medical Association

515 North State Street
Chicago, IL 60654
Toll-Free: 800-621-8335
Website: www.ama-assn.org

American Social Health Association

P.O. Box 13827
Research Triangle Park, NC 27709
Phone: 919-361-8400
Fax: 919-361-8425
Websites: www.ashastd.org;
www.iwannaknow.org
E-mail: info@ashastd.org

American Psychiatric Association

1000 Wilson Boulevard
Suite 1825
Arlington, VA 22209
Toll-Free: 888-35-PSYCH
(357-7924)
Website: www.psych.org
E-mail: apa@psych.org

American Psychological Association

750 First Street, NE
Washington, DC 20002-4242
Toll-Free: 800-374-2721
Phone: 202-336-5500
TDD/TTY: 202-336-6123
Website: www.apa.org

Anxiety Disorders Association of America

8730 Georgia Avenue
Silver Spring, MD 20910
Phone: 240-485-1001
Fax: 240-485-1035
Website: www.adaa.org

Candlelighters Childhood Cancer Foundation

American Childhood Cancer Organization
P.O. Box 498
Kensington, MD 20895-0498
Toll-Free: 800-366-CCCF
(366-2223)
Phone: 301-962-3520
Fax: 301-962-3521
Website: www.candlelighters.org
E-mail: staff@acco.org

Center for Young Women's Health

333 Longwood Avenue
Fifth Floor
Boston, MA 02115
Phone: 617-355-2994
Fax: 617-730-0186
Website: www.
youngwomenshealth.org

Child and Adolescent Bipolar Foundation

820 Davis Street
Suite 520
Evanston, IL 60201
Phone: 847-492-8519
Website: www.bpkids.org
E-mail: cabf@bpkids.org

Cincinnati Children's Hospital Medical Center
3333 Burnet Avenue
Cincinnati, OH 45229-3039
Toll-Free: 800-344-2462
Phone: 513-636-4200
TTY: 513-636-4900
Website: www
.cincinnatichildrens.org

Cleveland Clinic
9500 Euclid Avenue
Cleveland, OH 44195
Toll-Free: 800-223-2273
TTY: 216-444-0261
Website: my.clevelandclinic.org

Crimes Against Children Research Center
University of New Hampshire
20 College Road
126 Horton Social Science
Center
Durham, NH 03824
Phone: 603-862-1888
Fax: 603-862-1122
Website: www.unh.edu
E-mail: kelly.foster@unh.edu

Depression and Bipolar Support Alliance
730 North Franklin Street
Suite 501
Chicago, IL 60654-7225
Toll-Free: 800-826-3632
Fax: 312-642-7243
Website: www.dbsalliance.org
E-mail: info@dbsalliance.org

Guttmacher Institute
125 Maiden Lane
Seventh Floor
New York, NY 10038
Toll-Free: 800-355-0244
Phone: 212-248-1111
Fax: 212-248-1951
Website: www.guttmacher.org

The Hormone Foundation
8401 Connecticut Avenue
Suite 900
Chevy Chase, MD 20815-5817
Toll-Free: 800-HORMONE
(467-6663)
Fax: 301-941-0259
Website: www.hormone.org
E-mail: hormone@endo-society
.org

Immunization Action Coalition
1573 Selby Avenue
Suite 234
St. Paul, MN 55104
Phone: 651-647-9009
Fax: 651-647-9131
Website: www.immunize.org
E-mail: admin@immunize.org

International OCD (Obsessive-Compulsive Disorder) Foundation
P.O. Box 961029
Boston, MA 02196
Phone: 617-973-5801
Fax: 617-973-5803
Website: www.ocfoundation.org
E-mail: info@ocfoundation.org

Juvenile Arthritis Alliance

Arthritis Foundation
P.O. Box 7669
Atlanta, GA 30357-0669
Toll-Free: 800-283-7800
Website: www.arthritis
.org/ja-alliance-main.php

Juvenile Diabetes Research Foundation International

26 Broadway
New York, NY 100004
Toll-Free: 800-533-CURE
(533-2873)
Fax: 212-785-9595
Website: www.jdrf.org
E-mail: info@jdrf.org

Henry J. Kaiser Family Foundation

2400 Sand Hill Road
Menlo Park, CA 94025
Phone: 650-854-9400
Fax: 650-854-4800
Website: www.kff.org

Mayo Clinic

Website: www.mayoclinic.org

Mental Health America

2000 North Beauregard Street
Sixth Floor
Alexandria, VA 22311
Toll-Free: 800-969-6642
Phone: 703-684-7722
Fax: 703-684-5968
Website: www.nmha.org
E-mail: infoctr@
mentalhealthamerica.net

National Adolescent Health Information Center

LHTS Suite 245
Box 0503
San Francisco, CA 94143-0503
Phone: 415-502-4856
Fax: 415-502-4858
Website: nahic.ucsf.edu
E-mail: nahic@ucsf.edu

National Alliance on Mental Illness

3803 North Fairfax Drive
Suite 100
Arlington, VA 22203
Toll-Free: 800-950-NAMI
(950-6264)
Phone: 703-524-7600
Fax: 703-524-9094
Website: www.nami.org

National Campaign to Prevent Teen Pregnancy

1776 Massachusetts Avenue, NW
Suite 200
Washington, DC 20036
Phone: 202-478-8500
Fax: 202-478-8588
Website: www.
thenationalcampaign.org

National Center for Missing and Exploited Children

Charles B. Wang International
Children's Building
699 Prince Street
Alexandria, Virginia 22314-3175
Toll-Free: 800-THE-LOST
(843-5678)
Phone: 703-224-2150
Fax: 703-224-2122
Website: www.missingkids.com

National Child Traumatic Stress Network
University of California
Los Angeles
11150 West Olympic Boulevard
Suite 650
Los Angeles, CA 90064
Phone: 310-235-2633
Fax: 310-235-2612
Website: www.nctsn.org

National Eating Disorders Association
603 Stewart Street
Suite 803
Seattle, WA 98101
Toll-Free: 800-931-2237
Phone: 206-382-3587
Fax: 206-829-8501
Website: www.
nationaleatingdisorders.org
E-mail: info@
NationalEatingDisorders.org

National Safety Council
1121 Spring Lake Drive
Itasca, IL 60143-3201
Toll-Free: 800-621-7615
Website: www.nsc.org
E-mail: info@nsc.org

National Scoliosis Foundation
5 Cabot Place
Stoughton, MA 02072
Toll-Free: 800-NSF-MYBACK
(673-6922)
Website: www.scoliosis.org
E-mail: NSF@scoliosis.org

National Youth Network
42165 Turqueries Avenue
Palm Desert, CA 92211
Website: www.nationalyouth
.com

Nemours Foundation Center for Children's Health Media
1600 Rockland Road
Wilmington, DE 19803
Phone: 302-651-4000
Website: www.teenshealth.org
E-mail: info@teenshealth.org

Palo Alto Medical Foundation
Website: www.pamf.org/teen

Parents, Families, and Friends of Lesbians and Gays
1828 L Street, NW
Suite 660
Washington, DC 20036
Phone: 202-467-8180
Fax: 202-467-8194
Website: community.pflag.org
E-mail: info@pflag.org

Partnership for a Drug-Free America
405 Lexington Avenue
Suite 1601
New York, NY 10174
Phone: 212-922-1560
Fax: 212-922-1570
Website: www.drugfree.org

Pew Internet and American Life Project
The Pew Research Center
1615 L Street, NW
Suite 700
Washington, DC 20036
Phone: 202-419-4500
Fax: 202-419-4505
Website: www.pewinternet
.org/default.aspx
E-mail: info@pewresearch.org

Planned Parenthood
434 West 33rd Street
New York, NY 10001
Toll-Free: 800-230-PLAN
(230-7526)
Phone: 212-541-7800
Fax: 212-245-1845
Website: www
.plannedparenthood.org

Sex, Etc.
Center for Applied Psychology
Rutgers University
41 Gordon Road, Suite C
Piscataway, NJ 08854
Phone: 732-445-7929
Fax: 732-445-5333
Website: www.sexetc.org
E-mail: sexetc@rci.rutgers.edu

Sexuality Information and Education Council of the United States
90 John Street
Suite 704
New York, NY 10038
Phone: 212-819-9770
Fax: 212-819-9776
Website: www.siecus.org

Society for Adolescent Health and Medicine
111 Deer Lake Road
Suite 100
Deerfield, IL 60015
Phone: 847-753-5226
Fax: 847-480-9282
Website: www.adolescenthealth
.org
E-mail: info@adolescenthealth
.org

Students Against Destructive Decisions
255 Main Street
Marlborough, MA 01752
Toll-Free: 877-SADD-INC
(723-3462)
Fax: 508-481-5759
Website: www.sadd.org
E-mail: info@sadd.org

Suicide Awareness Voices of Education
8120 Penn Avenue South
Suite 470
Bloomington, MN 55431
Toll-Free: 800-273-8255
Phone: 952-946-7998
Website: www.save.org

TeenGrowth
11274 West Hillsborough Avenue
Tampa, FL 33635
Website: www.teengrowth.com

World Health Organization
Avenue Appia 20
1211 Geneva 27
Switzerland
Phone: + 41 22 791 21 11
Fax: + 41 22 791 31 11
Website: www.who.int/topics/
adolescent_health/en
E-mail: info@who.int

Young Men's Health
333 Longwood Avenue
Fifth Floor
Boston, MA 02115
Website: www.
youngmenshealthsite.org

Hotlines and Referral Services for Teens: General Help

Covenant House
Toll-Free: 800-999-9999
Website: nineline.org

Girls and Boys Town National Hotline
Toll-Free: 800-448-3000
Website: www.girlsandboystown
.org

Hotlines and Referral Services for Teens: Assistance for Specific Concerns

Al-Anon and AlaTeen
Toll-Free: 888-4AL-ANON
(425-2666)
Website: www.al-anon.org

America's Pregnancy Helpline
Toll-Free: 866-942-6466
Website: www.thehelpline.org

Centers for Disease Control and Prevention Sexually Transmitted Disease Hotline
Toll-Free: 800-CDC-INFO
(232-4636)
Website: www.cdc.gov/std

National Clearinghouse for Alcohol and Drug Information
Toll-Free: 800-729-6686
(English)
Toll-Free: 877-767-8432
(Spanish)
Website: www.ncadi.samhsa.gov

National Domestic Violence Hotline
Toll-Free: 800-799-SAFE
(799-7233)
Toll-Free TTY: 800-787-3224
Website: www.ndvh.org

National Runaway Switchboard
Toll-Free: 800-RUNAWAY
(786-2929)
Website: www.nrscrisisline.org

National Suicide Hotline
Toll-Free: 800-SUICIDE
(784-2433)
Website: www.hopeline.com

Planned Parenthood
Toll-Free: 800-230-PLAN
(230-7526)
Website: www.
plannedparenthood.org

Rape, Abuse, and Incest National Network
Toll-Free: 800-656-HOPE
(656-4673)
Website: www.rainn.org

SAFE (Self-Abuse Finally Ends)
Toll-Free: 800-DONT-CUT
(366-8288)
Website: www.selfinjury.com

Index

Index

Page numbers followed by 'n' indicate a footnote. Page numbers in *italics* indicate a table or illustration.

Health Reference Series
Complete Catalog
List price $93 per volume. School and library price $84 per volume.

Adolescent Health Sourcebook, 3rd Edition

Basic Consumer Health Information about Adolescent Growth and Development, Puberty, Sexuality, Reproductive Health, and Physical, Emotional, Social, and Mental Health Concerns of Teens and Their Parents, Including Facts about Nutrition, Physical Activity, Weight Management, Acne, Allergies, Cancer, Diabetes, Growth Disorders, Juvenile Arthritis, Infections, Substance Abuse, and More

Along with Information about Adolescent Safety Concerns, Youth Violence, a Glossary of Related Terms, and a Directory of Resources

Edited by Amy L. Sutton. 600 pages. 2010. 978-0-7808-1140-9.

Adult Health Concerns Sourcebook

Basic Consumer Health Information about Medical and Mental Concerns of Adults, Including Facts about Choosing Healthcare Providers, Navigating Insurance Options, Maintaining Wellness, Preventing Cancer, Heart Disease, Stroke, Diabetes, and Osteoporosis, and Understanding Aging-Related Health Concerns, Including Menopause, Cognitive Changes, and Changes in the Coronary and Vascular Systems

Along with Tips on Caring for Aging Parents and Dealing with Health-Related Work and Travel Issues, a Glossary, and a Directory of Resources for Additional Help and Information

Edited by Sandra J. Judd. 648 pages. 2008. 978-0-7808-0999-4.

"Provides a thorough list of topics that are important to adult health and for caregivers."
—*CHOICE, Nov '08*

"Written in easy-to-understand language... the content is well-organized and is intended to aid adults in making health care-related decisions."
—*AORN Journal, Dec '08*

AIDS Sourcebook, 4th Edition

Basic Consumer Health Information about Human Immunodeficiency Virus (HIV) and Acquired Immunodeficiency Syndrome (AIDS), Featuring Updated Statistics and Facts about Risks, Prevention, Screening, Diagnosis, Treatments, Side Effects, and Complications, and Including a Section about the Impact of HIV/ AIDS on the Health of Women, Children, and Adolescents

Along with Tips on Managing Life with AIDS, Reports on Current Research Initiatives and Clinical Trials, a Glossary of Related Terms, and Resource Directories for Further Help and Information

Edited by Ivy L. Alexander. 680 pages. 2008. 978-0-7808-0997-0.

SEE ALSO *Contagious Diseases Sourcebook, 2nd Edition*

Alcoholism Sourcebook, 3rd Edition

Basic Consumer Health Information about Alcohol Use, Abuse, and Dependence, Featuring Facts about the Physical, Mental, and Social Health Effects of Alcohol Addiction, Including Alcoholic Liver Disease, Pancreatic Disease, Cardiovascular Disease, Neurological Disorders, and the Effects of Drinking during Pregnancy

Along with Information about Alcohol Treatment, Medications, and Recovery Programs, in Addition to Tips for Reducing the Prevalence of Underage Drinking, Statistics about Alcohol Use, a Glossary of Related Terms, and Directories of Resources for More Help and Information

Edited by Joyce Brennfleck Shannon. 600 pages. 2010. 978-0-7808-1141-6.

SEE ALSO *Drug Abuse Sourcebook, 3rd Edition*

Allergies Sourcebook, 3rd Edition

Basic Consumer Health Information about Allergic Disorders, Such as Anaphylaxis, Hives,

Eczema, Rhinitis, Sinusitis, and Conjunctivitis, and Their Triggers, Including Pollen, Mold, Dust Mites, Animal Dander, Insects, Chemicals, Food, Food Additives, and Medications

Along with Advice about the Diagnosis and Treatment of Allergy Symptoms, a Glossary of Related Terms, a Directory of Resources for Help and Information, and Suggestions for Additional Reading

Edited by Amy L. Sutton. 588 pages. 2007. 978-0-7808-0950-5.

SEE ALSO Asthma Sourcebook, 2nd Edition

Alzheimer Disease Sourcebook, 4th Edition

Basic Consumer Health Information about Alzheimer Disease, Other Dementias, and Related Disorders, Including Multi-Infarct Dementia, Dementia with Lewy Bodies, Frontotemporal Dementia (Pick Disease), Wernicke-Korsakoff Syndrome (Alcohol-Related Dementia), AIDS Dementia Complex, Huntington Disease, Creutzfeldt-Jacob Disease, and Delirium

Along with Information about Coping with Memory Loss and Forgetfulness, Maintaining Skills, and Long-Term Planning for People with Dementia, and Suggestions Addressing Common Caregiver Concerns, Updated Information about Current Research Efforts, a Glossary of Related Terms, and Directories of Sources for Additional Help and Information

Edited by Karen Bellenir. 603 pages. 2008. 978-0-7808-1001-3.

"An invaluable resource for persons who have received a diagnosis, for caregivers, and for family members dealing with this insidious disease. It is recommended for public, community college, and ready-reference sections in academic libraries."
—American Reference Books Annual, 2009

SEE ALSO Brain Disorders Sourcebook, 3rd Edition

Arthritis Sourcebook, 3rd Edition

Basic Consumer Health Information about the Risk Factors, Symptoms, Diagnosis, and

Treatment of Osteoarthritis, Rheumatoid Arthritis, Juvenile Arthritis, Gout, Infectious Arthritis, and Autoimmune Disorders Associated with Arthritis

Along with Facts about Medications, Surgeries, and Self-Care Techniques to Manage Pain and Disability, Tips on Living with Arthritis, a Glossary of Related Terms, and Resources for Additional Help and Information

Edited by Amy L. Sutton. 600 pages. 2010. 978-0-7808-1077-8.

Asthma Sourcebook, 2nd Edition

Basic Consumer Health Information about the Causes, Symptoms, Diagnosis, and Treatment of Asthma in Infants, Children, Teenagers, and Adults, Including Facts about Different Types of Asthma, Common Co-Occurring Conditions, Asthma Management Plans, Triggers, Medications, and Medication Delivery Devices

Along with Asthma Statistics, Research Updates, a Glossary, a Directory of Asthma-Related Resources, and More

Edited by Karen Bellenir. 581 pages. 2006. 978-0-7808-0866-9.

SEE ALSO Lung Disorders Sourcebook; Respiratory Disorders Sourcebook, 2nd Edition

Attention Deficit Disorder Sourcebook

Basic Consumer Health Information about Attention Deficit/Hyperactivity Disorder in Children and Adults, Including Facts about Causes, Symptoms, Diagnostic Criteria, and Treatment Options Such as Medications, Behavior Therapy, Coaching, and Homeopathy

Along with Reports on Current Research Initiatives, Legal Issues, and Government Regulations, and Featuring a Glossary of Related Terms, Internet Resources, and a List of Additional Reading Material

Edited by Dawn D. Matthews. 447 pages. 2002. 978-0-7808-0624-5.

"Recommended reference source."
—Booklist, Jan '03

SEE ALSO Learning Disabilities Sourcebook, 3rd Edition

Autism and Pervasive Developmental Disorders Sourcebook

Basic Consumer Health Information about Autism Spectrum and Pervasive Developmental Disorders, Such as Classical Autism, Asperger Syndrome, Rett Syndrome, and Childhood Disintegrative Disorder, Including Information about Related Genetic Disorders and Medical Problems and Facts about Causes, Screening Methods, Diagnostic Criteria, Treatments and Interventions, and Family and Education Issues

Along with a Glossary of Related Terms, Tips for Evaluating the Validity of Health Claims, and a Directory of Resources for Additional Help and Information

Edited by Sandra J. Judd. 603 pages. 2007. 978-0-7808-0953-6.

"This book provides a current overview of disorders on the autism spectrum and information about various therapies, educational resources, and help for families with practical issues such as workplace adjustments, living arrangements, and estate planning. It is a useful resource for public and consumer health libraries."
—American Reference Books Annual, 2009

SEE ALSO *Learning Disabilities Sourcebook, 3rd Edition*

Back and Neck Disorders Sourcebook, 2nd Edition

Basic Consumer Health Information about Spinal Pain, Spinal Cord Injuries, and Related Disorders, Such as Degenerative Disk Disease, Osteoarthritis, Scoliosis, Sciatica, Spina Bifida, and Spinal Stenosis, and Featuring Facts about Maintaining Spinal Health, Self-Care, Pain Management, Rehabilitative Care, Chiropractic Care, Spinal Surgeries, and Complementary Therapies

Along with Suggestions for Preventing Back and Neck Pain, a Glossary of Related Terms, and a Directory of Resources

Edited by Amy L. Sutton. 607 pages. 2004. 978-0-7808-0738-9.

"Recommended... An easy to use, comprehensive medical reference book."
—E-Streams, Sep '05

"For anyone who has back or neck problems, this book is ideal. Its easy-to-understand language and variety of topics makes this sourcebook a worthwhile read. The price... is reasonable for the amount of information contained in the book"
—Occupational Therapy in Health Care, 2007

Blood & Circulatory Disorders Sourcebook, 3rd Edition

Basic Consumer Health Information about Blood and Circulatory System Disorders, Such as Anemia, Leukemia, Lymphoma, Rh Disease, Hemophilia, Thrombophilia, Other Bleeding and Clotting Deficiencies, and Artery, Vascular, and Venous Diseases, Including Facts about Blood Types, Blood Donation, Bone Marrow and Stem Cell Transplants, Tests and Medications, and Tips for Maintaining Circulatory Health

Along with a Glossary of Related Terms and a List of Resources for Additional Help and Information

Edited by Sandra J. Judd. 600 pages. 2010. 978-0-7808-1081-5.

SEE ALSO *Leukemia Sourcebook*

Brain Disorders Sourcebook, 3rd Edition

Basic Consumer Health Information about Acquired and Traumatic Brain Injuries, Brain Tumors, Cerebral Palsy and Other Genetic and Congenital Brain Disorders, Infections of the Brain, Epilepsy, and Degenerative Neurological Disorders Such as Dementia, Huntington Disease, and Amyotrophic Lateral Sclerosis (ALS)

Along with Information on Brain Structure and Function, Treatment and Rehabilitation Options, a Glossary of Terms Related to Brain Disorders, and a Directory of Resources for More Information

Edited by Joyce Brennfleck Shannon. 600 pages. 2010. 978-0-7808-1083-9.

SEE ALSO *Alzheimer Disease Sourcebook, 4th Edition*

Breast Cancer Sourcebook, 3rd Edition

Basic Consumer Health Information about Breast Health and Breast Cancer, Including Facts about Environmental, Genetic, and Other Risk Factors, Prevention Efforts, Screening and Diagnostic Methods, Surgical Treatment Options and Other Care Choices, Complementary and Alternative Therapies, and Post-Treatment Concerns

Along with Statistical Data, News about Research Advances, a Glossary of Related Terms, and Directories of Resources for Additional Information and Support

Edited by Karen Bellenir. 606 pages. 2009. 978-0-7808-1030-3.

"A very useful reference for people wanting to learn more about breast cancer and how to negotiate their care or the care of a loved one. The third edition is necessary as information/treatment options continue to evolve."

—*Doody's Review Service, 2009*

SEE ALSO *Cancer Sourcebook for Women, 3rd Edition, Women's Health Concerns Sourcebook, 3rd Edition*

Breastfeeding Sourcebook

Basic Consumer Health Information about the Benefits of Breastmilk, Preparing to Breastfeed, Breastfeeding as a Baby Grows, Nutrition, and More, Including Information on Special Situations and Concerns Such as Mastitis, Illness, Medications, Allergies, Multiple Births, Prematurity, Special Needs, and Adoption

Along with a Glossary and Resources for Additional Help and Information

Edited by Jenni Lynn Colson. 367 pages. 2002. 978-0-7808-0332-9.

SEE ALSO *Pregnancy and Birth Sourcebook, 3rd Edition*

Burns Sourcebook

Basic Consumer Health Information about Various Types of Burns and Scalds, Including Flame, Heat, Cold, Electrical, Chemical, and Sun Burns

Along with Information on Short-Term and Long-Term Treatments, Tissue Reconstruction, Plastic Surgery, Prevention Suggestions, and First Aid

Edited by Allan R. Cook. 604 pages. 1999. 978-0-7808-0204-9.

"This is an exceptional addition to the series and is highly recommended for all consumer health collections, hospital libraries, and academic medical centers."

—*E-Streams, Mar '00*

"This key reference guide is an invaluable addition to all health care and public libraries in confronting this ongoing health issue."

—*American Reference Books Annual, 2000*

SEE ALSO *Dermatological Disorders Sourcebook, 2nd Edition*

Cancer Sourcebook, 5th Edition

Basic Consumer Health Information about Major Forms and Stages of Cancer, Featuring Facts about Head and Neck Cancers, Lung Cancers, Gastrointestinal Cancers, Genitourinary Cancers, Lymphomas, Blood Cell Cancers, Endocrine Cancers, Skin Cancers, Bone Cancers, Metastatic Cancers, and More

Along with Facts about Cancer Treatments, Cancer Risks and Prevention, a Glossary of Related Terms, Statistical Data, and a Directory of Resources for Additional Information

Edited by Karen Bellenir. 1105 pages. 2007. 978-0-7808-0947-5.

"The 5th, updated edition of Cancer Sourcebook should be in every public and health lending library collection... An unparalleled discussion essential for any health collections considering an all-in-one basic general reference."

—*California Bookwatch, Aug '07*

SEE ALSO *Breast Cancer Sourcebook, 3rd Edition, Cancer Survivorship Sourcebook, Leukemia Sourcebook*

Cancer Sourcebook for Women, 4th Edition

Basic Consumer Health Information about Gynecologic Cancers and Other Cancers of Special Concern to Women, Including Cancers of the Breast, Cervix, Colon, Lung, Ovaries, Thyroid, and Uterus

Along with Facts about Benign Conditions of the Female Reproductive System, Cancer Risk

Factors, Diagnostic and Treatment Procedures, Side Effects of Cancer and Cancer Treatments, Women's Issues in Cancer Survivorship, a Glossary of Related Terms, and a Directory of Resources for Additional Help and Information

Edited by Karen Bellenir. 600 pages. 2010. 978-0-7808-1139-3.

SEE ALSO Breast Cancer Sourcebook, 3rd Edition, Women's Health Concerns Sourcebook, 3rd Edition

Cancer Survivorship Sourcebook

Basic Consumer Health Information about the Physical, Educational, Emotional, Social, and Financial Needs of Cancer Patients from Diagnosis, through Cancer Treatment, and Beyond, Including Facts about Researching Specific Types of Cancer and Learning about Clinical Trials and Treatment Options, and Featuring Tips for Coping with the Side Effects of Cancer Treatments and Adjusting to Life after Cancer Treatment Concludes

Along with Suggestions for Caregivers, Friends, and Family Members of Cancer Patients, a Glossary of Cancer Care Terms, and Directories of Related Resources

Edited by Karen Bellenir. 633 pages. 2007. 978-0-7808-0985-7.

"Well organized and comprehensive in coverage, the book speaks to issues encountered both during and after cancer treatment. Recommended for consumer health and public libraries."
—*Library Journal, Aug 1 '07*

"Cancer Survivorship Sourcebook will be useful to anyone who has a friend or loved one with a cancer diagnosis."
—*American Reference Books Annual, 2008*

SEE ALSO *Cancer Sourcebook, 5th Edition, Disease Management Sourcebook*

Cardiovascular Disorders Sourcebook, 4th Edition

Basic Consumer Health Information about Heart and Blood Vessel Diseases and Disorders, Such as Angina, Heart Attack, Heart Failure, Cardiomyopathy, Arrhythmias, Valve Disease, Atherosclerosis, Aneurysms, and

Congenital Heart Defects, Including Information about Cardiovascular Disease in Women, Men, Children, Adolescents, and Minorities

Along with Facts about Diagnosing, Managing, and Preventing Cardiovascular Disease, a Glossary of Related Medical Terms, and a Directory of Resources for Additional Information

Edited by Amy L. Sutton. 600 pages. 2010. 978-0-7808-1080-8.

Caregiving Sourcebook

Basic Consumer Health Information for Caregivers, Including a Profile of Caregivers, Caregiving Responsibilities and Concerns, Tips for Specific Conditions, Care Environments, and the Effects of Caregiving

Along with Facts about Legal Issues, Financial Information, and Future Planning, a Glossary, and a Listing of Additional Resources

Edited by Joyce Brennfleck Shannon. 583 pages. 2001. 978-0-7808-0331-2.

"Essential for most collections."
—*Library Journal, Apr 1 '02*

"An ideal addition to the reference collection of any public library. Health sciences information professionals may also want to acquire the Caregiving Sourcebook for their hospital or academic library for use as a ready reference tool by health care workers interested in aging and caregiving."
—*E-Streams, Jan '02*

Child Abuse Sourcebook, 2nd Edition

Basic Consumer Health Information about the Physical, Sexual, and Emotional Abuse of Children, Neglect, Münchhausen Syndrome by Proxy (MSBP), and Shaken Baby Syndrome, and Featuring Facts about Withholding Medical Care, Corporal Punishment, Child Maltreatment in Youth Sports, and Parental Substance Abuse

Along with Information about Child Protective Services, Foster Care, Adoption, Parenting Challenges, Abuse Prevention Programs, and Intervention, Treatment, and Recovery Guidelines, a Glossary of Related Terms, and Resources for Additional Help and Information

Edited by Joyce Brennfleck Shannon. 600 pages. 2009. 978-0-7808-1037-2.

SEE ALSO *Domestic Violence Sourcebook, 3rd Edition*

Childhood Diseases and Disorders Sourcebook, 2nd Edition

Basic Consumer Health Information about the Physical, Mental, and Developmental Health of Pre-Adolescent Children, Including Facts about Infectious Diseases, Asthma, Allergies, Diabetes, and Other Acute and Chronic Conditions Affecting the Gastrointestinal Tract, Ears, Nose, Throat, Liver, Kidneys, Heart, Blood, Brain, Muscles, Bones, and Skin

Along with Reports on Recommended Childhood Vaccinations, Wellness Guidelines, a Glossary of Related Medical Terms, and a List of Resources for Parents

Edited by Sandra J. Judd. 694 pages. 2009. 978-0-7808-1031-0.

"The strength of this source is the wide range of information given about childhood health issues... It is most appropriate for public libraries and academic libraries that field medical questions."
—*American Reference Books Annual, 2009*

SEE ALSO *Healthy Children Sourcebook*

Colds, Flu and Other Common Ailments Sourcebook

Basic Consumer Health Information about Common Ailments and Injuries, Including Colds, Coughs, the Flu, Sinus Problems, Headaches, Fever, Nausea and Vomiting, Menstrual Cramps, Diarrhea, Constipation, Hemorrhoids, Back Pain, Dandruff, Dry and Itchy Skin, Cuts, Scrapes, Sprains, Bruises, and More

Along with Information about Prevention, Self-Care, Choosing a Doctor, Over-the-Counter Medications, Folk Remedies, and Alternative Therapies, and Including a Glossary of Important Terms and a Directory of Resources for Further Help and Information

Edited by Chad T. Kimball. 622 pages. 2001. 978-0-7808-0435-7.

"A good starting point for research on common illnesses. It will be a useful addition to public and consumer health library collections."
—*American Reference Books Annual, 2002*

"Will prove valuable to any library seeking to maintain a current, comprehensive reference collection of health resources... Excellent reference."
—*The Bookwatch, Aug '01*

SEE ALSO Contagious Diseases Sourcebook, 2nd Edition

Communication Disorders Sourcebook

Basic Information about Deafness and Hearing Loss, Speech and Language Disorders, Voice Disorders, Balance and Vestibular Disorders, and Disorders of Smell, Taste, and Touch

Edited by Linda M. Ross. 533 pages. 1996. 978-0-7808-0077-9.

"This is skillfully edited and is a welcome resource for the layperson. It should be found in every public and medical library."
—*Booklist Health Sciences Supplement, Oct '97*

Complementary & Alternative Medicine Sourcebook, 4th Edition

Basic Consumer Health Information about Ayurveda, Acupuncture, Aromatherapy, Chiropractic Care, Diet-Based Therapies, Guided Imagery, Herbal and Vitamin Supplements, Homeopathy, Hypnosis, Massage, Meditation, Naturopathy, Pilates, Reflexology, Reiki, Shiatsu, Tai Chi, Traditional Chinese Medicine, Yoga, and Other Complementary and Alternative Medical Therapies

Along with Statistics, Tips for Selecting a Practitioner, Treatments for Specific Health Conditions, a Glossary of Related Terms, and a Directory of Resources for Additional Help and Information

Edited by Amy L. Sutton. 600 pages. 2010. 978-0-7808-1082-2.

Congenital Disorders Sourcebook, 2nd Edition

Basic Consumer Health Information about Nonhereditary Birth Defects and Disorders

Related to Prematurity, Gestational Injuries, Congenital Infections, and Birth Complications, Including Heart Defects, Hydrocephalus, Spina Bifida, Cleft Lip and Palate, Cerebral Palsy, and More

Along with Facts about the Prevention of Birth Defects, Fetal Surgery and Other Treatment Options, Research Initiatives, a Glossary of Related Terms, and Resources for Additional Information and Support

Edited by Sandra J. Judd. 619 pages. 2007. 978-0-7808-0945-1.

"Congenital Disorders Sourcebook provides an excellent, non-technical overview of many aspects of pregnancy with the focus on congenital disorders."
—*American Reference Books Annual,*
2008

"An excellent readable reference aimed at the lay public for difficult to understand medical problems. An excellent starting point for the interested parent or family member who may then be motivated to seek more information."
—*Doody's Review Service,*
2007

SEE ALSO Pregnancy and Birth Sourcebook,
3rd Edition

Contagious Diseases Sourcebook, 2nd Edition
Basic Consumer Health Information about Diseases Spread from Person to Person through Direct Physical Contact, Airborne Transmissions, Sexual Contact, or Contact with Blood or Other Body Fluids, Including Pneumococcal, Staphylococcal, and Streptococcal Diseases, Colds, Influenza, Lice, Measles, Mumps, Tuberculosis, and Others

Along with Facts about Self-Care and Over-the-Counter Medications, Antibiotics and Drug Resistance, Disease Prevention, Vaccines, and Bioterrorism, a Glossary, and a Directory of Resources for More Information

Edited by Joyce Brennfleck Shannon. 600 pages. 2010. 978-0-7808-1075-4.

SEE ALSO AIDS Sourcebook, 4th Edition,
Hepatitis Sourcebook

Cosmetic and Reconstructive Surgery Sourcebook, 2nd Edition
Basic Consumer Information about Plastic Surgery and Non-Surgical Appearance-Enhancing Procedures, Including Facts about Botulinum Toxin, Collagen Replacement, Dermabrasion, Chemical Peels, Eyelid Surgery, Nose Reshaping, Lip Augmentation, Liposuction, Breast Enlargement and Reduction, Tummy Tucking, and Other Skin, Hair, Facial, and Body Shaping Procedures

Along with Information about Reconstructive Procedures for Congenital Disorders, Disfiguring Diseases, Burns, and Traumatic Injuries, a Glossary of Related Terms, and a Directory of Additional Resources

Edited by Karen Bellenir. 483 pages. 2007. 978-0-7808-0951-2.

"A comprehensive source for people considering cosmetic surgery... also recommended for medical students who will perform these procedures later in their careers; and public librarians and academic medical librarians who may assist patrons interested in this information."
—*Medical Reference Services Quarterly,*
Fall '08

"A practical guide for health care consumers and health care workers... This easy-to-read reference guide would be useful for novice and veteran health care consumers, surgical technology students, nursing students, and perioperative nurses new to plastic and reconstructive surgery. It also may be helpful for medical-surgical nurses as a guide for patient teaching in their practices."
—*AORN Journal, Aug '08*

SEE ALSO Surgery Sourcebook, 2nd Edition

Death and Dying Sourcebook, 2nd Edition
Basic Consumer Health Information about End-of-Life Care and Related Perspectives and Ethical Issues, Including End-of-Life Symptoms and Treatments, Pain Management, Quality-of-Life Concerns, the Use of Life Support, Patients' Rights and Privacy Issues, Advance Directives, Physician-Assisted Suicide, Caregiving, Organ and Tissue Donation, Autopsies, Funeral Arrangements, and Grief

Along with Statistical Data, Information about the Leading Causes of Death, a Glossary, and Directories of Support Groups and Other Resources

Edited by Joyce Brennfleck Shannon. 626 pages. 2006. 978-0-7808-0871-3.

Dental Care and Oral Health Sourcebook, 3rd Edition

Basic Consumer Health Information about Dental Care and Oral Health Throughout the Lifespan, Including Facts about Cavities, Bad Breath, Cold and Canker Sores, Dry Mouth, Toothaches, Gum Disease, Malocclusion, Temporomandibular Joint and Muscle Disorders, Oral Cancers, and Dental Emergencies

Along with Information about Mouth Hygiene, Crowns, Bridges, Implants, and Fillings, Surgical, Orthodontic, and Cosmetic Dental Procedures, Pain Management, Health Conditions that Impact Oral Care, a Glossary of Related Terms, and a Directory of Additional Resources

Edited by Amy L. Sutton. 619 pages. 2008. 978-0-7808-1032-7.

"Could serve as turning point in the battle to educate consumers in issues concerning oral health. Tightly written in terms the average person can understand, yet comprehensive in scope and authoritative in tone, it is another excellent sourcebook in the Health Reference Series... Should be in the reference department of all public libraries, and in academic libraries that have a public constituency."
—American Reference Books Annual, 2009

Depression Sourcebook, 2nd Edition

Basic Consumer Health Information about Unipolar Depression, Bipolar Disorder, Dysthymia, Seasonal Affective Disorder, Postpartum Depression, and Other Depressive Disorders, Including Facts about Populations at Special Risk, Coexisting Medical Conditions, Symptoms, Treatment Options, and Suicide Prevention

Along with Statistical Data, a Glossary of Related Terms, and a Directory of Resources for Additional Help and Information

Edited by Sandra J. Judd. 646 pages. 2008. 978-0-7808-1003-7.

"Recommended for public libraries."
—American Reference Books Annual, 2009

SEE ALSO *Mental Health Disorders Sourcebook, 4th Edition*

Dermatological Disorders Sourcebook, 2nd Edition

Basic Consumer Health Information about Conditions and Disorders Affecting the Skin, Hair, and Nails, Such as Acne, Rosacea, Rashes, Dermatitis, Pigmentation Disorders, Birthmarks, Skin Cancer, Skin Injuries, Psoriasis, Scleroderma, and Hair Loss, Including Facts about Medications and Treatments for Dermatological Disorders and Tips for Maintaining Healthy Skin, Hair, and Nails

Along with Information about How Aging Affects the Skin, a Glossary of Related Terms, and a Directory of Resources for Additional Help and Information

Edited by Amy L. Sutton. 617 pages. 2006. 978-0-7808-0795-2.

"Well organized... presents a plethora of information in a manner that is appropriate in style and readability for the intended audience."
—Physical Therapy, Nov '06

"Helpfully brings together... sources in one convenient place, saving the user hours of research time."
—American Reference Books Annual, 2006

SEE ALSO *Burns Sourcebook*

Diabetes Sourcebook, 4th Edition

Basic Consumer Health Information about Type 1 and Type 2 Diabetes Mellitus, Gestational Diabetes, Monogenic Forms of Diabetes, and Insulin Resistance, with Guidelines for Lifestyle Modifications and the Medical Management of Diabetes, Including Facts about Insulin, Insulin Delivery Devices, Oral Diabetes Medications, Self-Monitoring of Blood Glucose, Meal Planning, Physical Activity Recommendations, Foot Care, and Treatment Options for People with Kidney Failure

Along with a Section about Diabetes Complications and Co-Occurring Conditions, a Glossary

of Related Terms, and Directories of Resources for Additional Help and Information

Edited by Karen Bellenir. 627 pages. 2008. 978-0-7808-1005-1.

"Completely and comprehensively covering almost everything a student or physician would need to know... well worth the investment."
— *Internet Bookwatch, Dec '08*

SEE ALSO *Endocrine and Metabolic Disorders Sourcebook, 2nd Edition*

Diet and Nutrition Sourcebook, 3rd Edition

Basic Consumer Health Information about Dietary Guidelines and the Food Guidance System, Recommended Daily Nutrient Intakes, Serving Proportions, Weight Control, Vitamins and Supplements, Nutrition Issues for Different Life Stages and Lifestyles, and the Needs of People with Specific Medical Concerns, Including Cancer, Celiac Disease, Diabetes, Eating Disorders, Food Allergies, and Cardiovascular Disease

Along with Facts about Federal Nutrition Support Programs, a Glossary of Nutrition and Dietary Terms, and Directories of Additional Resources for More Information about Nutrition

Edited by Joyce Brennfleck Shannon. 605 pages. 2006. 978-0-7808-0800-3.

"A valuable resource tool for any individual."
— *Journal of Dental Hygiene, Apr '07*

"From different recommended eating habits to reduce disease and common ailments to nutrition advice for those with specific conditions, Diet and Nutrition Sourcebook is especially important because so much is changing in this area, and so rapidly."
— *California Bookwatch, Jun '06*

SEE ALSO *Eating Disorders Sourcebook, 2nd Edition, Vegetarian Sourcebook*

Digestive Diseases and Disorders Sourcebook

Basic Consumer Health Information about Diseases and Disorders that Impact the Upper and Lower Digestive System, Including Celiac Disease, Constipation, Crohn's Disease, Cyclic Vomiting Syndrome, Diarrhea, Diverticulosis and Diverticulitis, Gallstones, Heartburn, Hemorrhoids, Hernias, Indigestion (Dyspepsia), Irritable Bowel Syndrome, Lactose Intolerance, Ulcers, and More

Along with Information about Medications and Other Treatments, Tips for Maintaining a Healthy Digestive Tract, a Glossary, and Directory of Digestive Diseases Organizations

Edited by Karen Bellenir. 323 pages. 2000. 978-0-7808-0327-5.

"An excellent addition to all public or patient-research libraries."
— *American Reference Books Annual, 2001*

"Recommended reference source."
— *Booklist, May '00*

SEE ALSO *Gastrointestinal Diseases and Disorders Sourcebook, 2nd Edition*

Disabilities Sourcebook

Basic Consumer Health Information about Physical and Psychiatric Disabilities, Including Descriptions of Major Causes of Disability, Assistive and Adaptive Aids, Workplace Issues, and Accessibility Concerns

Along with Information about the Americans with Disabilities Act, a Glossary, and Resources for Additional Help and Information

Edited by Dawn D. Matthews. 602 pages. 2000. 978-0-7808-0389-3.

"A must for libraries with a consumer health section."
— *American Reference Books Annual, 2002*

"A much needed addition to the Omnigraphics Health Reference Series. A current reference work to provide people with disabilities, their families, caregivers or those who work with them, a broad range of information in one volume, has not been available until now... It is recommended for all public and academic library reference collections."
— *E-Streams, May '01*

"An excellent source book in easy-to-read format covering many current topics; highly recommended for all libraries."
— *CHOICE, Jan '01*

Disease Management Sourcebook

Basic Consumer Health Information about Coping with Chronic and Serious Illnesses, Navigating the Health Care System, Communicating with Health Care Providers, Assessing Health Care Quality, and Making Informed Health Care Decisions, Including Facts about Second Opinions, Hospitalization, Surgery, and Medications

Along with a Section about Children with Chronic Conditions, Information about Legal, Financial, and Insurance Issues, a Glossary of Related Terms, and Directories of Additional Resources

Edited by Joyce Brennfleck Shannon. 621 pages. 2008. 978-0-7808-1002-0.

"Consumers need to know how to manage their health care the same way they manage anything else in their lives. The text is very readable and is written for the layperson and consumer. The cost is not prohibitive. This book should be in all collections of health care libraries and public libraries."
— *American Reference Books Annual, 2009*

"The information is very current, and the selection of font and layout make the book easy to read. A hardback that will stand up to much usage, this is an excellent resource for consumers... Recommended. General readers."
—*CHOICE, Nov '08*

"Intended for lay readers, this resource clarifies the many confusing and overwhelming details associated with chronic disease care. Meticulous and clearly explained, the book even includes diagrams intended to ease comprehension of over-the-counter medication labels. An essential guide to navigating the health-care rapids."
—*Library Journal, Aug '08*

Domestic Violence Sourcebook, 3rd Edition

Basic Consumer Health Information about Warning Signs, Risk Factors, and Health Consequences of Intimate Partner Violence, Sexual Violence and Rape, Stalking, Human Trafficking, Child Maltreatment, Teen Dating Violence, and Elder Abuse

Along with Facts about Victims and Perpetrators, Strategies for Violence Prevention, and Emergency Interventions, Safety Plans, and Financial and Legal Tips for Victims, a Glossary of Related Terms, and Directories of Resources for Additional Information and Support

Edited by Joyce Brennfleck Shannon. 634 pages. 2009. 978-0-7808-1038-9.

"A recommended pick for any library interested in consumer health and social issues... A 'must' for any serious health collection."
—*California Bookwatch, Jul '09*

SEE ALSO *Child Abuse Sourcebook, 2nd Edition*

Drug Abuse Sourcebook, 3rd Edition

Basic Consumer Health Information about the Abuse of Cocaine, Club Drugs, Hallucinogens, Heroin, Inhalants, Marijuana, and Other Illicit Substances, Prescription Medications, and Over-the-Counter Medicines

Along with Facts about Addiction and Related Health Effects, Drug Abuse Treatment and Recovery, Drug Testing, Prevention Programs, Glossaries of Drug-Related Terms, and Directories of Resources for More Information

Edited by Joyce Brennfleck Shannon. 600 pages. 2010. 978-0-7808-1079-2.

SEE ALSO *Alcoholism Sourcebook, 3rd Edition*

Ear, Nose, and Throat Disorders Sourcebook, 2nd Edition

Basic Consumer Health Information about Disorders of the Ears, Hearing Loss, Vestibular Disorders, Nasal and Sinus Problems, Throat and Vocal Cord Disorders, and Otolaryngologic Cancers, Including Facts about Ear Infections and Injuries, Genetic and Congenital Deafness, Sensorineural Hearing Disorders, Tinnitus, Vertigo, Ménière Disease, Rhinitis, Sinusitis, Snoring, Sore Throats, Hoarseness, and More

Along with Reports on Current Research Initiatives, a Glossary of Related Medical Terms, and a Directory of Sources for Further Help and Information

Edited by Sandra J. Judd. 631 pages. 2007. 978-0-7808-0872-0.

"A resource book for the general public that provides comprehensive coverage of basic up-to-date medical information about the causes, symptoms, diagnosis, and treatment of diseases and disorders that affect the ears, nose, sinuses, throat, and voice... The majority of information is presented in question and answer format, much like questions a patient might ask of a health care provider. An extensive index facilitates the reader's ability to easily access information on any specific topic."
—*Journal of Dental Hygiene, Oct '07*

"A handy compilation of information on common and some not so common ailments of the ears, nose, and throat."
—*Doody's Review Service, 2007*

Eating Disorders Sourcebook, 2nd Edition

Basic Consumer Health Information about Anorexia Nervosa, Bulimia, Binge Eating, Compulsive Exercise, Female Athlete Triad, and Other Eating Disorders, Including Facts about Body Image and Other Cultural and Age-Related Risk Factors, Prevention Efforts, Adverse Health Effects, Treatment Options, and the Recovery Process

Along with Guidelines for Healthy Weight Control, a Glossary, and Directories of Additional Resources

Edited by Joyce Brennfleck Shannon. 557 pages. 2007. 978-0-7808-0948-2.

"Recommended for the reference collection of large public libraries."
—*American Reference Books Annual, 2008*

"A basic health reference any health or general library needs."
—*Internet Bookwatch, Jun '07*

SEE ALSO *Diet and Nutrition Sourcebook, 3rd Edition, Mental Health Disorders Sourcebook, 4th Edition*

Emergency Medical Services Sourcebook

Basic Consumer Health Information about Preventing, Preparing for, and Managing Emergency Situations, When and Who to Call for Help, What to Expect in the Emergency Room, the Emergency Medical Team,

Patient Issues, and Current Topics in Emergency Medicine

Along with Statistical Data, a Glossary, and Sources of Additional Help and Information

Edited by Jenni Lynn Colson. 472 pages. 2002. 978-0-7808-0420-3.

"Handy and convenient for home, public, school, and college libraries. Recommended."
—*CHOICE, Apr '03*

"This reference can provide the consumer with answers to most questions about emergency care in the United States, or it will direct them to a resource where the answer can be found."
—*American Reference Books Annual, 2003*

SEE ALSO *Injury and Trauma Sourcebook*

Endocrine and Metabolic Disorders Sourcebook, 2nd Edition

Basic Consumer Health Information about Hormonal and Metabolic Disorders that Affect the Body's Growth, Development, and Functioning, Including Disorders of the Pancreas, Ovaries and Testes, and Pituitary, Thyroid, Parathyroid, and Adrenal Glands, with Facts about Growth Disorders, Addison Disease, Cushing Syndrome, Conn Syndrome, Diabetic Disorders, Multiple Endocrine Neoplasia, Inborn Errors of Metabolism, and More

Along with Information about Endocrine Functioning, Diagnostic and Screening Tests, a Glossary of Related Terms, and Directories of Additional Resources

Edited by Joyce Brennfleck Shannon. 597 pages. 2007. 978-0-7808-0952-9.

SEE ALSO *Diabetes Sourcebook, 4th Edition*

Environmental Health Sourcebook, 3rd Edition

Basic Consumer Health Information about the Environment and Its Effects on Human Health, Including Facts about Air, Water, and Soil Contamination, Hazardous Chemicals, Foodborne Hazards and Illnesses, Household Hazards Such as Radon, Mold, and Carbon Monoxide, Consumer Hazards from Toxic Products and Imported Goods, and Disorders

Linked to Environmental Causes, Including Chemical Sensitivity, Cancer, Allergies, and Asthma

Along with Information about the Impact of Environmental Hazards on Specific Populations, a Glossary of Related Terms, and Resources for Additional Help and Information.

Edited by Laura Larsen. 600 pages. 2010. 978-0-7808-1078-5

Ethnic Diseases Sourcebook

Basic Consumer Health Information for Ethnic and Racial Minority Groups in the United States, Including General Health Indicators and Behaviors, Ethnic Diseases, Genetic Testing, the Impact of Chronic Diseases, Women's Health, Mental Health Issues, and Preventive Health Care Services

Along with a Glossary and a Listing of Additional Resources

Edited by Joyce Brennfleck Shannon. 648 pages. 2001. 978-0-7808-0336-7.

"Not many books have been written on this topic to date, and the Ethnic Diseases Sourcebook is a strong addition to the list. It will be an important introductory resource for health consumers, students, health care personnel, and social scientists. It is recommended for public, academic, and large hospital libraries."

— American Reference Books Annual, 2002

"Will prove valuable to any library seeking to maintain a current, comprehensive reference collection of health resources... An excellent source of health information about genetic disorders which affect particular ethnic and racial minorities in the U.S."

—The Bookwatch, Aug '01

Eye Care Sourcebook, 3rd Edition

Basic Consumer Health Information about Eye Care and Eye Disorders, Including Facts about the Diagnosis, Prevention, and Treatment of Refractive Disorders, Cataracts, Glaucoma, Macular Degeneration, and Problems Affecting the Cornea, Retina, and Lacrimal Glands

Along with Advice about Preventing Eye Injuries and Tips for Living with Low Vision or

Blindness, a Glossary of Related Terms, and Directories of Resources for More Help and Information

Edited by Amy L. Sutton. 646 pages. 2008. 978-0-7808-1000-6.

"A solid reference tool for eye care and a valuable addition to a collection."
—American Reference Books Annual, 2009

Family Planning Sourcebook

Basic Consumer Health Information about Planning for Pregnancy and Contraception, Including Traditional Methods, Barrier Methods, Hormonal Methods, Permanent Methods, Future Methods, Emergency Contraception, and Birth Control Choices for Women at Each Stage of Life

Along with Statistics, a Glossary, and Sources of Additional Information

Edited by Amy Marcaccio Keyzer. 503 pages. 2001. 978-0-7808-0379-4.

"Recommended for public, health, and undergraduate libraries as part of the circulating collection."
—E-Streams, Mar '02

"Will prove valuable to any library seeking to maintain a current, comprehensive reference collection of health resources... Excellent reference."
—The Bookwatch, Aug '01

SEE ALSO Pregnancy and Birth Sourcebook, 3rd Edition

Fitness and Exercise Sourcebook, 3rd Edition

Basic Consumer Health Information about the Physical and Mental Benefits of Fitness, Including Cardiorespiratory Endurance, Muscular Strength, Muscular Endurance, and Flexibility, with Facts about Sports Nutrition and Exercise-Related Injuries and Tips about Physical Activity and Exercises for People of All Ages and for People with Health Concerns

Along with Advice on Selecting and Using Exercise Equipment, Maintaining Exercise Motivation, a Glossary of Related Terms, and a Directory of Resources for More Help and Information

Edited by Amy L. Sutton. 635 pages. 2007. 978-0-7808-0946-8.

"Updates the consumer information on the physical and mental benefits of physical activity throughout the lifespan offered in earlier editions... Recommended. All readers; all levels."
—*CHOICE, Oct '07*

"An exceptionally well-rounded coverage perfect for any concerned about developing and understanding a fitness program."
—*California Bookwatch, Jun '07*

SEE ALSO *Sports Injuries Sourcebook, 3rd Edition*

Food Safety Sourcebook

Basic Consumer Health Information about the Safe Handling of Meat, Poultry, Seafood, Eggs, Fruit Juices, and Other Food Items, and Facts about Pesticides, Drinking Water, Food Safety Overseas, and the Onset, Duration, and Symptoms of Foodborne Illnesses, Including Types of Pathogenic Bacteria, Parasitic Protozoa, Worms, Viruses, and Natural Toxins

Along with the Role of the Consumer, the Food Handler, and the Government in Food Safety, a Glossary, and Resources for Additional Help and Information

Edited by Dawn D. Matthews. 327 pages. 1999. 978-0-7808-0326-8.

"Recommended reference source."
—*Booklist, May '00*

"This book takes the complex issues of food safety and foodborne pathogens and presents them in an easily understood manner. [It does] an excellent job of covering a large and often confusing topic."
— *American Reference Books Annual, 2000*

Forensic Medicine Sourcebook

Basic Consumer Information for the Layperson about Forensic Medicine, Including Crime Scene Investigation, Evidence Collection and Analysis, Expert Testimony, Computer-Aided Criminal Identification, Digital Imaging in the Courtroom, DNA Profiling, Accident Reconstruction, Autopsies, Ballistics, Drugs and Explosives Detection, Latent Fingerprints,

Product Tampering, and Questioned Document Examination

Along with Statistical Data, a Glossary of Forensics Terminology, and Listings of Sources for Further Help and Information

Edited by Annemarie S. Muth. 574 pages. 1999. 978-0-7808-0232-2.

"Given the expected widespread interest in its content and its easy to read style, this book is recommended for most public and all college and university libraries."
—*E-Streams, Feb '01*

"A wealth of information, useful statistics, references are up-to-date and extremely complete. This wonderful collection of data will help students who are interested in a career in any type of forensic field. It is a great resource for attorneys who need information about types of expert witnesses needed in a particular case. It also offers useful information for fiction and nonfiction writers whose work involves a crime. A fascinating compilation. All levels."
—*CHOICE, Jan '00*

"There are several items that make this book attractive to consumers who are seeking certain forensic data... This is a useful current source for those seeking general forensic medical answers."
—*American Reference Books Annual, 2000*

Gastrointestinal Diseases and Disorders Sourcebook, 2nd Edition

Basic Consumer Health Information about the Upper and Lower Gastrointestinal (GI) Tract, Including the Esophagus, Stomach, Intestines, Rectum, Liver, and Pancreas, with Facts about Gastroesophageal Reflux Disease, Gastritis, Hernias, Ulcers, Celiac Disease, Diverticulitis, Irritable Bowel Syndrome, Hemorrhoids, Gastrointestinal Cancers, and Other Diseases and Disorders Related to the Digestive Process

Along with Information about Commonly Used Diagnostic and Surgical Procedures, Statistics, Reports on Current Research Initiatives and Clinical Trials, a Glossary, and Resources for Additional Help and Information

Edited by Sandra J. Judd. 654 pages. 2006. 978-0-7808-0798-3.

"The text is designed for the general reader seeking information on prevention, disease warning signs, diagnostic and therapeutic questions... It is an excellent resource for the general reader to conveniently locate credible, coordinated and indexed information... The sourcebook will prove very helpful for patients, caregivers and should be available in every physician waiting room."
—*Doody's Review Service, 2006*

SEE ALSO *Diet and Nutrition Sourcebook, 3rd Edition, Digestive Diseases and Disorders Sourcebook*

Genetic Disorders Sourcebook, 4th Edition

Basic Consumer Health Information about Hereditary Diseases and Disorders, Including Facts about the Human Genome, Genetic Inheritance Patterns, Disorders Associated with Specific Genes, Such as Sickle Cell Disease, Hemophilia, and Cystic Fibrosis, Chromosome Disorders, Such as Down Syndrome, Fragile X Syndrome, and Turner Syndrome, and Complex Diseases and Disorders Resulting from the Interaction of Environmental and Genetic Factors, Such as Allergies, Cancer, and Obesity

Along with Facts about Genetic Testing, Suggestions for Parents of Children with Special Needs, Reports on Current Research Initiatives, a Glossary of Genetic Terminology, and Resources for Additional Help and Information

Edited by Sandra J. Judd. 600 pages. 2010. 978-0-7808-1076-1.

Head Trauma Sourcebook

Basic Information for the Layperson about Open-Head and Closed-Head Injuries, Treatment Advances, Recovery, and Rehabilitation

Along with Reports on Current Research Initiatives

Edited by Karen Bellenir. 414 pages. 1997. 978-0-7808-0208-7.

Headache Sourcebook

Basic Consumer Health Information about Migraine, Tension, Cluster, Rebound and Other Types of Headaches, with Facts about the Cause and Prevention of Headaches, the Effects of Stress and the Environment, Headaches during Pregnancy and Menopause, and Childhood Headaches

Along with a Glossary and Other Resources for Additional Help and Information

Edited by Dawn D. Matthews. 342 pages. 2002. 978-0-7808-0337-4.

"Highly recommended for academic and medical reference collections."
—*Library Bookwatch, Sep '02*

SEE ALSO *Pain Sourcebook, 3rd Edition*

Healthy Aging Sourcebook

Basic Consumer Health Information about Maintaining Health through the Aging Process, Including Advice on Nutrition, Exercise, and Sleep, Help in Making Decisions about Midlife Issues and Retirement, and Guidance Concerning Practical and Informed Choices in Health Consumerism

Along with Data Concerning the Theories of Aging, Different Experiences in Aging by Minority Groups, and Facts about Aging Now and Aging in the Future; and Featuring a Glossary, a Guide to Consumer Help, Additional Suggested Reading, and Practical Resource Directory

Edited by Jenifer Swanson. 537 pages. 1999. 978-0-7808-0390-9.

"Recommended reference source."
—*Booklist, Feb '00*

SEE ALSO *Adult Health Sourcebook, Physical and Mental Issues in Aging Sourcebook*

Healthy Children Sourcebook

Basic Consumer Health Information about the Physical and Mental Development of Children between the Ages of 3 and 12, Including Routine Health Care, Preventative Health Services, Safety and First Aid, Healthy Sleep, Dental Care, Nutrition, and Fitness, and Featuring Parenting Tips on Such Topics as Bedwetting, Choosing Day Care, Monitoring TV and Other Media, and Establishing a Foundation for Substance Abuse Prevention

Along with a Glossary of Commonly Used Pediatric Terms and Resources for Additional Help and Information.

Edited by Chad T. Kimball. 624 pages. 2003. 978-0-7808-0247-6.

"Should be required reading for parents and teachers."
—E-Streams, Jun '04

"It is hard to imagine that any other single resource exists that would provide such a comprehensive guide of timely information on health promotion and disease prevention for children aged 3 to 12."
—American Reference Books Annual, 2004

"This easy-to-read volume is a tremendous resource."
—AORN Journal, May '05

SEE ALSO Childhood Diseases and Disorders Sourcebook, 2nd Edition

Healthy Heart Sourcebook for Women

Basic Consumer Health Information about Cardiac Issues Specific to Women, Including Facts about Major Risk Factors and Prevention, Treatment and Control Strategies, and Important Dietary Issues

Along with a Special Section Regarding the Pros and Cons of Hormone Replacement Therapy and Its Impact on Heart Health, and Additional Help, Including Recipes, a Glossary, and a Directory of Resources

Edited by Dawn D. Matthews. 321 pages. 2000. 978-0-7808-0329-9.

"A good reference source and recommended for all public, academic, medical, and hospital libraries."
—Medical Reference Services Quarterly, Summer '01

"Contains very important information about coronary artery disease that all women should know. The information is current and presented in an easy-to-read format. The book will make a good addition to any library."
—American Medical Writers Association Journal, Summer '00

SEE ALSO Cardiovascular Diseases and Disorders Sourcebook, 4th Edition, Women's Health Concerns Sourcebook, 3rd Edition

Hepatitis Sourcebook

Basic Consumer Health Information about Hepatitis A, Hepatitis B, Hepatitis C, and Other Forms of Hepatitis, Including Autoimmune Hepatitis, Alcoholic Hepatitis, Nonalcoholic Steatohepatitis, and Toxic Hepatitis, with Facts about Risk Factors, Screening Methods, Diagnostic Tests, and Treatment Options

Along with Information on Liver Health, Tips for People Living with Chronic Hepatitis, Reports on Current Research Initiatives, a Glossary of Terms Related to Hepatitis, and a Directory of Sources for Further Help and Information

Edited by Sandra J. Judd. 570 pages. 2006. 978-0-7808-0749-5.

"The breadth of information found in this one book would not be readily found in another source. Highly recommended."
—American Reference Books Annual, 2006

SEE ALSO Contagious Diseases Sourcebook, 2nd Edition

Household Safety Sourcebook

Basic Consumer Health Information about Household Safety, Including Information about Poisons, Chemicals, Fire, and Water Hazards in the Home

Along with Advice about the Safe Use of Home Maintenance Equipment, Choosing Toys and Nursery Furniture, Holiday and Recreation Safety, a Glossary, and Resources for Further Help and Information

Edited by Dawn D. Matthews. 587 pages. 2002. 978-0-7808-0338-1.

"As a sourcebook on household safety this book meets its mark. It is encyclopedic in scope and covers a wide range of safety issues that are commonly seen in the home."
—E-Streams, Jul '02

Hypertension Sourcebook

Basic Consumer Health Information about the Causes, Diagnosis, and Treatment of High Blood Pressure, with Facts about Consequences, Complications, and Co-Occurring Disorders, Such as Coronary Heart Disease, Diabetes, Stroke, Kidney Disease, and Hypertensive Retinopathy, and Issues in Blood Pressure

Control, Including Dietary Choices, Stress Management, and Medications

Along with Reports on Current Research Initiatives and Clinical Trials, a Glossary, and Resources for Additional Help and Information

Edited by Dawn D. Matthews and Karen Bellenir. 588 pages. 2004. 978-0-7808-0674-0.

"Academic, public, and medical libraries will want to add the Hypertension Sourcebook to their collections."

—E-Streams, Aug '05

"The strength of this source is the wide range of information given about hypertension."

—American Reference Books Annual, 2005

SEE ALSO Stroke Sourcebook, 2nd Edition

Immune System Disorders Sourcebook, 2nd Edition

Basic Consumer Health Information about Disorders of the Immune System, Including Immune System Function and Response, Diagnosis of Immune Disorders, Information about Inherited Immune Disease, Acquired Immune Disease, and Autoimmune Diseases, Including Primary Immune Deficiency, Acquired Immunodeficiency Syndrome (AIDS), Lupus, Multiple Sclerosis, Type 1 Diabetes, Rheumatoid Arthritis, and Graves' Disease

Along with Treatments, Tips for Coping with Immune Disorders, a Glossary, and a Directory of Additional Resources

Edited by Joyce Brennfleck Shannon. 643 pages. 2005. 978-0-7808-0748-8.

"Highly recommended for academic and public libraries."

—American Reference Books Annual, 2006

"The updated second edition is a 'must' for any consumer health library seeking a solid resource covering the treatments, symptoms, and options for immune disorder sufferers... An excellent guide."

—MBR Bookwatch, Jan '06

SEE ALSO AIDS Sourcebook, 4th Edition, Arthritis Sourcebook, 3rd Edition

Infant and Toddler Health Sourcebook

Basic Consumer Health Information about the Physical and Mental Development of Newborns, Infants, and Toddlers, Including Neonatal Concerns, Nutrition Recommendations, Immunization Schedules, Common Pediatric Disorders, Assessments and Milestones, Safety Tips, and Advice for Parents and Other Caregivers

Along with a Glossary of Terms and Resource Listings for Additional Help

Edited by Jenifer Swanson. 570 pages. 2000. 978-0-7808-0246-9.

"As a reference for the general public, this would be useful in any library."

—E-Streams, May '01

"Recommended reference source."

—Booklist, Feb '01

Infectious Diseases Sourcebook

Basic Consumer Health Information about Non-Contagious Bacterial, Viral, Prion, Fungal, and Parasitic Diseases Spread by Food and Water, Insects and Animals, or Environmental Contact, Including Botulism, E. Coli, Encephalitis, Legionnaires' Disease, Lyme Disease, Malaria, Plague, Rabies, Salmonella, Tetanus, and Others, and Facts about Newly Emerging Diseases, Such as Hantavirus, Mad Cow Disease, Monkeypox, and West Nile Virus

Along with Information about Preventing Disease Transmission, the Threat of Bioterrorism, and Current Research Initiatives, with a Glossary and Directory of Resources for More Information

Edited by Karen Bellenir. 610 pages. 2004. 978-0-7808-0675-7.

"This reference continues the excellent tradition of the Health Reference Series in consolidating a wealth of information on a selected topic into a format that is easy to use and accessible to the general public."

—American Reference Books Annual, 2005

"Recommended for public and academic libraries."

—E-Streams, Jan '05

SEE ALSO Environmental Health Sourcebook, 3rd Edition

Injury and Trauma Sourcebook

Basic Consumer Health Information about the Impact of Injury, the Diagnosis and Treatment of Common and Traumatic Injuries, Emergency Care, and Specific Injuries Related to Home, Community, Workplace, Transportation, and Recreation

Along with Guidelines for Injury Prevention, a Glossary, and a Directory of Additional Resources

Edited by Joyce Brennfleck Shannon. 675 pages. 2002. 978-0-7808-0421-0.

"Practitioners should be aware of guides such as this in order to facilitate their use by patients and their families."
— *Doody's Health Sciences Book Review Journal, Sep-Oct '02*

"Recommended reference source."
— *Booklist, Sep '02*

"Highly recommended for academic and medical reference collections."
— *Library Bookwatch, Sep '02*

SEE ALSO *Emergency Medical Services Sourcebook, Sports Injuries Sourcebook, 3rd Edition*

Learning Disabilities Sourcebook, 3rd Edition

Basic Consumer Health Information about Dyslexia, Auditory and Visual Processing Disorders, Communication Disorders, Dyscalculia, Dysgraphia, and Other Conditions That Impede Learning, Including Attention Deficit/ Hyperactivity Disorder, Autism Spectrum Disorders, Hearing and Visual Impairments, Chromosome-Based Disorders, and Brain Injury

Along with Facts about Brain Function, Assessment, Therapy and Remediation, Accommodations, Assistive Technology, Legal Protections, and Tips about Family Life, School Transitions, and Employment Strategies, a Glossary of Related Terms, and Directories of Additional Resources

Edited by Joyce Brennfleck Shannon. 613 pages. 2009. 978-0-7808-1039-6.

"Intended to be a starting point for people who need to know about learning disabilities. Each chapter on a specific disability includes readable,

well-organized descriptions... The book is well indexed and a glossary is included. Chapters on organizations and helpful websites will aid the reader who needs more information."
— *American Reference Books Annual, 2009*

"This book provides the necessary information to better understand learning disabilities and work with children who have them... It would be difficult to find another book that so comprehensively explains learning disabilities without becoming incomprehensible to the average parent who needs this information."
— *Doody's Review Service, 2009*

SEE ALSO *Attention Deficit Disorder Sourcebook, Autism and Pervasive Developmental Disorders Sourcebook*

Leukemia Sourcebook

Basic Consumer Health Information about Adult and Childhood Leukemias, Including Acute Lymphocytic Leukemia (ALL), Chronic Lymphocytic Leukemia (CLL), Acute Myelogenous Leukemia (AML), Chronic Myelogenous Leukemia (CML), and Hairy Cell Leukemia, and Treatments Such as Chemotherapy, Radiation Therapy, Peripheral Blood Stem Cell and Marrow Transplantation, and Immunotherapy

Along with Tips for Life During and After Treatment, a Glossary, and Directories of Additional Resources

Edited by Joyce Brennfleck Shannon. 564 pages. 2003. 978-0-7808-0627-6.

"Unlike other medical books for the layperson... the language does not talk down to the reader... This volume is highly recommended for all libraries."
— *American Reference Books Annual, 2004*

"A fine title which ranges from diagnosis to alternative treatments, staging, and tips for life during and after diagnosis."
— *The Bookwatch, Dec '03*

SEE ALSO *Blood & Circulatory Disorders Sourcebook, 3rd Edition, Cancer Sourcebook, 5th Edition*

Liver Disorders Sourcebook

Basic Consumer Health Information about the Liver and How It Works; Liver Diseases, Including Cancer, Cirrhosis, Hepatitis, and

Toxic and Drug Related Diseases; Tips for Maintaining a Healthy Liver; Laboratory Tests, Radiology Tests, and Facts about Liver Transplantation

Along with a Section on Support Groups, a Glossary, and Resource Listings

Edited by Joyce Brennfleck Shannon. 580 pages. 2000. 978-0-7808-0383-1.

"This title is recommended for health sciences and public libraries with consumer health collections."
—E-Streams, Oct '00

"Recommended reference source."
—Booklist, Jun '00

SEE ALSO *Gastrointestinal Diseases and Disorders Sourcebook, 2nd Edition, Hepatitis Sourcebook*

Lung Disorders Sourcebook

Basic Consumer Health Information about Emphysema, Pneumonia, Tuberculosis, Asthma, Cystic Fibrosis, and Other Lung Disorders, Including Facts about Diagnostic Procedures, Treatment Strategies, Disease Prevention Efforts, and Such Risk Factors as Smoking, Air Pollution, and Exposure to Asbestos, Radon, and Other Agents

Along with a Glossary and Resources for Additional Help and Information

Edited by Dawn D. Matthews. 657 pages. 2002. 978-0-7808-0339-8.

"Highly recommended for academic and medical reference collections."
—Library Bookwatch, Sep '02

SEE ALSO *Asthma Sourcebook, 2nd Edition, Respiratory Disorders Sourcebook, 2nd Edition*

Medical Tests Sourcebook, 3rd Edition

Basic Consumer Health Information about X-Rays, Blood Tests, Stool and Urine Tests, Biopsies, Mammography, Endoscopic Procedures, Ultrasound Exams, Computed Tomography, Magnetic Resonance Imaging (MRI), Nuclear Medicine, Genetic Testing, Home-Use Tests, and More

Along with Facts about Preventive Care and Screening Test Guidelines, Screening and

Assessment Tests Associated with Such Specific Concerns as Cancer, Heart Disease, Allergies, Diabetes, Thyroid Disfunction, and Infertility, a Glossary of Related Terms, and a Directory of Resources for Additional Help and Information

Edited by Karen Bellenir. 627 pages. 2008. 978-0-7808-1040-2

"This volume has a wide scope that makes it useful... Can be a valuable reference guide."
—American Reference Books Annual, 2009

"Would be a valuable contribution to any consumer health or public library."
—Doody's Book Review Service, 2009

Men's Health Concerns Sourcebook, 3rd Edition

Basic Consumer Health Information about Wellness in Men and Gender-Related Differences in Health, With Facts about Heart Disease, Cancer, Traumatic Injury, and Other Leading Causes of Death in Men, Reproductive Concerns, Sexual Dysfunction, Disorders of the Prostate, Penis, and Testes, Sex-Linked Genetic Disorders, and Other Medical and Mental Concerns of Men

Along with Statistical Data, a Glossary of Related Terms, and a Directory of Resources for Additional Information

Edited by Sandra J. Judd. 632 pages. 2009. 978-0-7808-1033-4.

"A good addition to any reference shelf in academic, consumer health, or hospital libraries."
—ARBAOnline, Oct '09

SEE ALSO *Prostate and Urological Disorders Sourcebook*

Mental Health Disorders Sourcebook, 4th Edition

Basic Consumer Health Information about the Causes and Symptoms of Mental Health Problems, Including Depression, Bipolar Disorder, Anxiety Disorders, Posttraumatic Stress Disorder, Obsessive-Compulsive Disorder, Eating Disorders, Addictions, and Personality and Psychotic Disorders

Along with Information about Medications and Treatments, Mental Health Concerns in

Children, Adolescents, and Adults, Tips on Living with Mental Health Disorders, a Glossary of Related Terms, and a Directory of Resources for Additional Help and Information

Edited by Amy L. Sutton. 680 pages. 2009. 978-0-7808-1041-9.

"Mental health concerns are presented in everyday language and intended for patients and their families as well as the general public... This resource is comprehensive and up to date... The easy-to-understand writing style helps to facilitate assimilation of needed facts and specifics on often challenging topics."
—*ARBAOnline, Oct '09*

"No health collection should be without this resource, which will reach into many a general lending library as well."
—*Internet Bookwatch, Oct '09*

SEE ALSO Depression Sourcebook, 2nd Edition, Stress-Related Disorders Sourcebook, 2nd Edition

---

Mental Retardation Sourcebook

Basic Consumer Health Information about Mental Retardation and Its Causes, Including Down Syndrome, Fetal Alcohol Syndrome, Fragile X Syndrome, Genetic Conditions, Injury, and Environmental Sources

Along with Preventive Strategies, Parenting Issues, Educational Implications, Health Care Needs, Employment and Economic Matters, Legal Issues, a Glossary, and a Resource Listing for Additional Help and Information

Edited by Joyce Brennfleck Shannon. 627 pages. 2000. 978-0-7808-0377-0.

"Public libraries will find the book useful for reference and as a beginning research point for students, parents, and caregivers."
—*American Reference Books Annual, 2001*

"The strength of this work is that it compiles many basic fact sheets and addresses them for further information in one volume. It is intended and suitable for the general public."
—*E-Streams, Nov '00*

"An invaluable overview."
—*Reviewer's Bookwatch, Jul '00*

Movement Disorders Sourcebook, 2nd Edition

Basic Consumer Health Information about the Symptoms and Causes of Movement Disorders, Including Parkinson Disease, Amyotrophic Lateral Sclerosis, Cerebral Palsy, Muscular Dystrophy, Multiple Sclerosis, Myasthenia, Myoclonus, Spina Bifida, Dystonia, Essential Tremor, Choreatic Disorders, Huntington Disease, Tourette Syndrome, and Other Disorders That Cause Slowed, Absent, or Excessive Movements

Along with Information about Surgical and Nonsurgical Interventions, Physical Therapies, Strategies for Independent Living, a Glossary of Related Terms, and a Directory of Resources for Additional Help and Information

Edited by Amy L. Sutton. 618 pages. 2009. 978-0-7808-1034-1.

"The second updated edition of Movement Disorders Sourcebook is a winner, providing the latest research and health findings on all kinds of movement disorders in children and adults... a top pick for any health or general lending library's health reference collection."
—*California Bookwatch, Aug '09*

SEE ALSO Muscular Dystrophy Sourcebook

Multiple Sclerosis Sourcebook

Basic Consumer Health Information about Multiple Sclerosis (MS) and Its Effects on Mobility, Vision, Bladder Function, Speech, Swallowing, and Cognition, Including Facts about Risk Factors, Causes, Diagnostic Procedures, Pain Management, Drug Treatments, and Physical and Occupational Therapies

Along with Guidelines for Nutrition and Exercise, Tips on Choosing Assistive Equipment, Information about Disability, Work, Financial, and Legal Issues, a Glossary of Related Terms, and a Directory of Additional Resources

Edited by Joyce Brennfleck Shannon. 553 pages. 2007. 978-0-7808-0998-7.

Muscular Dystrophy Sourcebook

Basic Consumer Health Information about Congenital, Childhood-Onset, and Adult-Onset

Forms of Muscular Dystrophy, Such as Duchenne, Becker, Emery-Dreifuss, Distal, Limb-Girdle, Facioscapulohumeral (FSHD), Myotonic, and Ophthalmoplegic Muscular Dystrophies, Including Facts about Diagnostic Tests, Medical and Physical Therapies, Management of Co-Occurring Conditions, and Parenting Guidelines

Along with Practical Tips for Home Care, a Glossary, and Directories of Additional Resources

Edited by Joyce Brennfleck Shannon. 552 pages. 2004. 978-0-7808-0676-4.

"This book is highly recommended for public and academic libraries as well as health care offices that support the information needs of patients and their families."
—E-Streams, Apr '05

"Excellent reference."
—The Bookwatch, Jan '05

SEE ALSO Movement Disorders Sourcebook, 2nd Edition

Obesity Sourcebook

Basic Consumer Health Information about Diseases and Other Problems Associated with Obesity, and Including Facts about Risk Factors, Prevention Issues, and Management Approaches

Along with Statistical and Demographic Data, Information about Special Populations, Research Updates, a Glossary, and Source Listings for Further Help and Information

Edited by Wilma Caldwell and Chad T. Kimball. 360 pages. 2001. 978-0-7808-0333-6.

"The book synthesizes the reliable medical literature on obesity into one easy-to-read and useful resource for the general public."
—American Reference Books Annual, 2002

"Well suited for the health reference collection of a public library or an academic health science library that serves the general population."
—E-Streams, Sep '01

Osteoporosis Sourcebook

Basic Consumer Health Information about Primary and Secondary Osteoporosis and Juvenile Osteoporosis and Related Conditions, Including Fibrous Dysplasia, Gaucher Disease, Hyperthyroidism, Hypophosphatasia,

Myeloma, Osteopetrosis, Osteogenesis Imperfecta, and Paget's Disease

Along with Information about Risk Factors, Treatments, Traditional and Non-Traditional Pain Management, a Glossary of Related Terms, and a Directory of Resources

Edited by Allan R. Cook. 568 pages. 2001. 978-0-7808-0239-1.

"This resource is recommended as a great reference source for public, health, and academic libraries, and is another triumph for the editors of Omnigraphics."
—American Reference Books Annual, 2002

"Will prove valuable to any library seeking to maintain a current, comprehensive reference collection of health resources... From prevention to treatment and associated conditions, this provides an excellent survey."
—The Bookwatch, Aug '01

SEE ALSO Healthy Aging Sourcebook, Women's Health Concerns Sourcebook, 3rd Edition

Pain Sourcebook, 3rd Edition

Basic Consumer Health Information about Acute and Chronic Pain, Including Nerve Pain, Bone Pain, Muscle Pain, Cancer Pain, and Disorders Characterized by Pain, Such as Arthritis, Temporomandibular Muscle and Joint (TMJ) Disorder, Carpal Tunnel Syndrome, Headaches, Heartburn, Sciatica, and Shingles, and Facts about Diagnostic Tests and Treatment Options for Pain, Including Over-the-Counter and Prescription Drugs, Physical Rehabilitation, Injection and Infusion Therapies, Implantable Technologies, and Complementary Medicine

Along with Tips for Living with Pain, a Glossary of Related Terms, and a Directory of Additional Resources

Edited by Joyce Brennfleck Shannon. 644 pages. 2008. 978-0-7808-1006-8.

"Excellent for ready-reference users and can be used for beginning students in health fields... appropriate for the consumer health collection in both public and academic libraries."
—American Reference Books Annual, 2009

SEE ALSO Arthritis Sourcebook, 3rd Edition; Back and Neck Sourcebook, 2nd Edition;

Headache Sourcebook; Sports Injuries Sourcebook, 3rd Edition

Pediatric Cancer Sourcebook

Basic Consumer Health Information about Leukemias, Brain Tumors, Sarcomas, Lymphomas, and Other Cancers in Infants, Children, and Adolescents, Including Descriptions of Cancers, Treatments, and Coping Strategies

Along with Suggestions for Parents, Caregivers, and Concerned Relatives, a Glossary of Cancer Terms, and Resource Listings

Edited by Edward J. Prucha. 575 pages. 1999. 978-0-7808-0245-2.

"An excellent source of information. Recommended for public, hospital, and health science libraries with consumer health collections."
—*E-Streams, Jun '00*

"A valuable addition to all libraries specializing in health services and many public libraries."
—*American Reference Books Annual, 2000*

SEE ALSO *Childhood Diseases and Disorders Sourcebook, 2nd Edition, Healthy Children Sourcebook*

Physical and Mental Issues in Aging Sourcebook

Basic Consumer Health Information on Physical and Mental Disorders Associated with the Aging Process, Including Concerns about Cardiovascular Disease, Pulmonary Disease, Oral Health, Digestive Disorders, Musculoskeletal and Skin Disorders, Metabolic Changes, Sexual and Reproductive Issues, and Changes in Vision, Hearing, and Other Senses

Along with Data about Longevity and Causes of Death, Information on Acute and Chronic Pain, Descriptions of Mental Concerns, a Glossary of Terms, and Resource Listings for Additional Help

Edited by Jenifer Swanson. 660 pages. 1999. 978-0-7808-0233-9.

"This is a treasure of health information for the layperson."
—*CHOICE Health Sciences Supplement, May '00*

"Recommended for public libraries."
—*American Reference Books Annual, 2000*

SEE ALSO *Healthy Aging Sourcebook*

Podiatry Sourcebook, 2nd Edition

Basic Consumer Health Information about Disorders, Diseases, and Deformities that Affect the Foot and Ankle, Including Sprains, Corns, Calluses, Bunions, Plantar Warts, Plantar Fasciitis, Neuromas, Clubfoot, Flat Feet, Achilles Tendonitis, and Much More

Along with Information about Selecting a Foot Care Specialist, Foot Fitness, Shoes and Socks, Diagnostic Tests and Corrective Procedures, Financial Assistance for Corrective Devices, a Glossary of Related Terms, and a Directory of Resources for Additional Help and Information

Edited by Ivy L. Alexander. 516 pages. 2007. 978-0-7808-0944-4.

"An excellent resource... Although there have been various types of 'foot books' published in the past, none are as comprehensive as this one. 5 Stars (out of 5)!"
—*Doody's Review Service, 2007*

"Perfect for both health libraries and general-interest lending collections."
—*Internet Bookwatch, Jul '07*

Pregnancy and Birth Sourcebook, 3rd Edition

Basic Consumer Health Information about Pregnancy and Fetal Development, Including Facts about Fertility and Conception, Physical and Emotional Changes during Pregnancy, Prenatal Care and Diagnostic Tests, High-Risk Pregnancies and Complications, Labor, Delivery, and the Postpartum Period

Along with Tips on Maintaining Health and Wellness during Pregnancy and Caring for Newborn Infants, a Glossary of Related Terms, and Directories of Resources for Additional Help and Information

Edited by Amy L. Sutton. 645 pages. 2009. 978-0-7808-1074-7.

SEE ALSO *Breastfeeding Sourcebook, Congenital Disorders Sourcebook, 2nd Edition, Family Planning Sourcebook, Women's Health Concerns Sourcebook, 3rd Edition*

Prostate and Urological Disorders Sourcebook

Basic Consumer Health Information about Urogenital and Sexual Disorders in Men, Including Prostate and Other Andrological Cancers, Prostatitis, Benign Prostatic Hyperplasia, Testicular and Penile Trauma, Cryptorchidism, Peyronie Disease, Erectile Dysfunction, and Male Factor Infertility, and Facts about Commonly Used Tests and Procedures, Such as Prostatectomy, Vasectomy, Vasectomy Reversal, Penile Implants, and Semen Analysis

Along with a Glossary of Andrological Terms and a Directory of Resources for Additional Information

Edited by Karen Bellenir. 604 pages. 2006. 978-0-7808-0797-6.

"Certain to be a popular pick among library reference holdings... No prior knowledge is assumed for any of the conditions or terms herein, making it a most accessible general-interest reference."
—*California Bookwatch, Apr '06*

SEE ALSO *Men's Health Concerns Sourcebook, 3rd Edition, Urinary Tract and Kidney Diseases and Disorders Sourcebook, 2nd Edition*

Prostate Cancer Sourcebook

Basic Consumer Health Information about Prostate Cancer, Including Information about the Associated Risk Factors, Detection, Diagnosis, and Treatment of Prostate Cancer

Along with Information on Non-Malignant Prostate Conditions, and Featuring a Section Listing Support and Treatment Centers and a Glossary of Related Terms

Edited by Dawn D. Matthews. 340 pages. 2001. 978-0-7808-0324-4.

"Recommended reference source."
—*Booklist, Jan '02*

"A valuable resource for health care consumers seeking information on the subject... All text is written in a clear, easy-to-understand language that avoids technical jargon. Any library that collects consumer health resources would strengthen their collection with the addition of the Prostate Cancer Sourcebook."
—*American Reference Books Annual, 2002*

SEE ALSO *Cancer Sourcebook, 5th Edition, Men's Health Concerns Sourcebook, 3rd Edition*

Rehabilitation Sourcebook

Basic Consumer Health Information about Rehabilitation for People Recovering from Heart Surgery, Spinal Cord Injury, Stroke, Orthopedic Impairments, Amputation, Pulmonary Impairments, Traumatic Injury, and More, Including Physical Therapy, Occupational Therapy, Speech/Language Therapy, Massage Therapy, Dance Therapy, Art Therapy, and Recreational Therapy

Along with Information on Assistive and Adaptive Devices, a Glossary, and Resources for Additional Help and Information

Edited by Dawn D. Matthews. 519 pages. 2000. 978-0-7808-0236-0.

"This is an excellent resource for public library reference and health collections."
—*American Reference Books Annual, 2001*

"Recommended reference source."
—*Booklist, May '00*

Respiratory Disorders Sourcebook, 2nd Edition

Basic Consumer Health Information about Infectious, Inflammatory, and Chronic Conditions Affecting the Lungs and Respiratory System, Including Pneumonia, Bronchitis, Influenza, Tuberculosis, Sarcoidosis, Asthma, Cystic Fibrosis, Chronic Obstructive Pulmonary Disease, Lung Abscesses, Pulmonary Embolism, Occupational Lung Diseases, and Other Bacterial, Viral, and Fungal Infections

Along with Facts about the Structure and Function of the Lungs and Airways, Methods of Diagnosing Respiratory Disorders, and Treatment and Rehabilitation Options, a Glossary of Related Terms, and a Directory of Resources for Additional Help and Information

Edited by Sandra L. Judd. 638 pages. 2008. 978-0-7808-1007-5.

"An excellent book for patients, their families, or for those who are just curious about respiratory disease. Public libraries and physician offices would find this a valuable resource as well. 4 Stars! (out of 5)"
—*Doody's Review Service, 2009*

"A great addition for public and school libraries because it provides concise health information... readers can start with this reference source and get satisfactory answers before proceeding to other medical reference tools for

more in depth information... A good guide for health education on lung disorders."
—*American Reference Books Annual, 2009*

SEE ALSO *Asthma Sourcebook, 2nd Edition, Lung Disorders Sourcebook*

Sexually Transmitted Diseases Sourcebook, 4th Edition

Basic Consumer Health Information about Chlamydial Infections, Gonorrhea, Hepatitis, Herpes, HIV/AIDS, Human Papillomavirus, Pubic Lice, Scabies, Syphilis, Trichomoniasis, Vaginal Infections, and Other Sexually Transmitted Diseases, Including Facts about Risk Factors, Symptoms, Diagnosis, Treatment, and the Prevention of Sexually Transmitted Infections

Along with Updates on Current Research Initiatives, a Glossary of Related Terms, and Resources for Additional Help and Information

Edited by Laura Larsen. 623 pages. 2009. 978-0-7808-1073-0.

"Extremely beneficial... The question-and-answer format along with the index and table of contents make this well-organized resource extremely easy to reference, read, and comprehend... an invaluable medical reference source for lay readers, and a highly appropriate addition for public library collections, health clinics, and any library with a consumer health collection"
—*ARBAOnline, Oct '09*

SEE ALSO *AIDS Sourcebook, 4th Edition, Contagious Diseases Sourcebook, 2nd Edition, Men's Health Concerns Sourcebook, 3rd Edition, Women's Health Concerns Sourcebook, 3rd Edition*

Sleep Disorders Sourcebook, 3rd Edition

Basic Consumer Health Information about Sleep Disorders, Including Insomnia, Sleep Apnea and Snoring, Jet Lag and Other Circadian Rhythm Disorders, Narcolepsy, and Parasomnias, Such as Sleep Walking and Sleep Talking, and Featuring Facts about Other Health Problems that Affect Sleep, Why Sleep Is Necessary, How Much Sleep Is Needed, the Physical and Mental Effects of Sleep Deprivation, and Pediatric Sleep Issues

Along with Tips for Diagnosing and Treating Sleep Disorders, a Glossary of Related Terms, and a List of Resources for Additional Help and Information

Edited by Sandra J. Judd. 600 pages. 2010. 978-0-7808-1084-6.

Smoking Concerns Sourcebook

Basic Consumer Health Information about Nicotine Addiction and Smoking Cessation, Featuring Facts about the Health Effects of Tobacco Use, Including Lung and Other Cancers, Heart Disease, Stroke, and Respiratory Disorders, Such as Emphysema and Chronic Bronchitis

Along with Information about Smoking Prevention Programs, Suggestions for Achieving and Maintaining a Smoke-Free Lifestyle, Statistics about Tobacco Use, Reports on Current Research Initiatives, a Glossary of Related Terms, and Directories of Resources for Additional Help and Information

Edited by Karen Bellenir. 595 pages. 2004. 978-0-7808-0323-7.

"Provides everything needed for the student or general reader seeking practical details on the effects of tobacco use."
—*The Bookwatch, Mar '05*

"Public libraries and consumer health care libraries will find this work useful."
—*American Reference Books Annual, 2005*

SEE ALSO *Respiratory Disorders Sourcebook, 2nd Edition*

Sports Injuries Sourcebook, 3rd Edition

Basic Consumer Health Information about Sprains and Strains, Fractures, Growth Plate Injuries, Overtraining Injuries, and Injuries to the Head, Face, Shoulders, Elbows, Hands, Spinal Column, Knees, Ankles, and Feet, and with Facts about Heat-Related Illness, Steroids and Sport Supplements, Protective Equipment, Diagnostic Procedures, Treatment Options, and Rehabilitation

Along with a Glossary of Related Terms and a Directory of Resources for Additional Help and Information

Edited by Sandra J. Judd. 623 pages. 2007. 978-0-7808-0949-9.

SEE ALSO Fitness and Exercise Sourcebook, 3rd Edition, Podiatry Sourcebook, 2nd Edition

Stress-Related Disorders Sourcebook, 2nd Edition

Basic Consumer Health Information about Stress and Stress-Related Disorders, Including Types of Stress, Sources of Acute and Chronic Stress, the Impact of Stress on the Body's Systems, and Mental and Emotional Health Problems Associated with Stress, Such as Depression, Anxiety Disorders, Substance Abuse, Posttraumatic Stress Disorder, and Suicide

Along with Advice about Getting Help for Stress-Related Disorders, Information about Stress Management Techniques, a Glossary of Stress-Related Terms, and a Directory of Resources for Additional Help and Information

Edited by Amy L. Sutton. 608 pages. 2007. 978-0-7808-0996-3.

"Accessible to the lay reader. Highly recommended for medical and psychiatric collections."
—*Library Journal, Mar '08*

"Well-written for a general readership, the 2nd Edition of Stress-Related Disorders Sourcebook is a useful addition to the health reference literature."
—*American Reference Books Annual, 2008*

SEE ALSO Mental Health Disorders Sourcebook, 4th Edition

Stroke Sourcebook, 2nd Edition

Basic Consumer Health Information about Stroke, Including Ischemic, Hemorrhagic, and Mini Strokes, as Well as Risk Factors, Prevention Guidelines, Diagnostic Tests, Medications and Surgical Treatments, and Complications of Stroke

Along with Rehabilitation Techniques and Innovations, Tips on Staying Healthy and Maintaining Independence after Stroke, a Glossary of Related Terms, and a Directory of Resources for Stroke Survivors and Their Families

Edited by Amy L. Sutton. 626 pages. 2008. 978-0-7808-1035-8.

"An encyclopedic handbook on stroke that is written in a language the layperson can understand... This is one of the most helpful, readable books on stroke. This volume is highly recommended and should be in every medical, hospital and public library; in addition, every family practitioner should have a copy in his or her office."
—*American Reference Books Annual, 2009*

SEE ALSO Brain Disorders Sourcebook, 3rd Edition, Hypertension Sourcebook

Surgery Sourcebook, 2nd Edition

Basic Consumer Health Information about Common Inpatient and Outpatient Surgeries, Including Critical Care and Trauma, Gastrointestinal, Gynecologic and Obstetric, Cardiac and Vascular, Neurologic, Ophthalmologic, Orthopedic, Reconstructive and Cosmetic, and Other Major and Minor Surgeries

Along with Information about Anesthesia and Pain Relief Options, Risks and Complications, Postoperative Recovery Concerns, and Innovative Surgical Techniques and Tools, a Glossary of Related Terms, and a Directory of Additional Resources

Edited by Amy L. Sutton. 645 pages. 2008. 978-0-7808-1004-4.

"Large public libraries and medical libraries would benefit from this material in their reference collections."
—*American Reference Books Annual, 2009*

SEE ALSO Cosmetic and Reconstructive Surgery Sourcebook, 2nd Edition

Thyroid Disorders Sourcebook

Basic Consumer Health Information about Disorders of the Thyroid and Parathyroid Glands, Including Hypothyroidism, Hyperthyroidism, Graves Disease, Hashimoto Thyroiditis, Thyroid Cancer, and Parathyroid Disorders, Featuring Facts about Symptoms, Risk Factors, Tests, and Treatments

Along with Information about the Effects of Thyroid Imbalance on Other Body Systems, Environmental Factors That Affect the Thyroid Gland, a Glossary, and a Directory of Additional Resources

Edited by Joyce Brennfleck Shannon. 573 pages. 2005. 978-0-7808-0745-7.

"Recommended for consumer health collections."
—*American Reference Books Annual, 2006*

"Highly recommended pick for Basic Consumer health reference holdings at all levels."
—*The Bookwatch, Aug '05*

SEE ALSO Endocrine and Metabolic Disorders Sourcebook, 2nd Edition

Transplantation Sourcebook

Basic Consumer Health Information about Organ and Tissue Transplantation, Including Physical and Financial Preparations, Procedures and Issues Relating to Specific Solid Organ and Tissue Transplants, Rehabilitation, Pediatric Transplant Information, the Future of Transplantation, and Organ and Tissue Donation

Along with a Glossary and Listings of Additional Resources

Edited by Joyce Brennfleck Shannon. 610 pages. 2002. 978-0-7808-0322-0.

"Recommended for libraries with an interest in offering consumer health information."
—*E-Streams, Jul '02*

"This is a unique and valuable resource for patients facing transplantation and their families."
—*Doody's Review Service, Jun '02*

Traveler's Health Sourcebook

Basic Consumer Health Information for Travelers, Including Physical and Medical Preparations, Transportation Health and Safety, Essential Information about Food and Water, Sun Exposure, Insect and Snake Bites, Camping and Wilderness Medicine, and Travel with Physical or Medical Disabilities

Along with International Travel Tips, Vaccination Recommendations, Geographical Health Issues, Disease Risks, a Glossary, and a Listing of Additional Resources

Edited by Joyce Brennfleck Shannon. 619 pages. 2000. 978-0-7808-0384-8.

"Recommended reference source."
—*Booklist, Feb '01*

"This book is recommended for any public library, any travel collection, and especially any collection for the physically disabled."
—*American Reference Books Annual, 2001*

SEE ALSO Worldwide Health Sourcebook

Urinary Tract and Kidney Diseases and Disorders Sourcebook, 2nd Edition

Basic Consumer Health Information about the Urinary System, Including the Bladder, Urethra, Ureters, and Kidneys, with Facts about Urinary Tract Infections, Incontinence, Congenital Disorders, Kidney Stones, Cancers of the Urinary Tract and Kidneys, Kidney Failure, Dialysis, and Kidney Transplantation

Along with Statistical and Demographic Information, Reports on Current Research in Kidney and Urologic Health, a Summary of Commonly Used Diagnostic Tests, a Glossary of Related Terms, and a Directory of Resources for Additional Help and Information

Edited by Ivy L. Alexander. 621 pages. 2005. 978-0-7808-0750-1.

"A good choice for a consumer health information library or for a medical library needing information to refer to their patients."
—*American Reference Books Annual, 2006*

SEE ALSO Prostate and Urological Disorders Sourcebook

Vegetarian Sourcebook

Basic Consumer Health Information about Vegetarian Diets, Lifestyle, and Philosophy, Including Definitions of Vegetarianism and Veganism, Tips about Adopting Vegetarianism, Creating a Vegetarian Pantry, and Meeting Nutritional Needs of Vegetarians, with Facts Regarding Vegetarianism's Effect on Pregnant and Lactating Women, Children, Athletes, and Senior Citizens

Along with a Glossary of Commonly Used Vegetarian Terms and Resources for Additional Help and Information

Edited by Chad T. Kimball. 337 pages. 2002. 978-0-7808-0439-5.

"Organizes into one concise volume the answers to the most common questions concerning vegetarian diets and lifestyles. This title is recommended for public and secondary school libraries."

—*E-Streams, Apr '03*

"**Invaluable reference for public and school library collections alike.**"
—*Library Bookwatch, Apr '03*

"**The articles in this volume are easy to read and come from authoritative sources. The book does not necessarily support the vegetarian diet but instead provides the pros and cons of this important decision... Recommended for public libraries and consumer health libraries.**"
—*American Reference Books Annual, 2003*

SEE ALSO *Diet and Nutrition Sourcebook, 3rd Edition*

Women's Health Concerns Sourcebook, 3rd Edition

Basic Consumer Health Information about Issues and Trends in Women's Health and Health Conditions of Special Concern to Women, Including Endometriosis, Uterine Fibroids, Menstrual Irregularities, Menopause, Sexual Dysfunction, Infertility, Cancer in Women, and Other Such Chronic Disorders as Lupus, Fibromyalgia, and Thyroid Disease

Along with Statistical Data, Tips for Maintaining Wellness, a Glossary, and a Directory of Resources for Further Help and Information

Edited by Sandra J. Judd. 679 pages. 2009. 978-0-7808-1036-5.

"**This useful resource provides information about a wide range of topics that will help women understand their bodies, prevent or treat disease, and maintain health... A detailed index helps readers locate information. This is a useful addition to public and consumer health library collections**"
—*ARBAOnline, Jun '09*

SEE ALSO *Breast Cancer Sourcebook, 3rd Edition, Cancer Sourcebook for Women, 4th Edition, Healthy Heart Sourcebook for Women*

Workplace Health and Safety Sourcebook

Basic Consumer Health Information about Workplace Health and Safety, Including the Effect of Workplace Hazards on the Lungs,

Skin, Heart, Ears, Eyes, Brain, Reproductive Organs, Musculoskeletal System, and Other Organs and Body Parts

Along with Information about Occupational Cancer, Personal Protective Equipment, Toxic and Hazardous Chemicals, Child Labor, Stress, and Workplace Violence

Edited by Chad T. Kimball. 610 pages. 2000. 978-0-7808-0231-5.

"**As a reference for the general public, this would be useful in any library.**"
—*E-Streams, Jun '01*

"**Provides helpful information for primary care physicians and other caregivers interested in occupational medicine... General readers; professionals.**"
—*CHOICE, May '01*

Worldwide Health Sourcebook

Basic Information about Global Health Issues, Including Malnutrition, Reproductive Health, Disease Dispersion and Prevention, Emerging Diseases, Risky Health Behaviors, and the Leading Causes of Death

Along with Global Health Concerns for Children, Women, and the Elderly, Mental Health Issues, Research and Technology Advancements, and Economic, Environmental, and Political Health Implications, a Glossary, and a Resource Listing for Additional Help and Information

Edited by Joyce Brennfleck Shannon. 597 pages. 2001. 978-0-7808-0330-5.

"**Named an Outstanding Academic Title.**"
—*CHOICE, Jan '02*

"**Yet another handy but also unique compilation in the extensive Health Reference Series, this is a useful work because many of the international publications reprinted or excerpted are not readily available. Highly recommended.**"
—*CHOICE, Nov '01*

SEE ALSO *Traveler's Health Sourcebook*